INVISIBLE LABOR

INVISIBLE LABOR

THE UNTOLD STORY OF THE CESAREAN SECTION

RACHEL SOMERSTEIN

An Imprint of HarperCollins*Publishers*

HarperCollins books may be purchased for educational, business, or sales promotional use. For information, please email the Special Markets Department at SPsales@harpercollins.com.

Ecco® and HarperCollins® are trademarks of HarperCollins Publishers.

FIRST EDITION

Designed by Alison Bloomer

Library of Congress Cataloging-in-Publication Data has been applied for.

ISBN 978-0-06-326441-0

24 25 26 27 28 LBC 5 4 3 2 1

TO MY FAMILY

CONTENTS

AUTHOR'S NOTE

THIS IS A WORK OF NONFICTION. THE EVENTS AND EXPERIENCES DE-
tailed here are all true and have been faithfully rendered as I have remembered them to the best of my ability. And though conversations come
from my recollection, emails, and journals, they are not always written
to represent word-for-word documentation. Where I haven't been able
to replicate exactly what was said, I've retold conversations in a way that
evokes their real feeling and meaning, in keeping with the true essence of
the mood and spirit of what took place.

This book uses the terms "pregnant women" and "pregnant people"
interchangeably, because not all people who are pregnant identify as
women. I use the term "women" not to leave anyone out, but because
mistreatment during pregnancy, labor, and birth comes in part from patriarchy and misogyny (as well as racism)—which are specifically and
explicitly anti-female. I use the term "mother" to refer to anyone who engages in mothering, regardless of gender identity, sexuality, or anatomy.

While some academic literature, particularly government resources,
uses the term "Hispanic," most people who fall into this category are not
predominantly of Spanish descent. "Latino" or "Latinx" are preferred
terms designated by these communities. Thus, I use the terms "Hispanic/
Latinx" for the sake of clarity and to recognize the many different backgrounds of people who fall into that category.

Last, at parents' request, I changed some names or used only first
names.

INVISIBLE LABOR

PROLOGUE

I DON'T REMEMBER WHO HELD THE PAPER UP TO MY FACE, BUT I'M sure I didn't read it. I'd been in labor for nearly twenty-four hours and was not in a state to read fine print. It was after midnight in a small town in upstate New York, in a hospital that suddenly seemed ill equipped to handle my first birth, which was rapidly careening toward an unplanned cesarean section. My daughter was having heart rate decelerations, and the labor nurse assigned to monitor her—the only person in the room I vaguely trusted—kept frowning as she tore papers from the machine spitting them out.

The anesthesiologist who had put in my epidural had a Jewish name. Initially I had taken this as a good omen; I assumed he was Jewish, like me, which gave me comfort, as if he'd do a good job if only because he wouldn't want to see a Jewish woman suffer. Pregnancy had brought out my irrational and romantic side, and I placed heavy stock in signs and symbols, perhaps even more than in research and evidence. But I didn't give enough weight to the signs that communicated unwelcome information—in this case, that he had had to redo my epidural three times to get it right.

It took some time to bring together the actors to operate on me. As I waited, I felt enormous terror. During pregnancy, no one had warned me that I might need a C-section. And I'd skipped the C-section parts of the birth books I'd read because I didn't think I'd need one, either. I'd done everything "right": I'd walked three miles a day through my third trimester. I'd done prenatal yoga. I'd hired a doula. And yet there it was, bearing down on me. I was certain that this left turn into unknown territory meant that the worst would happen—that I would die, that my baby would die.

Although the midwife, the nurse, the doula, and my husband assured me we would be okay, no one genuinely tended to my fear. The feeling, my husband told me later, was that I was hysterical. That I wasn't listening to what people were telling me, and that my fear was unreasonable. Really I was scared, exhausted, did not understand what was happening, and did not trust the people taking care of me.

Possibly, from my caregivers' perspective, I was getting all worked up for nothing about the world's most common surgery—one that was safe and routine, and likely wasn't even the first they'd performed that day. That's because in the US, as in the hospital where I gave birth, C-sections comprise one in three births, and one in four births for first-time moms who are at least thirty-seven weeks pregnant with one head-down baby, as I was.[1]

I have a flash of memory of being rolled on a gurney to the operating room. Nearly naked and freezing, I hunched over my belly and braced myself against the doula.

As the anesthesiologist tried to insert a new tube into my spine to deliver the anesthesia, my body continued to try to push out the baby. "Your belly looks totally different!" the doula said—the baby had already moved very far down, and I'd been pushing when they'd called the section—as if I hadn't noticed the contractions that had dominated me over the previous twenty-four hours. As with the epidural, the anesthesiologist struggled to place the needle correctly.

Someone may have strapped or held down my arms. The physician made the first cut.

"I felt that," I told him.

"You'll feel pressure," he said.

I felt it all: the separation of my rectus muscles; the scissors used to move my bladder; the scalpel, with which he "incised" my uterus.

Everyone in the room knew I was in pain. As the obstetrician later put in his notes: "The patient was having a great deal of difficulty, tolerating pain, was indicating that she was having a great deal of difficulty coping with the pain and was screaming from the pain."

My legs, as I remember, and as the doctor wrote, "were moving quite a bit." They were kicking high enough for me to see them above the drape, rigged so I wouldn't be able to see what was going on.

The leg-kicking: the body will react this way during torture. This is why, before the introduction of ether in 1846, specially trained people were employed to hold down the patient during an operation.[2] One for each limb.

The anesthesia had failed, and everyone knew it. Yet the operation continued. I was expected to bear the pain. Later, I would find scratches on my hips. From the nurses' nails, maybe, holding me down. I believe that's how, once the operation began, my body wasn't able to run itself off the bed. But it seems implausible that the nurses could have done that during the operation, because the obstetrician couldn't have reached me.

After my baby was born, the doctor held her up to my face. "Here's your baby!" he said. I don't remember this—my husband told me about it later—but that was our first meeting on this side of the veil. Then he ushered my husband out of the room with the baby, and the anesthesiologist put me under general anesthesia so the obstetrician could sew me up.

In recovery, the doula brought the baby to my breast to nurse. I heard her tell someone, "A good latch," in a tone that meant, *A mercy*. I don't remember anyone speaking to me or asking if I wanted to nurse. Perhaps they thought I was still unconscious.

But I didn't want to see my daughter. I was in too much pain. "I don't want to see her," I cried. "No, no, no, I can't see her. Take her away!"

I used to blame myself for rejecting my baby at her first hour of need. But now I see this as a moment of clarity, wisdom, one of my first, best acts as a mother: I didn't want to associate her with any more of my pain. She was already so bound up with it.

I WAS DETERMINED TO BREASTFEED despite the pain, and my daughter's poor weight gain, mostly to prove to myself that I could do it. Formula, lovingly given, would have been a better choice. But I refused. As a consequence, and because my daughter cluster-fed for several weeks from midnight until 4:00 a.m., I rarely slept. Though I was far from alone—problems breastfeeding after C-sections are quite common—I blamed myself.

Yet despite the days and nights we spent together, I didn't feel much toward my baby. There was no wave of oxytocin like the pregnancy websites said I'd feel. I did not want to cuddle. Instead, my body was so full of stress and electricity that I was afraid I would zap her. I'm sure she felt it; she used to eyeball me while nursing with an expression I took to mean, *I'm watching you. Don't run away.* None of this squared with my vision of being a new mom, which I thought vaguely consisted of taking long walks with the baby in a stroller while sipping iced coffee.

One day, when the doula came over to play with her, I watched them, totally detached. I remember thinking I would have been fine if she had taken my daughter with her when she left.

"Isn't this fun?" the doula said.

"Yeah," I agreed. I was still in such shock from the operation that I didn't know what else to say. I didn't even know how to get angry. "It's great."

I had a good poker face—still do—and if you didn't know me, you wouldn't have known that part of me had died on that operating table. But I was so shaken I couldn't even email a birth announcement. I didn't have any joy to share.

TWO MONTHS AFTER THE OPERATION, I had my last postpartum checkup. Though I was praised for looking great—I'd bought high-waisted leggings to contain my newly pooched abdomen, a forever gift from the operation—internally I was still raw. I tried to contract my core muscles during yoga but had lost all proprioception. My vulva was numb, yet sex hurt. A midwife suggested lube, which didn't work. ("It still hurts," I told her. "More lube," she said.) Later, through my own research, I'd find out that pelvic floor physical therapy probably would have helped. But at the time, the widespread belief that an operative birth "spares" your vagina and perineum—that, because I hadn't pushed out a baby, I wouldn't have needed pelvic floor PT—was yet another misperception about C-sections that I stumbled through alone.

Birth control was the only prescription my midwife offered regarding sex. I was to avoid getting pregnant for at least two years to give my body time to heal. Other problems, like burning around the incision and continued discomfort when I sneezed or coughed—evidently normal side effects—no one mentioned, so I never asked about them. C-sections, I was learning, presented a very long tail of complications that persist far beyond when the official "healing" is over, and that most people cope with alone.

But I didn't appreciate the most difficult part of my recovery until nearly two years after the operation. I was awaiting a colonoscopy, the first time I'd been in a hospital setting since the birth. I lay on a gurney in a surgical bay. The apparatuses of the OR surrounded me: an IV pole, a blood pressure cuff, supplemental oxygen. I started to shake and cry but couldn't explain to the nurse what was happening—because I didn't understand it, either. I was having a panic attack, something that had never happened to me before. Then the anesthesiologist came in to ask if I'd ever had any problems with anesthesia. Sobbing, I told him that I'd felt my C-section. This was the first time I'd spoken out loud about the experience to a stranger. It was so inconceivable to him that he didn't believe me. I repeated myself. Then he backed out of the room.

I don't remember what happened next. But on the drive home with my husband, I told him I didn't know if I'd ever recover enough to have another baby. Only then did I realize how seriously traumatized I'd been by the operation, and that I'd developed PTSD, something that isn't routinely screened for postpartum, though nearly one out of five mothers who are "high risk" develop PTSD after birth. High-risk mothers are those who have had a traumatic birth, like I did; a severe obstetric complication; "a history of sexual or physical violence or childhood abuse;" or who birth babies that are premature, a very low birth weight, or have "fetal [anomalies]."[3] Yet until I sought therapy on my own, several years later, no one suggested that I might be at risk for developing PTSD.

Friends encouraged me to file a malpractice lawsuit. I tried, buoyed by the changing winds in the culture to #BelieveWomen. I called around to local attorneys, but none would take the case. One asked what the big deal was. "How long did it really take?" he asked. "Five minutes?" Another insinuated I was suddenly hard up for money, which was why I'd waited so long to file a lawsuit. The most empathic one explained that payouts for pain and suffering are capped. Because my daughter and I hadn't been permanently physically injured, it didn't make financial sense to represent me. It was similar to what I'd heard since the baby's birth, even from people who were well-meaning: The baby's healthy; you're fine. What you went through doesn't matter. Forget it and move on.

I used to think hospitals were kind of exciting—the bustle of all these people, working together to save lives. Before I got pregnant, I'd even joked to my husband that maybe I'd leave academia, where I worked as an assistant professor of journalism, to go to med school. But now I had a panic attack when I went to the doctor, especially if I'd never met them before. At its worst, it was as if my brain would evacuate while my body stayed put, shaking, crying, blood pressure rocketing up. Sometimes, I'd seem normal on the outside, while inside I'd be so paralyzed that I couldn't think. I found the physiological experience of this panic unbearable. So I stopped going. I skipped physicals, the dentist.

Perhaps most terribly, most unfairly, I would bear my next pregnancy in the shadow of this operation, afraid that I would die, or my baby would die, but also largely dissociated from the body growing inside mine. "Maybe that's not a bad thing," my therapist said at the time, about how disconnected I felt from the baby inside me. "Maybe that's what you have to do to get through it."

OVER THE NEXT SEVERAL YEARS, to try to make sense of what had happened—how I could have been operated upon with no anesthesia in a hospital that boasted of its "expert" medical care—I first turned to literature: books about birth, becoming a mother, motherhood. Then, I turned to "the" literature: the academic medical literature on cesareans, surgical complications, and anesthesia. I felt nauseated to learn how many people are hurt, damaged, or killed during or after pregnancy or birth—harms borne disproportionately by mothers of color. And while I'd thought that what I'd experienced was highly unusual—so terrible, for many years it felt unspeakable—I found that breakthrough pain during C-sections isn't that rare, though researchers have only begun to investigate it. Moreover, the way that my providers dealt with my pain—or rather, didn't deal with it—isn't unusual, either: women's pain is regularly undercredited or outright ignored, throughout their lives and during childbirth in particular. Nor was my trauma unique; a large proportion of mothers—as many as 45 percent, per one study—feel traumatized by birth.[4] Though I'd felt isolated by my experience, I was far from alone in the ways that birth had hurt me.

As part of my healing, I also wanted to understand more about C-sections as a phenomenon: how they came to be the most common operation in the world. To my surprise, I found that although they may be a relatively simple operation for a new doctor to learn, the forces that have increased their numbers are incredibly complex. Follow one cause, like electronic fetal monitoring, and all sorts of problems within the US medical system fall into view: an emphasis on technology, not the patient; the lack of value accorded to human presence and human touch; hospital systems that seek ever-expanding profits; obstetricians' deep-seated fears of litigation; lack of trust in mothers' bodies; a belief that pregnancy and birth are disasters waiting to happen; mistrust between patients and providers; the US's dismantling of midwifery, which occurred at the beginning of the twentieth century, and which sets us apart from other high-income countries, where midwives attend a far greater percentage of births. These multifactorial and often overlapping causes are what make addressing C-sections so complicated. In that way, the number of them that we do, and the harms these potentially avoidable surgeries perpetuate, are symptoms of other, larger problems. At the same time, that complexity is what makes them such a fruitful lens through which to look at America: our values, priorities, weaknesses, economy, and deeply entrenched worldviews. C-sections run through all of this, a fault line exposing many often-difficult realities of our past and our present.

ONE OF THE MORE DAMAGING stories that I told myself was that the birth was my fault. That I hadn't done enough to stop it, to speak up for myself. And because this had happened, I must not be the strong, independent person I had believed myself to be. I can now see that I felt debased by the operation. So many people had watched what had happened but hadn't intervened. It was almost embarrassing—even though the people who froze, and the OB and the anesthesiologist, are the ones who should feel embarrassed. Nevertheless, I interpreted these facts as evidence of my worthlessness, which caused me to question the core of my identity.

Though it wasn't rational, this sense of personal responsibility caused me tremendous suffering and guilt. Now I can see that it was an inevitable response to cultural, political, and legal systems that tell mothers over and over that our success is our responsibility, that lead us to believe we alone are liable for a perfect baby, and that encourage us to look away from the underlying conditions that shape our outcomes.

This emphasis on mothers' individual responsibility is a relatively recent phenomenon. For much of the twentieth century, birth was considered a matter of public health in the US. Getting it right or making it better was the government's responsibility. To that end, beginning in the 1920s, an array of legislation and federal funding emerged, aimed at making birth safer—though with uneven effects.

Ultimately, what most effectively improved birth outcomes were medical innovations, particularly an understanding of germ transmission, the adoption of antiseptic techniques, the development of antibiotics, and blood banking.[5] As a result, birth got a lot safer in the US between 1940 and 1990. White women benefited the most from these improvements, while birth remained more dangerous for Black mothers.

Yet by the 1990s, collective efforts to make birth safer for everyone stalled. From a public-health angle, we couldn't seem to move the needle.

Then the needle did start to move—but in the wrong direction. Birth in the US started to become more dangerous. Where in 1990 the US's maternal mortality rate was twelve out of every one hundred thousand births, by 2008 it doubled to twenty-four out of one hundred thousand births, according to data compiled by the World Bank.[6]

It's important to note that birth seemed to get more dangerous in part because we started counting maternal deaths differently, Amy Metcalfe, an epidemiologist at the University of Calgary, told me. Beginning in 2003, states began including a checkbox on death certificates if a person was pregnant at the time of, or within a year of, death. States adopted the box piecemeal, over fourteen years; the last state, West Virginia, did so in 2017.[7] This new checkbox system includes maternal deaths that previously were not considered to be pregnancy-related, such as from accidents, suicide, violence, and drug overdoses.[8] It also counts deaths that occur up to a year postpartum. Still, even using the old system for assessing maternal mortality—one that *doesn't* include these new deaths—maternal mortality in forty-eight US states increased by an estimated 27 percent from 2000 to 2014, reaching 23.8 of every 100,000 live births, among the highest rates of all wealthy countries.[9]

And while birth became more dangerous for a variety of reasons, the country's increasing number of C-sections played a part, according to a 2007 review by the US Department of Health and Human Services. The rate of the operation more than doubled between 1996 and 2007, when it reached 31.8 percent of all births, a figure it has hovered around ever since.

As in the past, pregnancy and birth have persisted in being more dangerous for Black mothers than for white ones. The often-cited statistic today, that Black mothers are three to four times more likely to die during pregnancy than white mothers, isn't new; the CDC issued a bulletin decrying it in 2003.[10] Looking at historical data from the turn of the twentieth century shows that these disparities have persisted for more than one hundred years. Nor is the media attention on the Black maternal health emergency a revelation to the Black and Brown communities who have been living with inequitable outcomes for generations.

The stories that generate the most news coverage typically involve Black mothers who die during or just after birth. Often, these deaths occur because providers overlook or fail to listen to a mother's symptoms, pain, or concerns. These deaths are tragic and largely preventable, and the pain they cause radiates through each mother's family, into her community, and beyond.

But despite the prominence of such cases, and the corresponding narrative of who's dying and why, the new way of counting maternal deaths attests that suicide and drug overdoses are the leading causes of maternal mortality. While suicide and drug overdoses have typically occurred more often among white women, as researchers Kathleen Chin and colleagues assert, "there is a disturbing trend of increase" in suicide and intentions of self-harm among Black women, according to a 2021 study of nearly six hundred thousand women with private health insurance.[11] Such "deaths of despair," as researchers Anne Case and Angus Deaton have termed them, indict not just the healthcare system but our nation as a whole for failing to provide resources for expecting and new mothers' basic survival.[12]

Reporters, physicians, midwives, academics, activists, and many others are deeply concerned about the Black maternal health emergency, and frequently invoke such data to drive funding and attention. Yet over the past several years, as scholar Jennifer C. Nash observes in her book *Birthing Black Mothers*, "racial disparity in maternal mortality has not changed and might have even worsened."[13] In fact, she writes, the urgent discourse around this issue "often stands in for political work designed to ameliorate the very conditions that produce the 'crisis.'" In other words, there's a lot of talk, but not much "political labor to improve the lives of Black mothers and children."

Set against such entrenched, systemic failure, the expectation that individual mothers tailor their behavior to ensure a safe, even perfect birth is, at best, feeble. If you or someone you're close with has been pregnant recently, then you're familiar with the litany of restrictions: Limit or avoid caffeine, sushi, deli meat, alcohol, cigarettes, soft cheeses, too much exercise, too little exercise. Don't raise your hands above your head. Don't stress too much or carry anything heavy. The visibility of pregnancy means we hold one another to account, in ways that range from menacing to meddlesome. Don't, a neighbor told me when I was six months pregnant, rake. Don't, a stranger called to me from her car, around the same point in my pregnancy, walk uphill.

These precautions seem particularly absurd considering how little attention we pay, collectively, to the greatest danger to pregnant people's health: domestic violence. More pregnant people die from murder each year than from car accidents and complications of pregnancy combined. But policy tends to focus public attention on trying to persuade pregnant people to stop drinking or smoking, even though only 7 percent of pregnant people smoke, and only about 10 percent have a drink at any point during pregnancy.[14] Imagine if every pregnancy test sold in the US included a statement about how simply becoming pregnant raises a person's risk of being murdered by 16 percent. Imagine if—like the risks of alcohol and drugs during pregnancy—this was something you just knew.[15]

Even as pregnant people have been charged with individually ensuring that their pregnancies turn out well, women's bodily autonomy has become more and more narrowed over the past several decades. Most emblematic of that shift is the Supreme Court's decision on *Dobbs* in 2022, which eliminated the constitutional right to abortion. On its face, the relationship between abortion access and autonomy during pregnancy may not be evident—especially for people like me, who came of age in a mostly white feminist movement that emphasized the idea of reproductive rights strictly as they pertain to abortion and birth control. But defining reproductive rights largely in terms of access to contraception and pregnancy termination isn't sufficient; it overlooks the many ways that pregnant people also have their reproductive rights infringed upon.

Reproductive justice, as conceived by women of color, offers a more expansive definition of reproductive rights, to include safe and autonomous pregnancy, pregnancy prevention, abortion, and the right to parent autonomously. In that way, reproductive justice accounts both for the challenges of obtaining a safe and accessible abortion—a well-known story—and for the obstacles mothers face when they seek, for instance, "out-of-hospital births, vaginal births after cesareans (VBACs), or midwifery care," writes scholar Julia Chinyere Oparah in the introduction to *Birthing Justice: Black Women, Pregnancy, and Childbirth.*

This more holistic framework makes sense: the majority of people who have an abortion are already mothers. Or, as Lynn Paltrow, the founder and former executive director of Pregnancy Justice (previously the National Advocates for Pregnant Women), told me, "people seeking a VBAC, and people seeking an abortion, are the same people. Just at different moments in their lives."

Reproductive justice leaders have also long critiqued what Oparah calls the "individualist and consumerist" language of choice around reproductive rights. Slogans like "my body, my choice," and campaigns about the right to choose sound great—who doesn't want to choose bodily autonomy?—but belie the reality of people's lives, which are constrained by the systems in which we operate. For instance, like many expectant parents, because of the corporatization of medicine and the limitations of my insurance coverage, I had little "choice" about whom to see for prenatal care. I could theoretically have elected to have a home birth, but my insurance wouldn't have covered it, so it wasn't a choice that was open to me. At my birth I had no "choice" about how my obstetrician responded to the pain I felt, nor the power to stop the operation once it began. I had few options when it came to staying home after the birth or caring for my newborn; my employer called the shots even in those realms, because like most American women, I didn't have sufficient paid leave.

Such constraints on mothers' autonomy are well-documented in academic studies. Pregnant and laboring women consistently report being coerced into induction, epidurals, episiotomies, and cesareans. Providers do not always ask for a woman's consent before examining her (*Let's see how dilated you are*). Nor do all mothers elect a cesarean with true informed consent, whose legal and ethical definition supposes that physicians share a given procedure's risks, benefits, and alternatives.

It's easy to blame providers for these harms. And individual providers are responsible. But it's essential to recognize, as this book explores, the historic roots of such denials of pregnant women's autonomy. "We're a country that's founded on slavery," says Paltrow. "The idea that somebody can control [another person's] body or self-determination can apply to any group of people not in power, and that includes . . . all pregnant women." That denial of autonomy and selfhood is even more pronounced for Black women, writes Dorothy Roberts in *Killing the Black Body*. Because enslaved Black women's bodies were (ab)used to breed more enslaved people, she asserts, they have long been "marked. . . . as objects whose decisions about reproduction should be subject to social regulation rather than to their own will."[16] Roberts's observation bears out in C-sections' history in particular: in the US, the operation developed on enslaved and othered women. That legacy shapes the present: today, Black mothers are more likely to have C-sections than white women, even among groups with similar risk factors.

The reality is that we have not yet begun to see reproductive rights as human rights. Or, as Paltrow put it to me, to accept that pregnant people are human.

AS I'VE RAISED MY CHILDREN over the past seven years, birth has come up a lot in conversations with other parents, often in snatches between dispensing snacks or pushing a swing at the park. When they heard about the book I was working on, many mothers confessed to me about their C-sections, "Physically, I was fine, but emotionally, it was rough." Or, "I had postpartum depression, but was never diagnosed." Even when the surgery went well, some mothers confided that they believed the operation hurt their relationships with their children, that their bodies were defective, or that they never actually gave birth. And once I'd gotten better at sharing my medical trauma with providers—so that they could know how I was feeling, and why my heart rate and blood pressure would be up—I encountered a surprising number of "traumatic C-section" stories. "Oh, honey," one nurse told me, over the phone, "I know how you feel. I had an emergency C-section, lost so much blood, and even lost my uterus."

Talking with one such mother at day-care pickup, I thought of an observation that writer Iris Jacob makes in her essay about maternal loss: "I always thought I had entered a secret club when I became a mother, one that no one really talked about but whose rules every mother seemed to know. This was a different club—one that was really top secret, yet had more members than I could have imagined."[17] Though the mothers in the "secret club" I'd tumbled into weren't dealing with the kind of loss Jacob faced, that's what these interactions about C-sections felt like to me, too: a secret club with a seemingly infinite membership. There are just so many of us, throughout every echelon of society, looking like normal, well-adjusted people doing our thing, belying the traumatizing or otherwise unresolved C-section at the center. It is astonishing.

Through these conversations with other mothers, I also saw clearly the cultural expectation that a mother's pain should be negated by that triumphant moment of union with her baby. How we simply have no script for what to do with a mother's pain when it persists beyond that moment: when the baby is fine, but the mother is not. This is true all the more when a birth is surgical, given that, notes Erica Delaney, a nurse-midwife who had a traumatic cesarean, "we don't think about it as birth, [so] we don't talk about it as birth."

WHEN I CAME HOME FROM the hospital with my baby girl that sunny afternoon in February, I never could have imagined that one day I'd have recovered enough from the operation to write about it. Talking with midwives, physicians, sociologists, historians, doulas, therapists, and other parents helped me to better understand how what happened to me could have happened. When it got tough—and sometimes it did—I was driven by my desire to write a book that might help others who found themselves in similar emotional territory: shocked, alone, and traumatized by a birth that they never would have expected, even though they did everything "right."

This book is for mothers looking to see themselves reflected in the story of birth, and for those seeking to better understand the many reasons why their births may have unfolded the way they did. It's for family members and others engaged with the feminist project of maternal autonomy, who want to explore why birth often looks the way it does in the US at this point in time. It is also for providers who want to make birth better: the committed, hardworking, and courageous midwives, physicians, nurses, physical and occupational therapists, and doulas who find themselves in a broken system, but who, in the words of nurse-midwife Helena A. Grant, "are strong enough—energetically, spiritually, and mentally—to say, 'I will not become that.'"

The book accomplishes these goals partly by looking to the past: how C-sections first developed on dead or dying women, their perfection on the enslaved and the unfit, and the operation's long entanglement with sterilization. But I also look critically at the received history of C-sections, to try to identify the voices and the narratives that don't get told—those primarily belonging to mothers and midwives—because they weren't adequately recorded. As a writer, I'm interested in what the world was like before: before industrialization, before the medicalization of birth, when birth was in the domain of women and attended almost exclusively by midwives. These accounts show us what we've lost and also serve as inspiration about how to reimagine birth's future. To explore why C-sections are sometimes stigmatized, and why mothers who have them might feel as though they didn't really give birth, I investigate the ways that the life, health, and safety of the unborn are often promoted at the expense of mothers' lives. And to understand—and reverse—the conditions that make it more likely for Black mothers to have cesareans, I look at the ways systemic and structural racism shape healthcare, and share solutions conceived by Black and Brown communities.

I'm lucky. I have a loving and supportive family, health insurance, and skilled therapists who walked with me as I looked into the pit of my birth, a maelstrom of fear, rage, and grief that I sometimes pictured as a whirling sandstorm, into which I might disappear. I have more than many other mothers, some of whom must contend with more trauma and less support.

And yet, when I think about what I went through, and what I recovered from, I still feel astonished. At the same time, I carry this trauma with me. I'm not the person I was before the operation. It isn't "over." Even though I'm better, I'm different.

So: *Hineini*. Here I am. And here is the book.

1

THE STATE OF THE UTERUS

WHEN I ARRIVED IN MY HOSPITAL ROOM AFTER THE BIRTH, A TALL IV pole stood beside my bed. Its tubing snaked into a vein at the top of my hand. If I needed more pain medicine, someone explained, all I had to do was press a button.

This device is called a PCA, which stands for patient-controlled analgesia. It's used to treat severe pain from an operation, cancer, or sickle-cell anemia. In my opiate haze, I watched the bright numbers on the IV, which seemed to wink at me. I imagined it was trying to tell me that it was my new best friend. *I hate you*, I thought. *Get away from me.* I didn't even think I needed the machine. The physical pain was enormous, but tolerable. It was the shock of what had happened that overwhelmed me.

The next morning, after having my catheter removed, the labor nurse from the night before helped me to the bathroom. Blood ran down my legs. I panicked, thinking it was from the incision, then realized it was coming from between my legs. I couldn't bend over to clean myself; I could not even bend to sit on the toilet. Mortified, I mumbled, "I'm sorry, I'm sorry," as the nurse used a washcloth to sponge the blood off my thighs. "You have nothing to apologize for," she told me. I was thirty-three. I had never been mopped up so intimately in this way—certainly not since childhood, and definitely not by a stranger.

Four more days in the hospital, and we'd packed for one. It didn't matter, because I didn't get dressed.

Friday night: the "celebratory" dinner. Our first Shabbat as a family. But no staff there seemed to know what Shabbat meant to us. I barely ate: my throat felt sore and scratchy, deep into my esophagus, from being intubated.

The pain in my throat made it easier not to speak. I couldn't even tell my parents what had happened; I asked the doula to do so for me, which she did by phone in another room. My mother took notes that she put into a ziplock bag, as if they were evidence from a crime scene.

A photograph my husband took: My skin looks ashen, gray. My mouth, mournful. I'm alone in the bed. No baby.

The doula visited to get me out of bed and walk. At first I thought she was joking; I could barely get to the bathroom. Because of the incision, I could not stand up straight. I leaned on her, hunched, and shuffled down the hall. *How do people even do this?* I wondered. I didn't know that this kind of pain and disability was even possible after a cesarean.

Middle of the night: Baby woke me, crying, needing to eat. It had taken days for my milk to come in, a common side effect of the surgery, but no one had told me that at the time. My baby would lose more than a pound in the hospital, and the "good" latch I'd had right after the operation seemed to have evaporated. I dragged my body to an armchair in the corner of the room and rang for the nurse; I could not lift the baby from her bassinet. The kind nurse came again. She suggested I try the "football hold": nestle the baby close to my side, then plop my nipple into her mouth. I tried and tried but could not get her to latch. We struggled; she cried more. The nurse managed to get us going. I winced; the latching hurt in waves, the feeling akin to smashing my toe into a chair.

The next day, a hospital lactation consultant came to my bedside, but I was taking so much opiate pain medication that I couldn't stay awake to follow her instructions. "It's okay, you can close your eyes," she told me. I remember thinking, *Why does she think I need permission?* It wasn't a choice, falling asleep. More like an autonomous body function.

Nursing and doing skin-to-skin, but I just don't feel attached yet, I wrote to my best friend. *I just feel overwhelmed and so sad. And it's hard to bond when I feel like that. Trying to separate her from the pain.*

EMOTIONALLY, THE AFTERMATH OF MY C-section was exceptionally rough. But its physical impacts, as shocking as they were at the time, are standard fare: the difficulty of sitting up or down on a bed, chair, or toilet. How hard it is to walk. Searing pain through the abdomen—what one mother described to me as a "fiery dog collar" of pain. Swollen legs—a result not of weight gain, but of all of the fluids pumped into me during the operation. The dismal breastfeeding. These are routine physical conditions of being in the "secret club" of new C-section motherhood. Yet despite how common C-sections are, we don't talk about the debilitating physical difficulties they cause. And so for many mothers, especially those whose cesareans weren't planned, they come as a surprise.

That's notable, because there's plenty of advice about how to prepare for a recovery from vaginal birth: I made frozen "pancakes" from menstrual pads and witch hazel that I wrapped and stored in the freezer; ordered extra-large underwear to accommodate those pads; bought a sitz bath. If the silences about C-section recovery are any indication, it's that we tend as a society to look away from what cesareans really do to the body. In that sense, the drape that's rigged to keep a mother from seeing what's going on during surgery is a good metaphor for how we treat the operation: something we don't want to look at too closely.

In fact, rather than recognize how invasive C-sections are, most resources—especially back in 2016—diminish the operation as no big deal. As Keisha L. Goode, an assistant professor of sociology at SUNY Old Westbury, puts it, "It's major surgery and we treat it like it is, you know, putting a Band-Aid on." Advice for recovery I encountered included taking it easy, avoiding stairs, and getting someone else to do the laundry. Some publications even suggested C-section moms had it easier than ones who'd had vaginal births: "Instead of huffing, puffing, and pushing your baby into the world, you'll get to lie back and let everybody else do all the heavy lifting," offers *What to Expect When You're Expecting*, which bills itself as the nation's number one bestselling pregnancy book. I laughed bitterly that any publication could so breathlessly drain the severity out of abdominal surgery.

For mothers, recovering from C-sections in a culture that doesn't respect or even fully see surgical birth exacerbates how isolating and emotionally difficult the operation can be. "Nobody tells you" is the phrase used by a number of mothers I interviewed when talking about the operation and its aftermath. (To be fair, "nobody tells you" is something mothers who've had vaginal births say, too; at this point in history, most new mothers in the US are largely unprepared for birth, and motherhood, no matter how the baby gets born.) *Nobody tells you* that you might vomit or dry heave when the baby's born, or that afterward, the anesthesia might make your whole body shake. *Nobody tells you* that after, for a few days at least, you won't be able to sit up unassisted. *Nobody tells you* that for several weeks you won't be able to pick up the car seat, and *nobody tells you* how you'll haul the baby around to the pediatrician as a result. *Nobody tells you* to massage your scar. As a result, mothers bear the fallout of C-sections in the shadows—an experience that itself can be traumatizing.

In their paper on assessing the risks of hormonal birth control, Mauro Turrini and Catherine Bourgain, scholars of science, technology, health, and illness, assert, "Something is [only] visible when somebody recognizes it as relevant."[1] That what a C-section mother's body endures is so out of public view demonstrates that such physical impacts aren't recognized as relevant—that in the story of birth, what happens to the mother's body doesn't matter that much.

But the truth is that these experiences couldn't be more important. Not only because a person's body matters—but because the ways that it's been treated, and overlooked, affect so much else: how a woman pursues future pregnancies. How she chooses and interacts with future providers—for pregnancy and other kinds of care. The way she thinks about her own body and its capacities. How much she trusts herself. How she narrates the story of her motherhood, and—in what can be especially painful for C-section mothers whose operations weren't planned—what kind of mother her birth suggests she is destined to become.

IT'S NOT ONLY MOTHERS WHO are lacking a full view of cesareans. There's also a lot that researchers don't yet know about the operation. Data has only recently started to emerge about how the operation may affect babies throughout their lives—for example, its impact on a baby's microbiome. Because C-section babies do not come into contact with bacteria from the mother's body as they would during vaginal birth, they may be more likely to develop asthma or allergies later in life. Researchers have also just begun looking at whether the operation shortens a mother's life, a possible consequence of the health problems that a C-section can cause decades later, from adhesions of internal organs to an increased need for a hysterectomy. And it seems there's no research that has assessed how having an invasive surgery performed while you're awake can impact your brain, though this question—what did that do to my brain?—came up in more than a few conversations with mothers who'd had the operation.

It's not only the physical effects of C-sections that are out of view. There's so much else about the operation that's overlooked: its risks, why we do so many of them, why people may feel so bad for having had one, even when the operation is necessary and goes well. How many and which layers of tissue the physician cuts and which are simply spread apart. The long-term consequences of those incisions and separations. How much a C-section costs—especially if insurance covers it—or who gets paid and how much. The complications it can cause, such as an infection or a scar that heals poorly. Its longer-term physical and emotional impacts, the ways it shapes future pregnancies, the placental problems it can cause—so many of these aspects of the operation are out of public view.

Nor is there widespread agreement about what percentage of births should be by cesarean section, a concept in medicine called the "normalcy rate." Take a given surgeon who does appendectomies. What percentage of the appendices he removes are normal? If the answer is 100 percent, then "this guy needs to get yanked—he shouldn't be working," Dr. Vikas Saini, a cardiologist and founder of the Lown Institute, a nonprofit that evaluates hospitals, told me. But if it's "zero," said Saini, "that's bad, too. He's probably missing some."

With cesareans, it is difficult to know the "normalcy" rate. Too few cesareans, as in parts of Africa and Asia, lead to preventable maternal and infant deaths. But because of the risks they pose, too many C-sections also cause harm. And even as birth in the US has gotten more dangerous for mothers, it hasn't gotten safer for babies—though the safety of the baby is often cited as reasoning for a cesarean. Since the 1970s, rates of cerebral palsy and other developmental delays—said to be prevented by timely cesareans—have not dropped.[2] Numerous institutions, from the American College of Obstetrics and Gynecologists (ACOG) to the World Health Organization to the editorial board of the *Lancet* assert that we do too many C-sections in this country and that they are definitively causing more harm than good.

The World Health Organization puts the ideal C-section rate—what Saini might call the normalcy rate—at 10 to 15 percent of all births. The US's more conservative goal, for 2030, is 23.6 percent of all low-risk women who've never had a baby before.[3] To put these figures in perspective, it's worth pointing out that until 1970, the US C-section rate was 5.5 percent.[4] That means out of one hundred births, fewer than six were cesarean. The rate of C-sections grew by 455 percent between 1965 and 1987. In 2009, the C-section rate in the US peaked at 32.9 percent. It's hovered around there ever since: one in three births, or about 1.2 million operations per year.[5]

Childbirth is unusual in that it's all-encompassing, but also fleeting: it occupies—very much in the sense that it takes control of—a distinct portion of a person's life. But it doesn't do so for very long, or that often, for the average American woman who now has about 2.07 children.[6] And while 80 percent of women will get pregnant during their lifetimes, only a small percent of women in the US are pregnant at any one time. As a result, the problems posed by surgical birth can be easy to diminish or, indeed, overlook, because only a small percentage of the population is experiencing them at the same time.

Yet the way that we birth has tremendous effects that endure for the rest of our lives, and not only physically. As one obstetrician put it to me: your birth story—you never forget that. Especially if it's not the kind of story about birth that's usually told.

ONE KEY ASPECT ABOUT CESAREANS that's sometimes overlooked is that they fall into four categories.[7] The first is planned C-sections. In the medical literature, these are sometimes called "elective," even if they aren't actually the mother's choice. For instance, a mother who wants to try for vaginal birth after cesarean (VBAC) or a vaginal breech birth, but can't access a provider to attend such births, will be said to have an elective C-section. So will a mother who needs to give birth because she has high blood pressure, and who is discouraged from induction. Or a mother who's told she's growing a baby that will be too big to birth, even though ultrasonic estimations of a baby's size are unreliable. In such instances, the word "elective" is misleading; it conceals the story, the circumstances, of such births, and codes them as if they were a choice, freely made. When in fact the word "elective" refers more to the operating room's scheduling needs. (Notably, the word "elective" has a similarly confusing connotation in other surgeries as well; that's because it can denote an operation that's truly by choice, such as cosmetic surgery, as well as an operation that's urgent but not immediate, like scheduled gallbladder removal.)

Among unplanned cesareans, there are, roughly, three types: nonurgent cesareans, meaning that decision to incision should be within about an hour; urgent, which should occur within thirty minutes; and extremely urgent emergencies, when there is an immediate threat of death to mother or baby.* In these very rare situations—also known more terrifyingly as "crash" cesareans—a C-section can save the life of a mother or baby, which may be threatened by a prolapsed cord, for example, or a uterine rupture.

While many of the mothers I spoke with called their C-sections "emergencies"—a term I used to describe my C-section, too—the truth is that although they may feel like emergencies, most of them aren't quite that urgent. In an emergency C-section, one labor and delivery nurse told me, staff will quite literally pull the hospital bed away from the wall, cords flying, and run it down the hall to the OR. Typically, the anesthesiologist uses general anesthesia to put the mother to sleep immediately. In these exceptionally rare circumstances, a skilled obstetrician will get that baby out in less than a minute and save the lives of one or even two people.

In the US, the majority of cesareans aren't planned. The most common reason for a C-section is stalled labor, accounting for 35 percent of cesareans each year. Nonreassuring fetal heart rate, as indicated by electronic fetal monitoring, is the second-most-common reason. Together, these are the indications for 59 percent of all primary cesareans, which is a person's first cesarean.[8] And while providers will tell a laboring mother if either of these situations is cause to operate, the full reasons for the operation are not always evident, especially in the moment—and particularly among mothers who don't have college degrees, according to research that shows a mismatch between why mothers believe they needed a C-section and the

---

* These are suggestions, but there is no national guideline on specific timing for an operation; the level of urgency depends on each situation and what else is going on in the unit at the time, such as whether the operating room is available.

reasons in their hospital records.[9] That miscommunication is also clear from the confusion among many mothers who believe their C-sections were "emergencies." It was true for me, when my midwife called my cesarean; I remember not being really sure why she had. Labor wasn't going well, that was clear, but what exactly made the operation the next step wasn't.

Sometimes mothers don't even find out what may have contributed to their operation for years—if at all. Alicea Bahl, for instance, who lives in Florida, had planned a home birth in 2012. She transferred to the hospital after forty hours of labor, where staff tried Pitocin and gave her an epidural. Some fifty-four hours after labor had started, the team said it was time for a C-section. The "reason" for the C-section was clear: stalled labor.

But it wasn't until Bahl saw her operative report, years later, that she learned her baby had been OP, meaning occiput posterior, or sunny side up. An OP baby has its back to its mother's spine. It's a position that makes a baby difficult to birth vaginally, because of the angle of their chin and the outlet of a mother's pelvis. The position can also cause back labor, which is especially painful, because the baby's spine knocks against its mother's sacrum. "No one ever told me that. Like how messed up is that?" Bahl says. "If you had a knee surgery they'd come and explain every detail to you. And they didn't tell me, 'This is why she didn't come out.'"

TO BE FAIR, I DIDN'T have much space to contemplate the physical impacts of birth going sideways when I got pregnant at the end of my first year as an assistant professor at SUNY New Paltz. Like most women in the US, I worked for an institution that, at the time, did not offer paid family leave.[10] New York State didn't offer anything, either. I did the math with HR and calculated that I would have accumulated three weeks of sick time when the baby was due. That was it. Theoretically I could take unpaid leave, through the Family Medical Leave Act, but we couldn't afford it. My husband, a photographer, was freelancing as a photo assistant and art handler. We were barely a year out of grad school and had virtually no savings. I had spent my twenties writing for magazines, first on staff and then as a freelancer. I'd also spent seven years in graduate school, pursuing an MFA and then a PhD. This work, as well as adjuncting, and a stipend during my doctorate, had kept me afloat. But financially, I had been only one step ahead of the law for years, and New Paltz was the first full-time job I'd had since I was twenty-four. It paid less than $60,000 a year.

Making life more complicated, if I went on unpaid leave in February, when my baby was due, and stayed off until the semester ended in May, I would not be paid again until the following October. "You got pregnant at a bad time," someone from HR told me—hilariously, given that I was married, fully employed, and had health insurance.

Though I started negotiations in my first trimester, it took until I was thirty-six weeks pregnant, near the end of the fall semester, to finalize a plan for "reassigned time": projects that I could do, besides teaching, to stay on payroll after the baby came. Compared with the average American woman, who has two weeks off of work after giving birth, I had a pretty good deal. (I won't say that I was lucky; that good fortune was predetermined by my whiteness, class, and education, which together had made it more likely for me to have a job that allowed for such an arrangement.)

But that whole semester leading up to the baby, while we were negotiating the reassigned time, I thought about quitting, even though the tenure-track position I'd landed—one within driving distance of my family—is a unicorn of a job, especially for a writer. Then, as the pregnancy progressed, I didn't think I *could* leave; I didn't believe anyone would hire me.

When things got really desperate during these negotiations, I reached out to an employment lawyer with a colleague friend who was also pregnant at the time. At this point it struck me that what was happening was the kind of thing I'd read about: the ways that employers can make life miserable for expectant mothers and new parents; the slow-moving wreck of motherhood colliding with career. Call it ridiculous, but at the time I remember thinking, *Wow. It's real. Those statistics, all the stuff I've read. And now it's happening to me.*

Maybe it was because I was an academic, and not in the corporate world—you know, we study this stuff, so surely we could do better—that I thought I'd be immune to the ways that gender, pregnancy, and motherhood can be used to exploit or punish mothers. I'm sure my naivete was also the product of what scholar Peggy McIntosh calls the "invisible knapsack" of privilege that white people carry around. McIntosh explains that though white people might not be aware of that metaphorical knapsack, it contains "unearned assets," "special provisions . . . and blank checks" that I could "count on cashing in each day." In hindsight, there's a parallel between this and my attitude toward cesareans. Because I didn't think that a cesarean would come for me, either, as if my body was too elite for such an operation.

In these ways, pregnancy and early parenthood were a good entree into becoming a mother in the US: a place where, my friend Kara remarked during the pandemic, the system simply abandons you. Because where "other countries have social safety nets," the sociologist Jessica Calarco told *New York Magazine* in 2020, "the US has women." Until I became a mother, I didn't see this, either.

There is an important kindness to mention in this story of hardship, and a way that my pain was seen. About two weeks after the birth, a friend visited me at home—the one with whom I'd consulted that employment lawyer. I was still frozen and zappy; my nipples were bloody from nursing. We sat together with our babies on my sofa. The concern on her face reflected back to me what I knew but could not see: how desperately brutal the birth had been. "You should ask the union for more time off," she counseled me. I must have told her that I didn't even have it in me to make the ask, because she did it for me, a process that required reaching out to a bushel of administrators.

As a consequence, an email went out on the faculty-staff listserv explaining that an employee facing a "complex medical situation" had run out of sick leave. It did not reveal my identity, or the details of what had happened to me. People on my campus whose identities were also kept confidential donated their vacation days to me, which made it possible for me to stay home an extra four weeks with my baby. An anonymous giver, and anonymous receiver—that is the highest form of charity, my mother observed. (It's also a good example of how individuals, rather than institutions or the government, are expected to provide solutions for systemic problems that are destined to arise again and again.)

Still, this is one of the most beautiful things that happened during one of the darkest parts of my life, and shows what community can do: give without the expectation of being thanked. The unconditional support that all new mothers need.

BIRTH CLASSES AND ONLINE CONTENT don't often describe exactly what happens during a cesarean, which further contributes to the ways that the operation is misunderstood. (One person told me that when they asked the woman teaching their birth class what happened in a C-section, the teacher told everyone to lie on the floor, spread out their arms, and imagine the white light of the OR shining down—an exercise that this mother found terrifying.)

Unplanned or scheduled, the operation is usually the same: an anesthesiologist or nurse anesthetist uses spinal anesthesia (known colloquially as a spinal) or an epidural to anesthetize a mother regionally. Use of regional anesthesia is very important, not only because it means a mother can be awake during birth, but because it is much safer than general anesthesia. Then the surgeon uses a scalpel to cut open the abdomen above the mons pubis, slicing through layers of skin and fat and the fascia that covers the abdominal muscles. The physician parts—but does not cut—the rectus abdominis muscles (the "six-pack") with her hands. Then she cuts through the peritoneum, the layer of tissue that contains organs in the abdomen as if in a tightly sealed bag. She moves the bladder aside to reach the uterus, making yet another incision to open it. She presses on the uterus to push out the baby—the source of the "pressure" C-section moms are told they might expect during the operation. Once the baby is born, the surgeon removes the uterus from the patient's body—sometimes lifting it out completely, like a bowling ball—to sew it closed. Then she sutures the other layers of the patient's abdominal wall and, finally, closes the topmost layer.

For an operation that we did not perfect until the mid-1950s, it is both miraculous and straightforward. For a new OB, it is also easy to learn. "You can train a brand-new doctor to do one in a couple weeks," Dr. Neel Shah, an obstetrician, told me. As numerous physicians and midwives told me, on a mother who's never had a C-section before, it is usually an easy surgery and relatively quick. Still, even for first-time C-sections, vaginal birth is generally safer, Shah said. "You can't get surgical complications without doing surgery." Yet the operation's risks also aren't adequately clear before the surgery. A C-section mom is about 80 percent more likely to have a serious complication, like needing a blood transfusion or an emergency hysterectomy. And though it's rare in the

US, she is about three times more likely to die from a planned C-section than from a planned vaginal birth.[11]

Repeat cesareans are more complicated. "Obstetricians are the only surgeons that routinely cut in the same scar over and over again," Shah explains. "If a vascular surgeon or a neurosurgeon has to go back, it's like a bad day in their workweek. But for an obstetrician it's like a Tuesday." As a result, they encounter scar tissue from previous operations. And that scar tissue makes the surgery more "technically challenging," he explained. "The normal tissue planes go away. They fuse together." In a person who's already had a cesarean, tissue can resemble "concrete," according to another OB I talked with, or, as Shah put it, "a melted box of crayons." This thick scar tissue can cause the uterus and the bladder to fuse together. But the surgeon needs to move the bladder away from the uterus to be able to cut open the uterus and deliver the baby. And that, explained Shah, is "how you get organ injury."

The placenta can also get caught up in that scar tissue, Shah says, which is also dangerous. He describes the placenta as "a big bag of blood vessels—it's 25 percent of everything the heart is pumping. If it gets caught up in the scar tissue and doesn't detach properly, people bleed a lot and quickly." It's for these reasons—these elevated risks of dying, or needing a blood transfusion, or of organ injury, or hysterectomy—that the medical establishment has focused on trying to prevent that first cesarean. And preventing that first C-section makes a person much less likely to have a C-section at all. Because the mother most likely to have a vaginal birth isn't the first-time mom who is at least thirty-seven weeks pregnant, her one baby head-down—a person referred to in medical literature as NTSV, for nulliparous, term, singleton, vertex. It's the mother who's already had a vaginal birth—something that's not clear to most first-time moms, who have at least a one in four chance of having the operation—a likelihood that only increases with a woman's age.[12]

SOME MOMS I TALKED TO—USUALLY, people who'd had a scheduled C-section—described their recoveries as "easy." Sure, some said, the first week, sometimes the first two, are tough; you engage your abs getting up from the sofa or the bed, walking up or down stairs, and C-sections make all of that hard. And the incision hurts; you have to stay on top of the pain. (These mothers also didn't face the emotional complications of a C-section that's a surprise.) Yet what went on during the operation, the planes of tissue that need to knit back together—most mothers have no idea about any of that, of the depth of the incisions and suturing and spreading of their abdominal muscles.

In part, that's because the operation's effects on the uterus, peritoneum, abdominus rectus, fascia, and skin aren't readily evident from the outside. The uppermost incision is often shocking at first, but it is usually small once it heals. People "see this small scar and they don't realize how many layers have to be spread apart," says Carrie Pagliano, a pelvic floor physical therapist based in the Washington, DC, area. The incisions are also less material and sometimes hurt in less intimate places than common injuries after vaginal birth, like a first- or second-degree vaginal or perineal tear or incontinence. But though it's not visible, the technique of a cesarean has serious implications for a mother's bodily integrity. Cutting through the peritoneum, the casing that holds all of the abdominal organs, for instance, disrupts the pressure within "the abdominal canister," explains Karen Brandon, a pelvic floor physical therapist in California. "The abdominal canister is how you maintain pressure to support your back. Your ability to turn on your deep core muscles. It gives you spinal stability. If you disrupt it and never try to maintain it, you can get away with it"—until you can't, which can lead to urinary incontinence and back pain decades after the operation.

The lack of thorough postoperative, postpartum support further contributes to C-sections' underestimation. Absent any significant health issue, at the six- or eight-week postpartum appointment—the single postpartum appointment that insurance will cover—the OB typically will say, "You're fine. You're on the other side. Everything's fine," says Brandon. And that's the extent of typical postpartum care in the United States. That is, if a person can even attend that visit, which fewer than two-thirds of mothers do.

The physical recovery, the new identity of motherhood, and the often terrifying and overwhelming landscape of caring 24/7 for a newborn arrive quickly and all at once. In the overwhelm, it can be impossible to know what to think, what's normal, or who to turn to—especially if you weren't expecting a C-section. On the first night we were home with our baby, my body still so crumpled that I couldn't get in—or out—of bed on my own, my daughter cried until 4:00 a.m. Terrified to bring her into our bed, we relented at dawn. We laid her between us, our arms tucked close to our sides. But we were so scared of accidentally suffocating her, and our house that February was so cold, that we dressed in layers of sweatshirts and sweatpants so we could keep the duvet down at our feet. It was one of the worst nights of my life. Before dropping off to sleep, I remember wondering, sincerely, if she would cry until she went to college. Becoming a mother, I believed, had been a terrible mistake.

THERE IS ONE THING ABOUT cesareans that is recognized—but that reflects a profound misunderstanding of them: that they seem to signal what kind of mother a person will be, even how invested she is in parenthood, as if mode of birth could possibly determine or predict such a thing.

Shakti Castro, a PhD candidate in history at Columbia who had an unplanned C-section in New York in 2019, and then struggled to breastfeed, put it well: "I had a C-section and I gave my kid formula. It was like, 'Oh. You're one of those moms. Okay,'" she says. "It seemed like I don't care enough. I was never going to be able to bond with my baby because I couldn't do these things right for her."

I felt similarly to Shakti when I became a mother. Because despite the blaring-red warnings to avoid the cascade of interventions said to lead inevitably to a cesarean, I really only wanted to avoid the operation not because of its risks, or how it might affect me in the future, but because of the stigma around it. Because I didn't really see C-sections, I misunderstood them as a second-class way to birth, one somehow less honorable than vaginal birth. If pushed to explain, I probably would have said something about how a "natural" birth would lead to a more natural connection with my baby. These notions reflected my ideas of myself (I am "one of those moms" who has a natural birth), as well as a deeply entrenched misunderstanding that getting birth "right" would make me a good mother. They also reflected the reputation that's clung to cesareans that's a vestige of its origins, and its development on women largely derided as unfit mothers.

These misapprehensions are themselves interesting and speak to the ways that C-sections are so broadly misunderstood because their risks, their effects, and the reasons people have them are so widely overlooked. That is, until and unless you've had one, and the issues the operation sets into motion become your problem. In other words, what I could see about C-sections is just as compelling as what I couldn't.

The language used to talk about unplanned C-sections further obscures the many factors that contribute to surgical birth, and suggests that the mode of birth reflects a mother's character. Too often, when a mother has an unplanned C-section, her vaginal birth is said to be "unsuccessful" or "failed." The implication, says Caitlin Bradley, a neonatal intensive care unit nurse who had a C-section with her second child, is that people who have C-sections are "lazy, their body is misbehaving. . . . They're not willing [vaginal birth] to happen." That plays into expectations that mothers are individually responsible for their births, and suggests that C-sections are possibly, or partly, the result of a personal flaw—an idea circulated in obstetric textbooks a century ago.

That attitude—that C-sections are the lazy way to birth—is evident in popular and mainstream books that suggest C-sections are easy because the mother doesn't have to do much. "You won't be able to participate actively at a cesarean delivery the way you would at a vaginal one, and some would consider that a definite plus," states *What to Expect When You're Expecting*, still among the country's bestselling books about pregnancy. Framing cesareans to emphasize a mother's inability to "participate actively" negates everything that's hard about the operation—physically and emotionally.

It also raises the question of whether C-sections even "count" as birth, which many mothers I spoke to wondered about, including Anchorage mom Kate, who had an unplanned C-section in 2017. "I didn't feel like I gave birth," she told me. "I didn't do anything. He got taken out of me."

Kate had planned for an unmedicated birth with a midwife. But labor stalled, and because she had thrombocytopenia, her platelets were too low to have regional anesthesia safely. So she had a C-section under general anesthesia. After the birth, Kate woke to a nurse massaging her abdomen, to expel any bits of afterbirth. The pain, she says, was unendurable. The first time she told me about it, when her son Oliver was almost five, she was so choked with tears she could barely finish her sentence.

Physically, Kate healed quickly. But she also felt lasting shame about the birth: She believed she'd asked for the C-section. That she had needlessly given up. And she felt guilty that she didn't remember meeting Oliver. All of that shame made it hard for her to talk about his birth, she says. It's not dissimilar from the messaging around having an abortion, which, when I was growing up, was meant to be "safe, legal, and rare." A person who had an abortion was someone you pitied, the procedure evidence that you'd made a mistake, the attendant guilt deserved for your errors of judgment.

But at the same time, Kate also felt embarrassed that she had such a difficult time emotionally, especially because she'd seemed to heal so quickly. She wondered if she was making a big deal about nothing. If she shouldn't just get over it. Her emotional experience shouldn't have mattered as much as it did, she reasoned, because physically she was okay, and her baby was, too. In a society that largely doesn't present C-sections as a way that birth will turn out, then overlooks their physical impacts in a medical environment where people don't even fully understand what the operation does to their bodies, it only makes sense that Kate would wonder if she was making a big deal out of nothing. The message about C-sections is that they're not a big deal. To react the way she had, surely there must be something wrong with her. But at the time, Kate didn't see that, either.

I felt similarly to Kate after my birth: for a while, I resisted how much the birth had harmed me, because my body and my baby physically were okay. I wondered if there wasn't something wrong with me that it had hurt me so badly. I see now that these feelings, like Kate's, are also the inevitable response to a "bad" birth, given the messages women encounter beginning in childhood: the pain you feel is not as bad as you say it is; you are exaggerating; perhaps it's all in your head. These messages lodge deep under the skin. This is how a thoughtful, reflective person becomes recruited into the process of gaslighting herself during a physical experience as uniquely embodied as birth.

NOT EVERYONE WHO HAS A C-section feels traumatized by it or lesser than. A C-section isn't essentially or inherently upsetting. "Yes!" Rachel

Samuelson, a family medicine doctor, said when she found out she was going to be having a cesarean. (She felt similarly happy about it after the birth, too.) Nor is a vaginal birth inherently not traumatic: "For years I was embarrassed to tell you," said my friend Andrea, "that I found my birth traumatic." She'd had her son vaginally, nearly two weeks after her due date, after a long and painful labor. A historian of antiquity, she now understood, she told me, why the ancient Greeks had likened childbirth to war.

Still, the pervasiveness of shame and stigma regarding C-sections is especially notable given how common the operation is. Talking with mothers, the same ideas came up again and again: C-section mothers don't really give birth; it's their fault their births turn out as they do; they're going to be bad mothers, because they seemingly don't care enough to get birth right.

Something as simple as changing the language used to explain why a person needs a cesarean might help reduce some of that shame, says Caitlin Bradley, the NICU nurse and mother of two. Providers can be more precise, explaining, for instance, that because of the contractions, the amniotic fluid is gone, and baby doesn't have much buoyancy to move into a better position. Or they might say we are "'lucky to have this tool that we can use, and we do it to keep everybody safe. And these are the reasons we think this isn't safe anymore.' Or, 'with every contraction, the baby is getting less blood flow, and we see that in the objective signs.' If you say it like that," she says, the language doesn't suggest that a mother could control what's happening if only she tried harder or had more stamina. It doesn't make the birth a test that the mother has failed. And it would also provide more clarity about why the mother needed the section to begin with, so she could more deeply understand why she was consenting to the operation at all.*

THERE'S A PARTICULAR KIND OF hurt that some C-section moms face that's as important as any physical impact as it is overlooked: Often,

---

* One OB I spoke with noted that this "insensitive language" shows up in diagnostic codes, and that it's not necessarily how physicians speak to patients.

mothers and newborns are separated during the surgery, and a mother doesn't get the chance to hold the baby right away. It might be that the baby is sent to the NICU (neonatal intensive-care unit). Maybe the baby is okay, but is sent to the nursery or back to the room while you're getting stitched up. Maybe you aren't awake when your baby is born. Maybe your arms aren't free to hold her. Maybe you're feeling woozy or nauseated or are shivering too much to feel safe holding your baby. Maybe you did hold your baby, but you don't remember it. Maybe you get stuck in recovery, waiting to go back to your room, wondering—like one mother told me—*Where the hell is my family?*

Being separated from your baby, or feeling as if you didn't get the opportunity to meet her, can be deeply traumatizing. It's what happened to me. I have no distinct memory of "meeting" my daughter, probably because of the shock and the medications I received during and after surgery. Kate felt similarly. She told me that part of her wondered if she didn't leave an "imprint" on her son because she wasn't awake during his birth.

Popular and academic literature alike emphasize that at birth, mother and baby are strangers who must be introduced so that they can bond. On top of this, we're in a particular moment of societal adulation of "the golden hour," the newborn's first hour of life. Literature about pregnancy and birth emphasize the almost unparalleled importance of that particular expression of parental devotion, linking the personal significance of immediately welcoming your baby to the physiological benefits of holding the baby skin-to-skin.

Yet the notion that mother and baby are strangers, introduced by the doctor, simply isn't true. Birth, sociologist Barbara Katz Rothman points out, is "a moment of separation, not a moment of joining." It is not the "introduction," but a sundering, and the next phase of a relationship that's already begun.

It might seem easy to dismiss this idea, but the belief that mother and baby are strangers is far from universal. Traditional interpretations of Jewish law, for instance, see birth as a separation, one that is so "drastic," writes Rav DovBer Pinson—from the fetus's "being part of and within [the mother's] body"—that some rabbis interpret it as "a form of death." It is because she has had an encounter with death, he says, that a mother is in a state of ritual impurity following birth.

To be sure, mothers should be given the option to hold their babies after birth if they can and want to. And perhaps shifting the story about birth—from it being a beginning you have to start right to it being an ending—can bring mothers some comfort: My baby already knows me. I already know my baby. My baby has been inside of my body. This is the next chapter of a story that's already begun. Mothering, over the long haul, is about that: separating and coming together, and, over time, finding new ways to be separate people who spend time together. Seen a certain way, these ideas take the pressure off those first hours. There is already so much that your body has accomplished: growing a baby, growing a placenta, keeping that baby and yourself alive. All of that you've done together.

When I was pregnant with my daughter, and then my son, they felt alternately like extensions of my own body but also like individual beings. They kicked at movies I found exciting; they seemed lulled to sleep when I walked. But they also had their own agendas. They rolled and punched before dawn. My son had a habit of pianoing his fingers lightly inside of my body, as if he were tracing a drawing on a wall. Light as feathers, this sensation was also fundamentally distracting, pulling me from a conversation as if he were already on the outside and he needed to connect; it felt that he was telling me something he needed me to know.

And yet such a liminal state, as legal scholar Marie Ashe puts it, "to which we can apply no number known to us," is not the way that pregnancy is discussed in the mainstream American judicial or medical systems.[13] Which is another reason why recognizing that birth is not an introduction but actually a separation is so important: doing so casts light on a big idea that governs us—that a fetus is an entirely distinct entity from its mother.

Though it's at the core of such laws as the *Dobbs* decision, which overturned the right to abortion, the idea that a mother and fetus are entirely separate entities doesn't describe the reality of pregnancy. Nor are the pregnant person and their fetus one single organism. The truth is far more complex, almost beyond the limits of spoken language: a pregnant person, legal scholar Isabel Karpin proposed, is in fact "not-one-but-not-two."[14]

When does the not-one-but-not-two process of separation even end? Because as any new mother can attest, it's not at birth. Separating from the baby is a slow unfold, dawning on the baby, then the toddler, that your two bodies are not one. It's a process that unfolds slowly for the mother, too. There are physiological examples of this; many mothers experience a letdown (their breast milk starts to flow) when they hear their baby cry.[15] Especially during those early months, parenting—mothering—is a slow cleave.

Contemplating Karpin's ideas, I thought that perhaps this is another reason C-sections can be so vexing: they're an operation that happens to you, and to your baby, and to the self/other that is a pregnant person. Their impact is that much harder to articulate, given that we don't even have sufficient language for the liminality, the not-one-but-not-two state of being pregnant. Perhaps, too, that is why they can be so deeply felt. Their impact isn't additive—an operation on two people. It's exponential. But because pregnancy as not-one-but-not-two is underexplored and legally undercredited, this aspect of C-sections is also far from view.

WHEN I CAME BACK TO work, about eight weeks after the birth, one of my tasks for reassigned time was to report on a talk given by a prominent journalist at my campus. Under other circumstances, this opportunity could have been good for my career. The journalist had published several well-received books and wrote often for publications I hoped one day to publish in.

But the assignment was a setup for disaster. My daughter was so young, and there wasn't anyone I could leave her with; my husband was out of town for work. We didn't even have a babysitter yet. This meant I had to bring her with me.

I worried about how my daughter's presence would mark me, in a bad way, as a mother. I knew that during the evening she'd have to eat—and that I'd have to nurse. I dreaded her crying; I worried about how disruptive that would be; I thought I'd be so embarrassed. And I didn't know how I'd be able to write about the talk if I wasn't there to hear it.

A senior colleague and friend, Lisa, introduced me to the journalist. We sat off to the side for a few minutes before his lecture, and I asked him questions for my story. I can't remember where my daughter was; probably in a stroller nearby. At a certain point, he asked—kindly, and with real surprise evident in his voice—"Why are you here?"

I can't recall how much I told him, but I did tell him I didn't have paid leave. I stopped short at loudly critiquing the institution. Because I wasn't tenured, I feared that condemnation—to a journalist known for reporting on poor working conditions—would only get me in trouble.

Between this conversation and the start of his talk, I took my baby to my office to nurse her. I sat in my desk chair, unzipped my dress, and brought her to my breast. I was so engorged, the physical relief of nursing felt like peeing after holding it in. It was early spring, and dark, but bright in my office. I gazed out the large windows at the gloaming outside. Anyone could see us. We cut an unexpected, lonely image of a college professor on campus.

I hoped that, with a full belly, the baby would sleep through the lecture. For this, I had a plan: I put on a boba wrap, wrapping the material taut against my body, around each shoulder, and then tied it at the front. The wrap created a little pouch, and I slid my baby into it and gave her a pacifier. Then I slipped into the auditorium. Eventually, this stopped working—she made her sounds—and I put her in her stroller. I paced around the back of the auditorium, rocking her and taking notes. Senior colleagues and administrators heard us. Saw me.

When the talk ended, and the journalist made his way out of the room, he stopped to greet me. He made a comment about how surprising it was that I was there, given my baby's age. I can't be certain that senior administrators heard this, but my journalism colleague Lisa did. Some administrators cooed over my baby; so cute, one said. One person looked at me, and I felt in their gaze irritation at my presence. As if they would prefer I were invisible. I remember feeling that I, too, wished I could disappear. That the whole of my body—my leaking, bleeding, bloated body, and my mewling baby beside it—was an embarrassment to the university. Which it was. I shouldn't have been there. I was an inconvenient, messy reality that revealed how my institution treated new parents, which until the journalist had made visible, we'd all ignored and pretended to be acceptable.

Another person might have felt defiant in such a situation, or even proud. I was too ashamed of what I'd gone through to access those feelings. Instead, I felt humiliated, and worried about possible consequences, but also somewhat thankful that the journalist had spoken up—had said what I had been too afraid to say.

I now see that my body was a good metaphor for how our society treats C-sections more generally: we skim over their surface because we don't want to look closely at them. Looking at why I was at that lecture, why it was so difficult for me to be there, and why I'd brought my daughter required navigating complicated and uncomfortable legal, economic, and medical truths: the lack of paid leave, my family's financial precarity, the difficulty of C-section recovery, the trauma I'd endured, the lack of high-quality infant care. Likewise, looking closely at C-sections reveals much that's complicated, and uncomfortable, about how we treat women, pain, medicine, technology, people of color, and reproductive autonomy.

For sure, these are difficult topics. Which is why we must look at them straight on.

In order to do that, I turn to what seems obvious: why vaginal birth, and particularly unmedicated vaginal birth, is so deeply vaunted. Doing so is one way to get at cesareans. Because in order to better understand the operation, it's essential to look at what it's not: vaginal birth, which has earned the moniker of "natural."

2

"NATURAL" CHILDBIRTH
AND THE "NORMAL" WOMAN

THERE ARE TWO VERSIONS OF CHILDBIRTH THAT DOMINATE THE POPU-
lar conversation, especially for first-time mothers. The first perspective
is that unmedicated, natural birth is painful, scary, dangerous—even
primitive: "It's totally stone age *what happens to you*," a columnist wrote
recently in an Australian paper.[1] If this version of childbirth had a repre-
sentative it might be St. Margaret of Antioch, the patron saint of women
in labor. Though Margaret never bore children, the physical suffering
she endured—including being eaten by a dragon—made her relatable to
childbearing women in the Middle Ages, among whom she was evidently
extremely popular.

To counteract the pain and danger of childbirth, according to this way
of thinking, we need to throw everything we can at it. Modern medicine
delivered in a hospital—inductions, epidurals, C-sections—ensures babies' and their mothers' safety, even survival. Anything less is dangerous
and irresponsible.

The other perspective: birth is a natural, physiological event; if there's
anything to be feared, it's not labor and birth, but the consequences of
messing with nature. This version of birth has many patron saints, among
whom the midwife and author Ina May Gaskin may be the best known,
though she has many aspirants on social media.

According to this perspective, birth isn't about getting eaten by a
dragon; birth is about becoming the dragon, relishing the fullness of the

embodied experience. "You are the birthing goddess," writes natural-birth coach Saima Kara, who runs the Instagram account @livewildbirthfree; "Feeling every part of birth is a GIFT."[2]

When I prepared for my daughter's birth, most of the advice coming my way arrived from that second camp. Without being able to attribute it to anyone in particular, I understood unmedicated birth as morally and experientially superior. Although my doula suggested it, I didn't seriously consider home birth—that felt too dangerous, living twenty-five minutes from the closest hospital—but to the extent that I thought about C-sections at all, I believed a "natural" birth would help me avoid the operation; epidurals fell into the cascade of interventions that I understood ended inevitably with a cesarean, a fear my doula repeatedly emphasized.

So it only made sense that I'd forgo an epidural. In fact, this wasn't even so much a decision as the inevitable consequence of my views about bodies and motherhood, the kind of woman I thought I was and where I believed I belonged, culturally—beliefs that, because they felt so inherent, so natural, I didn't recognize as the product of a worldview at all.

I announced my intention to have a "natural" birth at Rosh Hashanah. I looked down the table at four generations of women, including my own mother. At thirty-three, I was the last grown-up woman among them to start a family. I can still see the restrained looks on their faces, these women who had birthed some twenty children over forty years, who'd changed thousands of diapers and cooked tens of thousands of meals, who'd seen children off to kindergarten and college—all while holding jobs outside the home—and who knew intimately about the many varieties of pain and love that comprise the ballad of the parent.

To their credit, the women said nothing. Possibly my reputation for making off-road decisions (i.e., moving to New Paltz, named the "hippiest" town in New York State, and not New York City; marrying a non-Jewish guy) weighed in my favor. Then my mother broke their polite silence. "Go for the drugs," she said with a laugh.

At the time, I remember feeling misunderstood, in what seems to me now an adolescent sort of way: *You don't get it, Mom.* For me, birth would be different. To be sure, my mother knew what she was talking about. She'd had two children. But she'd also once told me that birth was better than any orgasm you've ever had in your life. So an epidural—I was confident I wouldn't need one.

WHEN IT COMES TO BIRTH, the term "natural" is at once fuzzy and imprecise. Does it mean vaginal? Vaginal and unmedicated? At home? In the water? Regardless of the definition—which changes depending on who you ask—it most definitely doesn't include C-sections. Though it would not become a regular part of obstetric practice in America until the early 1900s, one of the earliest known mentions of cesarean birth, in the late thirteenth century, referred to it as "artificium," meaning artificial.[3] And so if natural birth is good—and, as we'll see, that "good" means closer to nature, more moral, and better for children—then C-sections are none of those. On multiple levels, the rhetoric around natural birth implies that C-sections are bad, and the mothers who have them are bad, too.

But to get at what "natural birth" means now, and why its power is among the reasons C-section mothers can feel cast out, we have to go back to its roots. That means visiting two people: Grantly Dick-Read, the British obstetrician who introduced the term "natural birth" to Americans; and Ina May Gaskin, credited as the latter-day mother of it all.

Dick-Read's books *Natural Childbirth* and *Childbirth Without Fear* appeared in the US in the early 1940s, introducing the term "natural birth" to the American lexicon. At the time, demand for medication to relieve labor pain was widespread in the US, among women and doctors both. Yet despite its popularity, obstetric anesthesia was inchoate; the epidural as we know it wouldn't become widely available until the late 1960s.[4]

Instead, many of the pain relievers used in the early and mid-twentieth century created more problems than they solved. Ether, for instance, increased risks of hemorrhage, lung irritation, and kidney damage for mothers and asphyxiation for babies. Morphine, another popular pain reliever, caused breathing problems in babies, who could be born needing to be resuscitated.[5] Other medications numbed the pelvis so completely that women could not feel how or when to push. That meant that obstetricians more often needed to use forceps to drag babies out.[6] Though forceps had been used since the 1700s to deliver stuck babies and save mothers' lives, in the wrong hands—for instance, among physicians who didn't really know how to use them—they could lacerate a mother and damage her baby, too.[7]

What's more, some of the labor medications especially popular at the time, like scopolamine, didn't relieve pain at all. They only served to cause amnesia so that women forgot birth altogether.[8] In fact, administered as part of twilight sleep, a labor management technique that was particularly popular in the US in the early twentieth century, women would often scream, thrash, and hallucinate.[9] Some even tried to climb out of windows.[10] As a result, hospital staff regularly tied women receiving twilight sleep to their beds.[11]

Twilight sleep quickly fell from favor after a New York woman receiving it died during childbirth in 1915. But physicians continued practices associated with it through the 1960s, such as using scopolamine, often with other drugs, "to erase women's memory of labor," writes historian Jacqueline H. Wolf in *Deliver Me from Pain*.[12] They also continued to restrain women during labor, which also lasted into the 1960s and beyond. My mother remembers having her wrists put in restraints as late as 1974.

In the search for how to relieve the pain of labor, Dick-Read's books stood out because he asserted that women could birth without the need for medicated pain relief—if they practiced calming their minds.[13] "Primitive" women, he wrote, knew instinctively to do this.[14] White women had forgotten how. But they could learn, he assured his readers. In that way he forged "natural" birth as a goal that white, middle-class women should pursue—a legacy that continues to this day. He also contributed to an extant division between white mothers and mothers of color, as if white women's exposure to "culture" had rewired their very biology.

For this technique to succeed, women needed continual male accompaniment during labor from their physicians and, in many cases, their husbands.[15] This was radical: at the time, women who gave birth in hospitals labored alone, their husbands banished to the waiting room. But it was also profoundly antifeminist: a calm, unmedicated labor wasn't something women could handle independently—they needed men to make it work.

Dick-Read also asserted that by being fully conscious and emotionally present for birth, women could achieve "the perfection of womanhood." Labor and childbirth were among the most important aspects of a woman's life. In that way, he yoked "natural," meaning unmedicated, labor to what he saw as women's biological imperative and the ultimate expression of female identity. Given how dangerous pain relief could be, it isn't surprising that Dick-Read's ideas found a receptive audience.

BUT IT WASN'T SIMPLY THE search for new ways to avoid labor pain that made Dick-Read's ideas enticing. By the middle of the twentieth century, a wider dissatisfaction was growing regarding the typical US hospital birth—a cultural moment similar to our own. A turning point came from a letter by a reader identified as "registered nurse" that was published in *Ladies' Home Journal* in November 1957. "I feel compelled to write you this letter asking you to investigate the tortures that go on in modern delivery rooms," she wrote.[16] She described women routinely "strapped down with cuffs around her arms and legs and steel clamps over her shoulders and chest;" a doctor who does episiotomies "without anesthetic because he almost lost a patient from an overdose some years ago"; women "strapped in the lithotomy position, with knees pulled far apart, for as long as eight hours."

When the magazine's editors asked readers to weigh in, to investigate the truth of the allegations, mothers, doctors, and nurses flooded the magazine with letters. While some refuted the charges, the responses widely corroborated "registered nurse's" claims. Notably, many letters echo the kind of bad experiences that plague birth today. For instance, although C-section rates were quite low at the time—less than 5 percent of births—some mothers still felt time pressure to birth their babies quickly.[17] Back in 1958, if doctors were in a rush, they'd "force the baby with forceps."[18] (Today, stalled labor is one of the most common reasons for a C-section.) Some mothers also birthed too fast for their doctor, who had other things to do, from patient rounds to dinner. In those cases, doctors slowed birth: they instructed nurses to administer ether or general anesthesia, or to hold women's legs closed.[19]

In such an environment, Dick-Read's ideas, along with other unmedicated approaches to managing labor such as the Bradley Method and Lamaze, started to become more popular among women in the US. In time, they became a sensation: they inspired radio and TV shows, newspaper and magazine articles, and books authored by women who'd employed the techniques to great effect: *Thank You, Dr. Lamaze: A Mother's Experience in Painless Childbirth* (1959) and *Six Practical Lessons for an Easier Childbirth* (1967) became bestsellers, with the latter selling a million copies.[20] By the 1970s, second-wave feminism claimed natural birth as part of the overall project for women seeking to reclaim autonomy over their bodies—right around the time Ina May Gaskin was cofounding the Farm, a commune and midwifery center in Tennessee that remains a destination for mothers seeking an unmedicated, "natural" birth.[21]

To a contemporary reader, what also stands out from *Ladies' Home Journal's* investigation is how women were often treated as an afterthought, a mere container for their babies. As one nurse wrote at the time: "So often a delivery seems to be 'job-centered'—that is, get the job done the easiest, quickest way possible with no thought to the patient's feelings. In too many cases, doctors and nurses lose sight of their primary concern—the *patient*."[22] I read that letter to my husband one chilly autumn morning while he was getting breakfast together for the kids. "Wait—is that from now?" he asked. It was one of many similar moments I had writing this book: articles from women's magazines published decades, even a century ago—from the US's high rate of maternal mortality, to inequitable infant mortality rates, to the often dismal experiences of hospital birth—felt eerily, and sadly, familiar.

IN THE LATE 1960S, STEPHEN Gaskin, a former professor of English at San Francisco State University, launched "Monday Night Class," a free lecture series open to anyone who wanted to come. His talks on spirituality, God, nonviolence, and anti-materialism eventually attracted upwards of 1,500 people a week. In 1970, Gaskin went on the road to deliver his sermons. Several hundred followers joined, packed into repurposed school buses and bread vans.[23] A pregnant Ina May and her young family were among them; that's how she and Stephen met.

To realize their dream of living collectively and in tune with the earth, the group of about three hundred people in the caravan decided to buy about a thousand acres near Summertown, Tennessee.[24] To join what would become known as the Farm, members had to take a vow of poverty and donate all of their money to the collective. They worked to sustain the collective through farming, cooking, teaching, and building homes. To minimize their impact on the environment, they ate only vegetarian food. ("Soybeans," children raised on the Farm remember. "We ate tons of soybeans.")

Ina May, along with other women, served as a midwife, attending births among the group and from a nearby Amish community. The need for midwifery grew quickly, because Stephen Gaskin had forbidden birth control; such is the outcome of "natural" family planning. In time, Ina May's influence on natural birth, and midwifery, would resonate throughout the US and even the world. Her 1975 book *Spiritual Midwifery*, initially published by the Farm's press, has since sold over five hundred thousand copies and been translated into six languages, according to historian Wendy Kline's 2015 study in the *Bulletin of the History of Medicine*.

The foundation of Gaskin's approach, and of some of its contemporary spin-offs, is that birth needn't—indeed shouldn't—be medicalized. Women's bodies are capable of birth, and most women can birth their babies without intervention. They need encouragement far more than they need drugs. Gaskin also writes that childbirth is only as painful as you expect it to be.[25] But unlike the pain of a C-section, an epidural headache, or an episiotomy, labor pain doesn't last beyond the birth.[26] It's pain that's "natural," productive, an almost good kind of pain. And it isn't something to fear, even if the "sensations" are intense.[27]

Gaskin is still largely credited as the "mother" of modern midwifery, as if she picked up and revived an ancient practice. For many of the mothers I interviewed who were—or are—interested in unmedicated, "natural" birth, her work served as an introduction. (Kate told me she was entranced, then frustrated, by Ina May's *Guide to Childbirth* and ultimately threw her copy of the book across the room.) Gaskin's fame is one reason why the image of midwifery is synonymous with a white woman in Birkenstocks, her hair in long braids.

But the image of the crunchy hippie midwife belies the reality of the midwifery workforce in the US. The vast majority of midwives here attend births in the hospital, not at home or in a community setting. That's because, unlike Gaskin, who is a certified professional midwife, most midwives in the US are certified nurse-midwives, or CNMs. CNMs are both registered nurses and hold a master's in midwifery, which entitles them to attend births in hospitals, in birth centers, and at home.* They not only tend to pregnant, laboring, and postpartum people, but provide a range of so-called well-woman care, including birth control, abortion, and gynecological exams. They can prescribe medicine, from antibiotics to Xanax to hormone replacement therapy, and can order tests, like pelvic ultrasounds and mammograms. Some CNMs even assist with cesareans.

By contrast, certified professional midwives (CPMs) like Gaskin do not have training in nursing. They learn the profession through accredited midwifery schools and a clinical apprenticeship that lasts at least two years. CPMs attend people who birth at home or in a birth center; they do not have hospital admitting privileges. Their training focuses exclusively on attending low-risk pregnant, laboring, and postpartum mothers.

These may seem like the kinds of distinctions that matter only within the profession—midwife to midwife. And indeed, the differences between these types of midwives often isn't legible to patients; I had no idea that there were different kinds of midwives until I started reporting this book. But these differently trained midwives have profound implications for birthing people, because of licensure regulations. For instance, each US state has its own rules governing CPMs' authority. Not all states even grant CPMs licenses, which means that in fourteen states, CPMs cannot practice legally, no matter their expertise.[28] Even in the states where they can practice, not all of them are reimbursed by Medicaid, which further limits who can access them. (Nationwide, more than 40 percent of all births are paid for by Medicaid.[29]) As chapter 5 explores, these constraints on CPMs are the legacy of state-driven efforts throughout the twentieth century to eradicate so-called lay midwives—who were predominantly Black, Indigenous, and immigrant women—and to replace them with the newly created designation of certified nurse-midwives, who were, and still are, predominantly white.

This history, and differences in respect and legitimacy, have led to animosity among some midwives of different training. Crucially, though, both types of midwives have one thing in common: lack of autonomy.

---

* Certified midwives (CMs) also hold a graduate degree in midwifery, but needn't have a degree in nursing.

Unlike the UK, the United States lacks a midwifery board to oversee and regulate midwives. Instead, both CNMs and CPMs—despite having their own accrediting organizations, despite their experience, and their training and knowledge—are overseen, at the state and hospital levels, by physicians.

READING INA MAY'S *Guide to Childbirth* when I was pregnant, I found the idea that pain was only pain because we called it that resonated with me. It made sense that fears around childbirth were overblown, and to some degree socially constructed, by a society that often stereotyped women as weak, hysterical, and incapable. I also believed myself to be outside mainstream US culture by dint of character and training. My dad had been born in a displaced persons camp in Germany and came to the US as a toddler. I grew up feeling as though my family had only one foot here, that we were still figuring out what it meant to be American, but that we were definitely not it. One long-running family joke was that when my father watched baseball on TV, wore a baseball hat, and—an extremely rare occurrence—drank a beer, he was "a real Amerikaner" (Yiddish for "American"). Gaskin's book hit the counterculture note in me, and also felt vaguely European (which it is; unlike the US, Western Europe never entirely forsook midwifery for obstetrics. Midwives attend a far greater percentage of births in Europe than they do in the US; our penchant for aggressive medical intervention, which goes back as far as colonial times, is one among many reasons for this).

In an email I wrote to a friend at the time—who was also pregnant—I gushed, *I don't feel scared of delivery in part because I read Ina May Gaskin's book on birthing (not* Spiritual Midwifery, *the other one). It has tons of birth stories and basically makes the point that we construct birth as something to fear in the US, and that doing so makes the process unnecessarily hard. I recommend reading it.*

I was an easy mark.

What also drew me to Gaskin—what attracts many people—was her exceptional birth outcomes. Of the more than 2,000 births on the Farm between 1970 and 2010, which included people who traveled there from all over the world, only 1.7 percent have been C-sections.[30] As Gaskin notes in her *Guide to Childbirth*, there were some 186 births before the Farm's first C-section, and that one was a baby who lay sideways and who would not be moved.[31]

Since 1970, seven babies born at the Farm have died, including Gaskin's own—the one she was pregnant with when she was traveling around by bus. The Farm has not lost a single mother.[32] To be sure, the people birthing at the Farm are self-selecting. And the midwives accept only low-risk pregnancies. But the data stand. And they beat the US's statistics. In 2020, 574 babies died in the US for every 100,000 births.[33] Some 23.8 mothers died per 100,000 births.[34] And our C-section rate, of course, is about one out of three.[35]

Too often, this data is interpreted as if there were something magical about Gaskin. If there is magic, it's what she and the other midwives offer at the Farm—noninterventionist, supportive, patient-centered and holistic care that midwives, who are experts in physiological vaginal birth, provide the world over. While this kind of care is often framed as an "alternative" to mainstream obstetrics, it isn't alternative at all, says P. Mimi Niles, an assistant professor of nursing at NYU, a CNM, and a practicing midwife. "We are not alternative—I'm not an alternative," she says. "I'm a legitimate, legible, independent practitioner" who possesses a body of knowledge particularly focused on pregnant and laboring people. Though physicians are reified as "the top of this knowledge pyramid," a general practitioner "is not going to know anything about . . . stimulating breasts to stimulate contractions," she points out. "Mainstream medicine does not speak to all the ways of knowing."

I DIDN'T SEE IT AT the time, but the natural-birth ideology Gaskin personifies leaves out a lot. Like so much of the culture around birth, it's used to emphasize what you, the individual, can do. How you can reject the medical model. How you can prepare your mind. How you can say no to intervention. "Your body is not a lemon," Gaskin writes.[36] "You are not a machine. The Creator is not a careless mechanic." The solution to the problem isn't to change society. It's to stick up for yourself. Never mind that when Black birthing people stick up for themselves by declining care, as a 2019 study by Laura B. Attanasio and Rachel R. Hardeman shows, they are more likely to be stigmatized "as non-compliant, aggressive or as the 'angry Black woman.'"[37]

That same insistence on focusing on yourself when facing adversity shows up in self-help books, women's magazines, and wellness culture. It sounds empowering, but when it comes to solving systemic problems like the overuse of C-sections, or structural racism, it's a losing battle. Scholars Rosalind Gill and Shani Orgad call it neoliberalism's "psychological turn."[38] They define this as a promotion of individual resilience that's reflective of and shaped by forty years of mostly Western governments enacting policies that promote individual responsibility in most realms of life. Wearing my daughter to the lecture, trying to parent a newborn while working at the same time, without any structural or organizational support for either one—that's an emblem of neoliberalism. And it's especially true for parenting; as education journalist Sarah Carr noted in a talk she gave in the fall of 2022, parents in the US don't have federally mandated paid family leave. No paid sick leave. No guaranteed basic income. No financial support for day care or preschool. The only thing parents have, she said, is public school. And that only starts at age five.

The imperative to manifest a good birth is seductive. And to be sure, getting yourself in the right headspace is important; labor and birth require tremendous mental persistence. It is important to believe that your body can birth safely and—if it's your intention—vaginally. But you can't think your way out of a broken system, or one that only appears to grant mothers freedom of choice. Believing that you can do so is a trap, especially when it turns out that you can't manifest the birth you want—no matter how smart or good at thinking you may be.

This focus on the individual getting it right also misses the mark for the kind of preparation needed to cope with the pain of labor. Because no matter how birth goes, and as chapter 9 explores, it will hurt. But the ways of coping that I knew of only vaguely—like HypnoBirthing, or other kinds of meditation—seemed ridiculous, easy to parody. (By the time I got pregnant again, I'd learned, and I listened to meditations in the months before birth.) In that way it's almost as if we've completely lost track of where and how birth actually happens, the very embodied experience it is—no matter whether you have an epidural, a C-section, or an unmedicated vaginal birth—as if it is something that you can will your way through simply with the power of your mind.

WHEN HELENA A. GRANT WAS a teenager growing up in New York, she wanted to be a singer, an actress, someone onstage. That gift to perform, you can feel it in her presence: she projects—her spirit and her voice—and brokers no bullshit. She knows that this doesn't always make her popular: "At my job I'm appreciated and not liked at the same time. And that's okay," she told me. "I feel that's what I'm called to do." She also has a big, beautiful smile, and though our conversations focus on deadly serious topics—maternal mortality, racism, health inequities—she flashes it frequently. She is also quite funny. (On the damaging message of Sheryl Sandberg's *Lean In*—to keep working through it all, to eschew recovery or rest—"I want to write a book that's *Lean the Fuck Out*," she says.)

Grant's father died two months shy of her sixteenth birthday. That changed her trajectory. "You're going to have to go to school and get a degree where you're going to get a job," her mother told her. "Although you have these other talents, you need the sure thing." Turning toward medicine was an easy pivot, and Grant enrolled in her BSN at Georgetown. There, a professor encouraged her to do her senior clinical rotation with midwives. Grant had always loved babies, and had initially contemplated becoming an OB-GYN. This was her first exposure to midwifery. Before that, Grant says, "I didn't know that midwifery even existed anymore, as most people in the United States of America do not. In Europe this is just a mainstay. In the United States of America, I say I'm a midwife—'You're a what? We still have those?'"

Grant wears large, black-framed glasses, her hair straightened. At home she's relaxed, in a sweatshirt; at work she wears a short strand of big pearls. A mother of three—one singleton and a set of twins—Grant has been a certified nurse-midwife since 1997. At the time of this writing, she was working as the director of midwifery services in the OB-GYN department at Brooklyn's Woodhull Medical Center, a hulking institution in south Brooklyn that primarily serves women of color. This isn't the Upper West Side, she told me; the mothers have every social determinant of health that you can imagine. Woodhull is also a popular transfer hospital among mothers planning to birth at home, because of its midwifery service. And it has among the lowest primary C-section rates in the city, Grant told me proudly.

The impacts of midwives like Grant are especially significant because the relaxed, community births celebrated on social media, and enshrined in *Spiritual Midwifery*, are much harder to access than they seem. For one, birthing in the hospital is the only financial choice for most people. Insurance covers hospital birth but only rarely covers home birth. If you want a home birth, you must pay in advance and out of pocket. For my C-section—sticker price $50,000—I paid less ($0) than I would have paid for a home birth, which cost $8,000 that my insurance wouldn't have reimbursed. Grant told me that, if they wanted to give birth to their own babies at home, the newer midwives in her hospital wouldn't be able to afford to; she's heard anecdotally that prices can be as high as $18,000. So while on the surface, the kind of birth that Gaskin represents seems open to anyone who'd like one—anyone courageous or independent enough to seek out a "natural" birth—in fact, it is out of reach for most people, especially women of color.

That's part of the reason that home and, by extension, natural birth are associated with white women: they're more likely to be able to afford a home birth.

At the same time, Grant knows about the trade-offs of birth in hospital, perhaps better than most people. She started her nursing career in labor and delivery at Cornell Medical Center. It was a highly medicalized space, she remembers, with a NICU, and high rates of interventions like cesareans and episiotomies. By the time she started her graduate training in midwifery, at SUNY Downstate, she says, "I was medicalized out of my mind." She had to learn to get into the "flow" of midwifery, and to see that not every birth is a potential emergency. So she focused her clinical experiences at less traditionally medicalized spaces: the Long Island Birth Center, which no longer exists, and in private practices. "By the time I graduated I was firmly in the middle," Grant says, between medicalized and "natural."

"I choose to practice in the middle. The women I want to serve are in the hospital. Most of the women who seek home birth are white and have the means to do so. Most people who have home births pay out of pocket and they can afford to do so. Women who are like me, who are working women, are going to always birth in a hospital. It is the American way. I wasn't going to brainfuck myself into believing that that is not the American way. We have socialized women to become comfortable [birthing in a hospital], and we've attached it to insurance."

And yet, she's well aware of the often dehumanizing parts of medicalized prenatal and pregnancy care. "We're talking about this whole maternal mortality and morbidity crisis, but forcing midwives and doctors to give this herd prenatal care, *go go go go*, where you're not even given the time to have a conversation, to develop a knowingness of the patient, and the patient a knowingness of you. To talk to the patient about options. To see what she wants, what her goals are, her dreams for her experience. Or to get to know her. It's not set up for that at all," she says. "You have to really fight for that in a hospital system."

As she learned the history of midwifery, and "how midwifery was taken" from Black communities, practicing as a nurse-midwife in a hospital resonated with Grant on another level. "It is my right to be there," she says. "My undeniable right to be there at all times. That's where I'm supposed to be, where I'm called to be, where I want to show up to serve."

GASKIN AND HER PEERS IN the environmentalist and counterculture movements of the 1970s saw "natural" birth as more than an experience that could be improved by rejecting medical intervention. Birthing outside the "techno-medical" complex also represented a coherence with the natural world and a rejection of the ways modernity had spoiled it.[39] Stephen Gaskin articulated the link with his explanation of the Farm's ethos: "If we had a platform, it was clean air, sane people, and healthy babies," a call that also advocated for "natural" motherhood.[40]

Newfound knowledge of humans' impact on the earth, and the dangers of pollution, had begun to attract attention in the mainstream, too. Rachel Carson's *Silent Spring* (1962) introduced readers to the effects of DDT on the environment and on animal and human health. A few years later, in 1969, Cleveland's Cuyahoga River famously caught fire. President Richard Nixon founded the Environmental Protection

Agency the following year. Concern about pollution and pesticides' impact on pregnant women and babies rippled through the culture.

By breastfeeding and making their own baby food, mothers could protect their babies from the dangers of the polluted world. And by embracing behaviors like co-sleeping and baby-wearing, they could also resist the soft harms perpetuated by contemporary society, like alienation, anxiety, and drug use. In turn, they believed that their children would grow up to become healthier, more physically robust, and more generous and loving adults.

But the environmental and social values that became attached to natural birth and parenting strategies added a moral component to what are, fundamentally, personal, cultural, and familial preferences of how to live. Now, to have a baby "naturally," and to babywear and feed it breast milk and swaddle it in pricey organic cotton blankets, is often understood as shorthand for the depth of your maternal love and the quality of your own character. To make natural choices is, at once, to be good to the planet, to be a good parent, and to be a good person.

We slip on these assumptions so easily in part because "participating in the marketplace" is the way women are socialized to express themselves, as Cornell University professor Brooke Erin Duffy writes in *(Not) Getting Paid to Do What You Love.*

I didn't see any of this when my daughter was little, though I absolutely bought into it. I remember keenly longing for a wool sleep sack that, in my mind, came from carefree sheep that scampered over sunlit New Zealand fields, leading a better life than I did. We were still so skint that dialing the heat up to seventy (actually, my husband reminds me, to sixty-five) caused me physical pain. (When I gazed at the floor registers near our drafty windows, I often felt as if I were throwing money out the window.) I worried constantly that our daughter was too cold.

But the wool sleepsack cost over $100, an exorbitant amount when we could barely keep the lights on. When, frankly, the monthly auto-payment of $45 worth of diapers threatened to plunge our bank account into negative territory.

What I couldn't have articulated at the time is that the sleep sack represented a more moral, authentic, and easy life: one in tune with nature, with the unadulterated land, with clean air and warm sunshine, where money was no object. This was the life I wanted to gift to my daughter, even if it wasn't one I was living myself. I believed that doing so was key to being a good mother.

To be sure, there's a lot to appreciate about low-intervention, "natural" approaches to pregnancy, birth, and parenting. Despite how time-consuming and sometimes irritating it is, for instance, I value making food from scratch for my kids: it's cheaper, but also a way to express love that feels meaningful. But it's hard—especially for a first-time parent—to disentangle the stuff we truly want to do from what the natural-birth culture makes us believe we should do. That's the magic of ideology, as well as the truly damaging aspect of late capitalism: it commodifies embodied experiences like birth, and intimate relationships like parenting, into seeming affirmations or denials of parental fitness and assessments of the depths of parental love.

SOCIETY'S EMBRACE OF "NATURAL" CHILDBIRTH began to wane during the 1980s and '90s, while induction and C-sections became more common, thanks partly to technological changes like external fetal monitoring, which measures a baby's heart rate.[41] In fact, C-sections became so popular—and seemed comparatively so free from risk—that the *New England Journal of Medicine* ran an editorial in 1985 by two obstetricians opining that perhaps all women should be offered C-sections at forty weeks, because, they claimed, it's safer for babies than going past their due dates.[42] The authors went so far as to suggest that physicians warn mothers about the dangers of attempting a vaginal birth after forty weeks, and require them to sign a consent form if they chose to do so. The only downsides to a C-section? They cost more, and were possibly fatal, they wrote. The authors neglected the same kinds of problems—secondary infertility, the emotional impact, placental problems, women's desires—that are still routinely overlooked with cesareans today. To be clear, the obstetricians' embrace of C-sections wasn't uniform; at the time, many obstetricians, midwives, and others voiced concern about the nation's growing percentage of C-sections, which by 1985 had reached 22.7 percent.[43]

Still, enthusiasm in the US for unmedicated birth had started to wane at this point. By 1992, about half of women in the US had an epidural, up from 22 percent of women in 1981.[44] In addition to enjoying pain re-lief, women began embracing technology, and medicalized birth, in part because hospitals had adopted some of the demands to make birth more humane. They permitted men in delivery rooms; they stopped using re-straints. These changes, along with overall cultural shifts away from the environmental and societal concerns of the 1970s, drained some of the fire from the birth revolution.

But as we know from the sizable minority of people who experience mistreatment during pregnancy and birth today—about 17 percent—the culture of hospital birth did not entirely transform.[45] In fact, critics say that most changes to labor and delivery units were superficial, like creating more spacious rooms with better views and more luxurious amenities—not unlike capitalism's usurpation of "natural" parenting.[46]

"Just let a few husbands into the delivery rooms and let them watch what goes on there. That's all it will take—they'll change it!" wrote one person to *Ladies' Home Journal*, back in 1958.[47] Look past the sexism baked in there, and you get to the real problem: witnessing didn't, can't, and won't reform an entire system. In fact, as rates of mistreatment and the dangers of birth attest, we're still waiting for the changes activists demanded in the 1950s. Only now, we've been distracted into thinking that we don't need to work together to demand them. We need only to dodge, to drop out.

"Want to avoid a cesarean? Plan to birth at home," writes Saima Kara (@livewildbirthfree), a natural-birth Instagram influencer. This is the ide-ology of capitalism, too: what matters is you, the individual. There's no investment in the collective project. What's especially depressing is that when it comes to birth, the collective project is us.

THE PENDULUM HAS SINCE SWUNG back. The current obsession with "natural" birth (and parenting, and pregnancy) started to take hold in the early 2000s. Home and birth-center births in the US have been rising since 2004, most significantly among white and college-educated women.[48] Ina May's *Guide to Childbirth* appeared in 2003; it is consistently among Ama-zon's top ten bestselling books on pregnancy and childbirth. Ricki Lake and Abby Epstein's 2008 documentary *The Business of Being Born*'s capitalist critique of hospital birth furthered the conversation advocating for nonmedicalized home birth.

One reason for the shift toward "natural" births is the sheer number of C-sections we're doing, and the reality that most first-time moms don't want surgical births. Embracing "the natural"—and the ways of being pregnant that go along with it—seems like a good (if not the only) way to avoid a C-section. Another reason for the newfound embrace of "natural" birth may be a response to the Anthropocene. Our disturbance of and impact on the natural world are now without dispute. Embracing "natural" birth is a way to reject the ways we have damaged the natural world, and to realign ourselves with nature. Where, for instance, mothers in the 1970s believed that they could protect their children from harmful substances by breastfeeding, we now know that so-called forever chemicals, and microplastics, make their way into breast milk and placentas.

More recently, coverage of the maternal health crisis has also pushed people away from the medical model. The media and popular culture have "been saying, especially to Black women, the hospital is bad, they're out to get you, there are white people in there who want to kill you," says Grant, the nurse-midwife. "They do this to you, they over-monitor you. If you over-monitor, what happens? You have to swing it the other [natural] way."

Then COVID hit, and home and birth-center births suddenly became so sought-after that midwives had to turn people away. While the surge has abated somewhat, home-birth rates have still gone up, especially among white women.[49] And the very fact that so many people pursued these options—even if they did so out of fear and desperation—shows that home births and birth centers seemed like viable places to birth. A fundamental acceptance, even adoption, of the natural-birth ideology, and all that it represents, was already ambient. It's evident in the way we talk about motherhood. Log on to virtually any social media site and you'll see that having a baby doesn't make you a mother or a mommy or a mom. It makes you a mama, the term that embodies the many contradictions embedded in being a good mother: at once crunchy and hip, youthful and experienced, authentic and authoritative, embodied and hot.

Even resources that might seem neutral, practical, or banal encode the natural-birth ideology. On the homepage of the *Birth Hour* podcast, billed as one of Spotify's top podcasts in parenting with some five million listeners, photographs evoke images we associate with natural birth: a pregnant woman in a lacy bra, reclining in a tub filled with flowers; a healthcare worker putting a newborn on a mother's chest, her eyes closed in exhaustion and relief, a washcloth on her forehead. The apparatuses of the hospital are not evident.

Then there are the silences, which don't offer divergent images of pregnancy and birth. TheBump.com, perhaps best known for sending out emails that compare a developing fetus's size to fruits and vegetables, offers resources on baby names, coping with pregnancy symptoms, and lots of articles, mixed in with ads, about what to buy to care for a baby and furnish a nursery. But on the actual birth part the site is strangely quiet. There isn't even a landing page for birth; the site goes from week forty-two of pregnancy to baby's development, week by week—as if, after the pregnancy, the mother disappears.

Even if you don't consider yourself a particularly crunchy person, the present pregnancy culture is awash with this stuff. It's the backdrop against which all of us are birthing, no matter where we plan to have the baby: what we might think of as "the wallpaper of consumer culture," as scholar Paul Frosh writes.[50] And it's no wonder that such a terroir would make C-section moms feel inadequate and personally responsible for the ways that their births turned out.

AT A MIDWIFERY MEETING IN Fort Worth, Texas, in 2017, a member of the audience asked Ina May Gaskin what could be done regarding the Black maternal health crisis. In her answer, Gaskin sidestepped mention of racism's impact on health and on birth outcomes. Instead, she touted the benefits to mothers of hard work, the dangers of drug use (and "drug overdose" as a reason for Black maternal mortality), and the importance of prayer. As critics pointed out, Gaskin's response effectively circulated racist stereotypes about Black women as lazy, drug-using, and immoral.[51] As bad mothers. She also connected good birth outcomes to personal responsibility, implying that if Black mothers made better choices, they'd have better outcomes. And, intended or not, she made an ugly insinuation: that her books, and her platform, even midwifery more broadly, are meant for "natural" types—i.e., women who are healthy and white.

Keisha L. Goode, the SUNY sociologist, points out that Gaskin was fundamentally the wrong person to answer the question. As she and many other Black birth workers and academics emphasized to me, the answers to the Black maternal health emergency are best given by Black mothers, birth workers, academics, policymakers, and community leaders: people from the communities most afflicted by it.

At the same time, Gaskin's response engaged a tacit, and white supremacist, ideology: that there's such a thing as an ideal, "normal," model woman out there who behaves in a certain way that makes her a good fit for the "natural" model of care. To some degree, midwives perpetuate this: they "hold the normal," only seeing patients with textbook pregnancies. Helena A. Grant satirizes this approach: "the woman has to be perfect, she has to come to all her appointments, [she's] never had a borderline blood pressure, she has to drink wheatgrass. The baby has to be damn near close to falling out." Midwives who only see these kinds of patients, she says, are "almost happy, in a way, to give up patients that have anything" going on, and "give them to the doctor."

That's not how Grant practices. "Every woman deserves the touch of a midwife. Every single one. If you're 'holding the normal,' on the perfect spectrum—good for you. If you had some issues, and your blood pressure's rising and you have preeclampsia—why can't I work with doctors to manage your blood pressure but still ensure you have a safe midwifery birth?" Niles made a similar observation: a person who has additional risks especially needs the continuity of care, and the relationship model, offered by midwifery. (American mothers enter pregnancy in poorer health than mothers in other countries, which providers stressed repeatedly in interviews, and which some pointed to as reason for the US's C-section rate.) Proponents of midwifery integration make the very same argument: midwives should be part of care for all pregnancies. That is because everyone can benefit from the midwifery model, which is holistic and emphasizes the "therapeutic use of human presence."[52]

What's more, Grant continued, the concept of a "normal woman" itself is problematic. "What the hell is a normal patient?" she asks. "Even if somebody is 'medically normal,' as a midwife you should know you may have to unpack people's trauma. Maybe their mother or their aunt told them a horrible birth story." Maybe there's something else going on in the background, from family tension to a history of sexual violence, she says.

Midwives who only hold the normal think of themselves as "practicing ancient midwifery," says Grant. But that's a fiction. In the time of "the midwife of ancient—there was no such thing as a doctor. You took care of everybody. You set bones. You were a surgeon. You were more like a family practice physician who also delivered babies," she says. "This is also part of this whole popular imagination that America has made where 'Oh, the mighty doctor has to take care of the pregnant woman because she can get sick at any minute,' and the midwife should only take care of the 'normal woman.'"

She pauses. "Whoever she is," she says. "I'm fifty, and I'm yet to meet a normal woman."

3

THE ORIGINS OF THE C-SECTION

GROWING UP, MY PARENTS KEPT A TARNISHED TIN CUP HANGING over our kitchen sink. We used it to perform a ritual handwashing on Shabbat and Jewish holidays. It had belonged to an American soldier. He gave it to my grandmother at my father's bris, in a Displaced Persons camp in Germany in 1946.

The soldier's cup is emblematic of the shadows I grew up lugging around, of all the people in my family who didn't make it out of Europe, whom Nazis shot in the streets or gassed at Belzec. My uncle—my grandmother's firstborn. My grandfather's brothers. His parents. Cousins. This past shaped how I saw the world and my place in it, my responsibility to my family to make something of myself, as the only daughter of the only son to survive in our family line.

I found myself thinking about this history often in the months after my daughter's birth. On the one hand, I reasoned, I was epigenetically prepared to withstand suffering—and to survive it. Other times I wondered if I hadn't inherited some divine curse that had tumbled down the generations of my family. Maybe, I thought, I had been destined to suffer. Perhaps only by invoking the past could I metabolize how something so brutal could happen in a shiny twenty-first-century American hospital. Regardless, I was on to something: whatever past we think our society has definitively left behind probably isn't past at all. It's ever-present.

The scholar Marianne Hirsch uses the term "postmemory" to describe atmospheres like the one I grew up in. Postmemory, she writes, "characterizes the experience of those who grow up dominated by narratives that preceded their birth."[1] Hirsch's concept helped me to understand my own life. Working on this book, I wondered if it might apply to contemporary obstetrics, too. Though it has been revolutionized by technology and modern understandings of germ theory, obstetrical history—its development on enslaved, impoverished, disabled, and othered women—continues to shape the contours of contemporary obstetric practice, and cesareans in particular. Moreover, as measured by the conversations that I had with Black women, this past is not past at all; obstetrics' development on enslaved women came up in nearly every conversation, even if we didn't set out to talk about the past.

In that sense, obstetrics is but one area in which all of us—doctors, patients, no matter what ethnicity—are living with what scholar Saidiya Hartman calls the "afterlife of slavery." Alicia D. Bonaparte, a Pitzer professor of sociology who shared Hartman's ideas with me, noted how very embodied the afterlife of slavery can be: from police use of deadly force, to the ways that missing women of color rarely make the news, "your lived experience [as a Black person] is a reminder of the fact that you are not even considered as a human, but as a body."

Understanding this present "afterlife of slavery" requires looking at the development of C-sections. And that story requires two looks: one that's straight on, relaying the story as it unfolds in the historical record; the other from the side, with attention to what wasn't recorded, and whose stories went untold. Such an approach to the past shows that this operation, though at its core meant to save both mothers and babies, has never been as simple as that.

C-SECTIONS DEVELOPED TO ADDRESS A tragic problem inherent to birth: some babies can't get born vaginally. They get stuck. In such circumstances, and without intervention, neither a baby nor its mother can survive.

Today, our notions of a baby's being "stuck" are much more all-encompassing than they once were. We might mean that labor has slowed or stalled. That you seem to have stopped dilating, before making it to full dilation. That the baby isn't descending. Or it could be that, during pushing, a baby's having a hard time making it through the vagina. Maybe her shoulder is caught on or behind the mother's pubic bone, or her head seems too large to get through.

But before the twentieth century, a stuck baby was one that quite literally could not fit through the birth canal—no matter how hard or long a person labored. That could happen if a woman had rickets, the result of vitamin D deficiency that deformed a woman's pelvis. Tumors could also block the uterus or prevent the cervix from dilating. Maybe the baby had hydrocephalus—an enlarged head—because of a birth defect. Still other women simply didn't dilate, for reasons that midwives and physicians couldn't understand.

Stuck babies weren't common. But they are so fundamental to birth that even the Mishnah, the compendium of Jewish law that comprises statements made by rabbis from 70 to 220 A.D., addressed them: "If a woman is having difficulty in giving birth [and her life is in danger], one cuts up the fetus within her womb and extracts it limb by limb, because her life takes precedence over that of the fetus."[2] Embryotomy, as this passage describes, was one way to rescue a woman from an otherwise hopeless birth. Craniotomy was another: inserting a crochet hook into the cervix and breaking up the infant's skull into smaller pieces, so that the mother could birth it. Both were arduous, horrific procedures, for mothers and birth attendants alike. And while the procedures were dangerous for mothers—they could cause deadly infection or permanent injury—without them, a woman's death was assured.

The desire to find an alternative to craniotomy and embryotomy, while simultaneously rescuing living mothers facing hopelessly obstructed labor, surely endured for much of human history. The Catholic Church played an important role in this: during the Counter-Reformation, which began in the middle of the sixteenth century, the Church frowned on craniotomy and embryotomy, and formally required that surgeons wait until the fetus died to do either procedure. That opprobrium, the gruesomeness of the procedures, and the desire to preserve newborns' lives encouraged physicians to devise other means of extracting a stuck fetus.[3]

Still, the widely accepted narrative about C-sections is that it wasn't until the 1700s that they were used to save a dying mother. Instead, beginning in at least the 500s, doctors, barbers, priests, and possibly midwives performed postmortem cesarean sections on dead or dying women in an effort to save their babies, spiritually or temporally—that is, to baptize them or to give them a chance, however remote, at life. (Midwives were long forbidden from doing surgery, but there is evidence that they were "prepared to use any instruments"; one eighteenth-century Milanese medical commission found midwives "equipped with iron tools and hooks of strange and rough workmanship."[4])

While in practice these babies were only rarely born alive after their mother's death, those who survived C-sections were considered special, lucky. Ancient English, Egyptian, Persian, Greek, Roman, Native American, Hindu, and other legends tell of babies born from their mothers' stomachs who grew up to become gods and heroes—from Buddha, depicted in sixth-century sculpture as being born through his mother's belly, to Asclepius, the Greek god of medicine. One father of a baby purportedly born alive after a C-section in 1610—one of the first such documented operations—named him "Fortunata," on account of his good fortune to survive.

And while Julius Caesar is said to have been born of a cesarean, the story is likely apocryphal, writes historian Katharine Park in her book *Secrets of Women: Gender, Generation, and the Origins of Human Dissection*: "There is no evidence that the Caesarean operation was ever actually performed in ancient Rome."[5] The tale, widely circulated in Italy and France in the late medieval age—and still in circulation today—was likely invented to do him honor. Instead, the operation may derive its name from Lex Cesarea—the emperor's law—adopted by Roman emperor Numa Pompilius in 715 B.C., which forbid burying a dead pregnant woman until her fetus had been removed and buried separately.[6] But even this attribution may be dubious; there is no description of postmortem cesareans in the writings left by physicians who addressed obstetrics, and historians speculate that even this historical "fact" may have been invented in the sixth century to legitimize postmortem cesareans, which "Christianity intended to promote."[7]

To that end, a public sermon from 1305, given in Florence, describes instances when "laypeople, rather than priests, might christen a child," writes Park. The friar told of a baby extracted from a woman's abdomen after her death, then baptized. "His soul was saved," the friar concluded.

But "many [souls] are lost in this way and are in Limbo, through your fault. [The women] should be opened up, and it is a great mercy."[8]

The expectation that surgeons do postmortem cesareans extended far beyond the Italian states. *La Grande Chirurgie*, an influential tome on surgery by Guy de Chauliac, a Frenchman and the so-called father of Western surgery, includes a description of such an operation.[9] Religious and royal edicts requiring physicians do postmortem cesareans existed in thirteenth-century Cologne, fifteenth-century Langres, and sixteenth-century Sens, among other places.[10] In the late 1700s, priests in New Spain and Peru also did "forced caesarean sections" in order to "save the souls of fetuses and not the lives of mothers," write Elizabeth O'Brien and Miriam Rich in the *Lancet*.[11] And in fact, through the nineteenth century Venice, Frankfurt, and Bavaria continued to require postmortem cesareans.[12]

The actual requirements for these surgeries varied from place to place: whether the fetus had to be of a certain age, for instance, or if the operation were to be done on any pregnant woman.[13] And while there is no way to know for certain how often physicians, barbers, priests, and surgeons complied with these rules—some scholars say that it happened only rarely—in Sicily and the kingdom of Greece they faced penalty of death if they did not.[14]

To be sure, church guidance advised physicians that they best be sure a woman really was dead before operating, which could be difficult to ascertain. A text from the 1600s instructs the surgeon to "[be] certainly assured, that the woman is dead, and that her kinsfolks, friends, and others that are present, doe all affirm and confesse, that her soule is departed" before attempting the operation. He must put "light feathers" on her mouth and nose, for even if her breath is faint "they will fly away." Such instruction suggests that physicians, barbers, or priests might perform a fetal extraction in too great haste, such that the cesarean was "promoted primarily by theological beliefs rather than by medical necessities," as a nineteenth-century German midwifery text put it.[15]

Despite its reach, it would be a mistake to suggest that the pressure for postmortem cesareans came only from the Church. Beginning in the 1500s, Protestant sources also advocated for postmortem sections because of the remote possibility that a baby would survive, and to improve the operation's technique. But some also urged caution: they were concerned that a postmortem cesarean could be performed on a mother who might not actually be dead.[16]

Fathers in noble families had another reason to hope for a living child: if a woman died but had had a living child, even if it lived only briefly, her widower kept her dowry. If she died without a child who'd lived, her dowry returned to her family.[17] For this reason, and to the extent that they occurred, postmortem C-sections were more common in noble families. Such were the institutional, economic, and religious forces that encouraged postmortem sections, to say nothing of the very human hope that, in a birth gone wrong, at least a baby might survive.

IT IS IMPOSSIBLE TO ASCERTAIN the "first" successful cesarean that both mother and baby definitively survived, though the literature is full of many such instances. Crumbling books and stained and brittle scientific journals relay tales from the fifteenth century on of men—a swine gelder, a dog shearer, an eighteenth-century physician—who had laboring wives who for whatever reason could not birth their babies vaginally and, after exhausting and lengthy labors, faced certain death.

What matters about these competing stories is that, taken together, they suggest that cesareans didn't exist as an operation meant to save a woman from dying in childbirth until medicine and male doctors invented it.

But Barbara Katz Rothman, a sociologist at CUNY who has published several books on midwifery and medicine, argues that midwives surely performed these operations as well. "It's inconceivable that the people who made dinner, so they knew how to cut animals apart, and sewed the clothing, so they know how to sew things—when a baby wasn't coming out, just let a mother and baby die," she told me.

This was one of the first things she said when we spoke by Zoom last year. My initial response was disbelief, though I didn't challenge her outwardly. *If midwives did surgery*, I remember thinking, *Then where's the proof? The primary source?* I was skeptical, even though—perhaps especially because—I wished it was true.

But the more I thought about it, the more I saw Rothman's argument as a larger commentary on the nature of received history: what gets recorded, and, consequently, whose stories get told. Who gets credit for innovation and for heroism. (Despite the primarily European reputation as the place that developed C-sections, for instance, there's evidence that they were practiced contemporaneously in Uganda.) The history of birth is full of silences, as Adrienne Rich points out, because "women did not write books. . . . Only after the Middle Ages, when male influence and the struggle for male control of midwifery were well underway, do we begin to hear of the 'heroes' of this branch of medicine. And indeed, there were some heroes, men who fought to save the lives of women in labor; but the names of the great midwives are mostly lost."[18] At the least, the narrative that men invented C-sections, that lifesaving operation, fit almost too neatly with the physician-dominated, heroic male history of obstetrics: men, and surgeons in particular, know best.

My knee-jerk rejection of Rothman's claim showed me that I had been mesmerized by the literature itself. I had not thought carefully enough about who'd written it, and about whose voices it didn't contain. "The archive dictates what can be said about the past," writes Saidiya Hartman, regarding her search for traces of enslaved people in her family, including her great-grandmother. It constrains "the kinds of stories that can be told about the persons catalogued, embalmed, and sealed away in box files and folios."[19] In other words, what's manifest in an archive obscures what isn't there—and it tells stories about people whose words haven't been preserved to tell the story themselves.

The Talmud's reference to babies born "through the wall" seems to support Rothman's argument, at least partially, because the text asks if women who birthed in this way were in a state of ritual impurity. This suggests women survived cesareans in antiquity—that it wasn't an operation invented by doctors in the 1700s. But Shana Schick, a Talmud scholar at Bar-Ilan University, dismissed this likelihood. The Talmud deals with hypothetical situations all the time, she said, because it is interested in argument—and not because the situations it discusses, like whether an animal can be used to form a wall of a sukkah, actually happened.

Still, some time later, after talking with Rothman, I found one of the earliest records of a successful cesarean, from Ireland in 1739. It was a midwife—a woman named Mary Donnelly—who'd saved her patient from certain death.[20]

UNTIL ABOUT TWO HUNDRED YEARS ago, obstetricians were split about whether to even attempt an operation as dangerous as cesarean section on a living woman. It was nearly always fatal, even if it meant to rescue a woman from death in birth. Many objected to it on "humanitarian grounds," and it was only rarely practiced; one late-nineteenth-century text found that, from between 1500 to 1769, there were only seventy-six cases of C-section in European literature that ended with a mother's survival.[21] Primarily, infection and hemorrhage claimed women's lives, the latter likely spurred on by physicians who initially declined to sew the uterus closed after delivering the baby.

But besides being dangerous to women and horrific for all involved, and in addition to the Catholic Church's rejection of them, craniotomies and embryotomies presented a key problem: they weren't always possible. Some women's cervixes didn't dilate at all—not even enough to permit the crochet hook or perforator. In Europe in the late 1700s and early 1800s, physicians debated the merits of attempting cesarean sections on such women. One text from 1801 relays the size of pelvic openings physicians encountered and what they did as a result, providing lengthy discussions of how many inches and lines a mother's pelvic inlet ("lines" being a unit of measurement then employed).

It's essential to recognize that saving mothers' lives was a key, driving reason why obstetricians performed the operation on living women in Europe in the 1700s, and certainly in the US in the 1800s. In fact, that's how physicians mostly defined the operation's success: even if her baby lived, but the mother died, the operation was a failure. One book about cesareans from the early 1800s cast a wide net to identify such "successful" operations in France, England, and Prussia, with the goal of demonstrating that a C-section wasn't inevitably fatal to the mother. Still, because the operation so often resulted in death for the mother, physicians of this period very nearly stopped practicing them. Jean-Louis Baudelocque, a leading obstetrician in Paris who championed the operation, was even accused of being an "assassin and a murderer" after a woman he'd operated on died.[22]

Physicians' egoistic desire to make history or showcase their skills also helped keep the operation in circulation. Textbooks like *Arts des Accouchements*, which Baudelocque wrote and that was widely used in Paris in the 1790s, touted the C-section as the most "supreme" obstetric procedure. From this description, the ambition to get this operation right—to become known for it—is almost palpable. Reading Baudelocque (in translation), I can almost smell his longing to make history.[23] "If the cesarean section be justly regarded as the grandest and the most dangerous operation of surgery," he wrote, "it must also appear much more important in its object than any other, since by exposing the life of a single individual to danger, it may preserve two and sometimes three lives." It's seductive, pioneering such medical frontiers. And it's not unlike the hero worship that still attends surgeons, the most widely respected, and often best compensated, purveyors of contemporary medicine.

Obstetric texts from the 1800s onward included directions about how to do a cesarean, indicating that the operation had begun to pass into a realm of medical practice that physicians might conceivably encounter, though they rarely did. In time, the operation evolved from one primarily performed on dead or dying women to a surgery of last resort that a woman might conceivably survive. Still, the chance of a mother's survival remained slim: Between 1838 and 1878, there were eighty-nine reported cesareans in the US; 62 percent of mothers died, as did 60 percent of their babies. The rates were even worse in Britain, where women died 90 percent of the time.[24] (Because recordkeeping wasn't standard, these rates differ slightly in different texts.)

In many cases, the women's names aren't recorded. Instead, they're defined in relation to their husbands' professions or the incredulity of their circumstances, like the woman on the Ohio frontier in the 1820s whose doctor operated during a storm so ferocious that his attendants held up blankets to keep the candles from blowing out.

It was difficult to read these stories: accountings in tepid prose of so many dead mothers. When the stories turned out well, I wanted to believe that the women survived not only because of their husbands' or doctors' desperation—their willingness to do whatever they could to keep these women alive—but because of their will to live. But that would be suggesting that the mothers who died did not wish for life hard enough. My friend Lisa calls me out on this: *There's that individualist belief about birth again*, she says. *If only you will it, you can manifest the birth you want.* To reject this way of thinking means accepting the painful truth about birth: no matter how much force of will we bring, no matter the expertise, no matter who is with us, sometimes birth's outcomes are beyond our control.

THE DRIVE TO SAVE MOTHERS from death during childbirth also had a critical, and today largely overlooked, wind at its back: the push to bring about more slaves. In the US, most early cesareans took place in the South, as they still do today; a disproportionate number of Black and enslaved women made up the subjects. Many of the physicians who developed the procedure were themselves slaveholders and worked at large plantations where they treated enslaved people. Their chief motivation for doing the operation, writes historian Deirdre Cooper Owens in her book *Medical Bondage*, was to grow their human property.

Childbearing, writes Cooper Owens, was "a centerpiece of the system of chattel slavery."[25] A colonial Virginia law passed in 1662 held that an enslaved woman's children would have the same "status" as their mother. Black women thus could "build capital for enslavers" through birth, which became even more important after the US banned the transatlantic slave trade in 1808.

That's why physicians and slaveholders were more likely to gamble on an enslaved woman's stuck baby and do a C-section; they had a chance of saving both baby and mother—and adding to their stable of enslaved people, Cooper Owens writes. They were willing to take this risk because enslaved people's lives were expendable, and because an enslaved woman's value was linked specifically to her capacity to bear children and enlarge her master's wealth.

Indeed, the physician who pioneered cesareans in the US was a French-born slavemaster named François-Marie Prevost. As Harriet Washington documents in her book *Medical Apartheid*, Prevost worked in Louisiana from 1800 to 1830, prior to the development of anesthesia.[26] He likely learned the procedure during medical school in Paris, from Baudelocque, the obstetrician who'd staked his reputation on C-sections.[27]

Prevost recorded four operations in Louisiana, two on the same woman; all the women were enslaved. The mothers survived, enduring the operation—from first cut to final suture—without anesthesia. Their babies all survived.[28] As evidence of how experimental the operation was, Prevost made an agreement with the owner of the first woman on whom he operated. If the woman survived, her baby was to be freed. The woman did live, and her owner gave her baby freedom. In a detail that further expresses the breadth of Prevost's power, he used his authority to name her: Cesarinne.

Prevost, who married twice but seems never to have had children, was no abolitionist, despite coming of age during a revolution whose motto called for *egalité, liberté, fraternité.*[29] At the time of his death, he owned forty-four people, ten of whom were children.

At the same time, the enslavers who agreed to these operations did so because the women's lives were endangered by vaginal birth. So the operation, while at once putting the women at grave risk, and though motivated to increase slaveholders' human property, may have also saved their lives. In fact, prior to the Civil War, the outcomes of cesareans in Louisiana were among the best in the nation, and most likely to save the mothers.[30] It's possible that the physicians and enslavers were motivated by the women's financial value; enslaved women who looked as if they would bear many children fetched high sums at slave markets. Alternatively, the obstetricians—many of whom attended medical school in France—may have been better trained than doctors elsewhere in the US.

Either way, fundamental assumptions about the differences between Black and white human bodies gave doctors and enslavers the cover under which to experiment on women of color and Black women in particular. Prevailing medical ideologies held that these women had less-developed nervous systems than whites. As a result, physicians and others believed that they did not feel pain as deeply as civilized, white women. (A twist on that belief would later inform Dick-Read's ideas that "primitive" women could bear labor more easily than whites.)

Because they were thought to experience less pain, and because they commanded less social value, physicians were ethically free to take risks on Black women's bodies. As physician J. Marion Sims's surgical experiments demonstrates, for example—he developed the operation to repair fistulas by practicing on enslaved women, also without anesthesia—cesarean sections were only one of the many procedures that white doctors practiced on them. "The bulk of medical practice in these plantation regions was among the slaves," writes Rudolph Matas in his glowing 1937 account of the history of C-section in Louisiana. Prevost, "like most of the country practitioners of that period, derived practically all of his experience and practice from them."[31] No white woman in Louisiana would have a C-section until 1867.

Physicians also did not ask for consent from enslaved women when operating on them. Instead, doctors asked for consent from their enslavers.[32] By contrast, before operating on whites, they obtained consent from everyone present, including the women. To be sure, in some cases they did railroad their white patients; one doctor in 1835, who in consultation with colleagues had decided in advance that his patient would need a cesarean, recalled that he "had some difficulty" obtaining her consent.[33] (He describes badgering her for several hours.) Today, women of all races and backgrounds report being coerced into obstetric interventions, including C-sections. But Black women are more likely to experience this particular form of browbeating.

Deceased female slaves may have also served as practice for white physicians learning the operation. Charles Hentz, who attended medical school in Louisville and went on to work as a physician on a cotton plantation in Florida, reported in his diary in 1860 that he "got from a [deceased] negro patient . . . a foetus of 3 or 4 mos" [en] "caul"—in the bag of waters—which he brought "home for a specimen."[34] He doesn't specify, but Hentz may have "got" that fetus by opening up its mother.

Nineteenth-century medical journals are littered with such accounts. Doctors and anatomists collected skulls, pelvises, and reproductive organs, primarily from the bodies of enslaved, nonwhite, and poor people for research and teaching, and also gifted them to medical schools and museums.[35]

These specimens served as more than prurient curiosities. Scientists, anthropologists, and doctors used these body parts to support the belief that different races—Blacks, Native Americans, whites, and others—

were separate species, created by God, with whites at the top of the social and moral hierarchy. This ideology, known as polygenesis, had by 1850 spread internationally, providing a theological defense of slavery and colonialism. Over the next several decades, a more thoroughly biological and seemingly scientific version of this racial hierarchy, eugenics, would help shape policies that called for the sterilization of women considered unfit mothers—including women who'd birthed through cesarean section.

NO. 14, 3 FT. 6/1/ 2″ , white . . . , a cripple and on crutches from early childhood.

Dwarf No. 16, . . . might have been saved if delivered with . . . promptness.

No. 18, white, 3 ft. 11 ½, stout, 115 pounds. . . . This woman was not only dwarfed, but her pelvis was nearly closed up by an exostosis growing from the sacrum.

A deformed and dwarfed mulatto, primipara, in her twentieth year, who had been confined to bed for fourteen years, during which period she had not been able to walk; she would probably have measured about four feet or four feet two inches.[36]

Enslaved women weren't the only ones in the 1800s who tended to have C-sections in disproportionate numbers. Physically disabled women, like those described above from nineteenth-century physician and researcher Robert P. Harris's list—which he compiled to help identify the conditions that would make C-section safer—also served as subjects. On the one hand it seems logical that these women were disproportionately candidates for the operation. Their disabilities—typically, contracted pelvises—made vaginal birth nearly impossible. Yet their disabilities also made these women "other," particularly when contrasted to dominant ideals of femininity, which favored "physical delicacy."[37] Because disabled women commanded less social power than women with able bodies, doctors may have been more likely to operate on them.[38]

Poverty was another factor that made a woman likely to have a cesarean.

Harris, the physician-researcher who devoted much of his life to gathering data on the operation, with the goal of discovering patterns to make it safer, noted that while "there are many women of the better class" with contracted pelvises, which would make vaginal birth of a live infant impossible, they "are far from requiring that the Caesarean operation should be performed."[39] Instead, these women could be persuaded to have their labors induced, so as to give birth to smaller babies who could fit through their pelvises.

By contrast, "the subjects of infantile rickets are usually of a different class," he wrote. They should be persuaded to have labor induced early or abort their fetuses altogether (abortion isn't something he suggests for women of a "better class"). But impoverished and nonwhite women do not have the "requisite degree of intelligence" to listen to their doctors, he scolds. They fail to recognize that they're too deformed to carry their babies to term and birth vaginally. By the time labor starts, they have no other choice but a cesarean.

In all, Harris concluded, women with pelvises so "badly deformed" that they necessitated cesareans "have hitherto been found almost always in foreigners, dwarfs, or negroes." By contrast, white women with "small pelves" might need forceps or craniotomy to birth their babies—techniques that were hardly benign, but suggested that they were more likely to be spared the risk of a cesarean. Important for the way that we think about C-sections today, Harris observed the link between C-sections and the social underclasses by virtue of race, class, or body. In a sense, it's no wonder that the operation is still stigmatized given that, historically, the people on whom it was predominantly practiced were stigmatized as well.

And yet—these operations saved some of these women's lives. They also saved some of their babies. Still, that their doctors were willing to do them may reflect their social and bodily value.

This operation has always lived in that tension. It is now, and has always been, both good and damaging. It saves lives even as it sunders them.

IN EARLY REPORTS ABOUT CESAREANS, doctors sometimes, though not always, also explicitly linked the need for a cesarean section to a woman's behavior, including lack of cleanliness and a "poor diet," as historian of medicine Jacqueline H. Wolf points out in her book *Cesarean Section: An*

American History of Risk, Technology, and Consequence. A woman's bad habits could also shape the operation's outcome. Harris, the researcher-physician, theorized that "beer drinking" among C-section mothers made the operation more fatal.[40] Similarly, some physicians blamed women's behavior for their deaths. In 1769, a thirty-seven-year-old woman died, five days post-op, "after some imprudent attempts to make her bed"; one nineteenth-century physician-researcher described a woman who died seven days after the operation "when, delighted at the prospects of recovery," she "jumped from bed, danced around, and swallowed a pint of brandy."[41]

Drinking and slovenliness stand out in light of prevailing notions of nineteenth-century femininity. The popular imagination held that women should be delicate, pure, moral, and submissive. Their domain wasn't the public sphere, but the domestic one. And their inherent morality granted them responsibility for their children's spiritual education and guardianship. In that way, the standards for good motherhood, and appropriate expressions of femininity, accrued to white middle- and upper-class women, who could afford (quite literally) to appear to behave in line with their gendered expectations.

On a number of fronts, from race to physical condition to class to behavior, C-section mothers fell beyond the parameters of either the good mother or the ideal woman. In that way, cesareans became linked with people who were unfit mothers, moored outside widely accepted standards of femininity and motherhood, a cultural space they, to some degree, still inhabit.

THESE HISTORIES LARGELY AREN'T PART of contemporary medical education. The most recent survey on the matter found that only 10 percent of medical schools teach even a rudimentary history of medicine. "Bioethics in the American understanding is often ahistoric," Harvard anatomy educator and associate professor of pediatrics Sabine Hildebrandt told me. "You're lucky if they go as far back as the Nuremberg code," the code of ethics formulated in 1947, and a key reference point for American medical researchers who perform experiments on human subjects. But that forgetting doesn't last. "There's something about the truth of history that—it sounds so unscientific—but it permeates our daily living," says Hildebrandt.

Recent research by Hildebrandt and others, on medical texts written and illustrated by Nazis, provides an example for how obstetrics might contend more publicly with its practice on enslaved and othered women. *The Pernkopf Anatomy*, a textbook on nerves considered among the best in the field, was written and illustrated by a Nazi doctor and Nazi artists, who almost certainly based their work—thorough illuminations of nerves, including in the face—using the bodies of executed political prisoners. The book's original edition, and some reprints, included swastikas and SS insignias in the authors' signatures. In later editions, however, these Nazi emblems disappeared. That was deliberate, to induce forgetting; when Hildebrandt visited Munich in 2019 to see the original version of the textbook, she found that someone seemed to have used a needle to pick out the ink from the swastika in the author's signature. As a consequence, physicians used these later editions of the book without knowing its provenance—to their horror, in some cases.

Thanks to recent ethics discussions among scholars like Hildebrandt, libraries that loan the *Pernkopf Anatomy* now include an insert from the Medical University of Vienna disclosing the book's provenance.

Imagine if the origins of C-sections were something we just knew. If *What to Expect When You're Expecting* included a section on the history of obstetrics. How might that shape how we talk about the operation, and how often, and in what scenarios, we'd be most likely to use it? Would we be so accustomed to thinking of women who'd had C-sections as somehow lesser than mothers who'd delivered vaginally?

Perhaps, I ventured in a conversation with midwife Helena A. Grant, if medical students learned this history, they'd be less likely to push Black women into interventions they didn't want, once becoming doctors.

Or maybe not. When talking about implicit biases, and whether they shape care, midwife Helena A. Grant tells me, "It's not about 'do they know,'" meaning people who say or do racist things to patients. "I don't think they care."

"The hubris is still within medicine," Hildebrandt says. "Unless the physician is always aware of the need of balancing certain invasive processes with empathy and true care for the patient, you end up with these kinds of terrible experiments," she says. "When you describe childbirth as experienced by women as enforced or unfree or not self-determined, that goes in the same direction."

To be sure, today, "none of the obstetricians or midwives involved in the process of delivery is truly 'comparable' to the Nazis," she cautions. "That's not where we're going with this. But the processes—if you overlook the agency that the patient should have, and the connection that those who care for the patient need to have for the patient to really care for them—then you can end up in a situation" where caregivers overlook patients' fundamental humanity.

SINCE THE SUPREME COURT RULED that the constitution does not protect the right to an abortion, it's felt even more difficult to imagine that physicians and the wider culture in the US so thoroughly agreed on prioritizing mothers' lives over their babies. That once-widespread agreement reflected a sad reality: motherless babies often didn't live long. Formula hadn't yet been developed and there wasn't much besides breast milk that was safe and nutritious for babies to eat. And even among affluent families who could afford a wet nurse, infant and child mortality were widespread—so much so that in the seventeenth and early eighteenth centuries, some of the most popular children's books in the US focused on death. Among the most widely circulated titles: *A Token for Children: Being an Exact Account of the Conversion, Holy and Exemplary Lives, and Joyful Deaths of Several Young Children.*[42]

By contrast, a woman had already made it to adulthood. She could theoretically go on to have more children. And she was needed by the ones she already had.

I have to remind myself that women's value hasn't been demoted, exactly, since the cesarean developed as a technique to save mothers. But we are accorded less autonomy than when I was born and *Roe v. Wade* was law; now, by measure of the *Dobbs* decision, we appear to have less right to assert ourselves over our unborn children than we did over one hundred years ago. "The position of a woman in society, her ties of relationship and friendship, and the associations which surround her, make her life far more important than that of an infant whose prospect of living to maturity, even under the most favorable circumstances, is very doubt-ful," argued Harris, the physician and obstetrics researcher, in 1871 at the first meeting of the Philadelphia Obstetrical Society. "We do not hesitate, however reluctantly, to sacrifice [an infant's life] for [its mother's] sake, and she in most instances prefers this decision to running any additional risk of her own life."[43]

BY THE END OF THE nineteenth century, surgical innovation had de-veloped to make cesarean safer. The Porro operation, developed in It-aly, made hemorrhage less likely by removing the uterus altogether. The Sanger technique, which Max Sanger pioneered in 1882 in Germany, involved suturing the uterus closed rather than leave an open wound. The Sanger technique became known as the so-called conservative cesarean, because it conserved a woman's fertility. And while it took decades for physicians to learn and implement these and other, subsequent surgical developments in hospitals throughout the US, by the 1920s, the cesarean largely replaced craniotomy as a means to address obstructed labor.[44]

At the same time as the operation's safety improved, obstetricians de-bated expanding the reasons that women should have a C-section. Where it was once only called for in cases where vaginal birth was physically im-possible, now eclampsia, tuberculosis, and small pelvises could be reason enough for the operation, according to some physicians. Even a person's emotional or psychological qualities could justify the operation: accord-ing to a 1921 textbook on cesareans by Harvard obstetrician Franklin S. Newell, women with an "unstable nervous equilibrium," or those who "have no reserve of nerve force and who are living up to their limits in their daily lives," and who might experience a "nervous breakdown" be-cause of labor, might be candidates for surgical birth—even if they had "normal pelves."[45]

This claim potentially expanded C-sections in terms of race and class. White, upper-class women were susceptible to being overly nervous, be-cause they were believed to be delicate and constitutionally unable to withstand pain.

On its surface, the possibility of applying C-sections to overly nervous white women who could birth vaginally doesn't make sense; the operation had otherwise largely been intended for the disabled and degenerate, and to address life-and-death situations in cases of hopelessly obstructed labor. But we see this contradiction today, too: on the one hand, the operation is associated with laziness, inadequacy, weakness—women who aren't strong or tough enough to make vaginal birth happen. And on the other, C-sections can be considered "designer deliveries," as one director of maternal fetal medicine put it. They're the preferred mode of birth for those too posh to push.

These categories of women appear to have nothing to do with each other. But at heart, the stereotypes around why they can't, or won't, birth vaginally share the same presumption: they're fundamentally inadequate. Either they're too physically or mentally weak, or too selfish to give themselves over to the process of labor and childbirth.

In the weeks after my operation, I was afraid to be alone with my baby. I believed I couldn't handle it because I was too damaged to handle her. The first time I was alone with her for a meaningful stretch I became so hysterical trying to calm her down that I frantically texted my husband, who was stuck in traffic between Manhattan and New Paltz. Alarmed, he called a friend to intervene. The friend arrived, snuggled my daughter, and sent me to bed. I lay awake, listening to my friend sitting in my kitchen, where she chatted to her husband and ate pizza like a normal person. I remember feeling profoundly outside of society and wondering if I'd ever be able to enter it again. I also felt like a terrible mother, as if there were something intrinsically wrong with me. My friend had made it seem so easy. What was my problem? I wondered. I'd been trying to get her to stop crying all afternoon; why couldn't I do that?

As the history of C-section shows, I belonged to a long line of women whose C-sections made their mothering suspect. Too posh to push, too deformed to birth; the conclusions about such women are the same, and similar to some of the worst thoughts I had about myself, those early days after the birth: we are undeserving of motherhood.

4

CASCADE OF CONSEQUENCES

I'D ONCE HOPED FOR THREE CHILDREN. THREE SOUNDED LIKE A PARTY. My husband was one of three. My brother, eight years older than me, had four. But three also meant a different car, a mentor (himself a father of three) cautioned me. Three college tuitions. Three, my husband said ominously, meant you were outnumbered.

Since the operation, though, my desire for more children seemed to have evaporated. I didn't know what I wanted. In fact, I didn't seem to want anything. I pictured myself as a walking question mark. I joked that I was a member of the Know-Nothing Party, a reference to an obscure nineteenth-century American political party that landed only with my nerdiest historian friends.

Beneath my not-knowing was fear. I was afraid of another C-section, I distrusted doctors, and I was anxious about hospitals. Still, as my daughter outgrew her clothes, I couldn't bring myself to get rid of them. Instead, I stuffed them into a dozen super-sturdy bags, each the size of a toddler. My friend Kiersten called it a "maybe baby" box: Maybe I'd have another baby. Maybe not. But to give all that stuff away meant that I was done having children, and I wasn't ready to make that call. So I entombed my daughter's things in the closets carved into the knee walls of our attic, where they gathered dust and symbolized the junk in my head I wasn't yet ready to sort out.

When my daughter was about two, I started to ask friends: *Should I have another baby?* I thought maybe they could tell me something that would help me decide what to do. Perhaps this was to audition whether they thought I'd sufficiently recovered emotionally, if they believed I could handle another birth. A better question was, *Did I want another baby?*

I asked my friend Diana, "How did you know you wanted another baby?"

"It's ineffable," she said. "It was as if there were someone else on the other side of the wall."

Did I feel that way? I had no idea. This feeling—or lack of feeling—is what drove me to therapy. Before long, the birth came up. I came to see that the blanket of not-knowing was my response to trauma. That the birth took up a lot of space in my brain, blotting out my wants. The birth was like a thick, gray, paralyzing haze. I couldn't see through it to picture the future.

A C-SECTION'S POTENTIAL IMPACT ON a person's reproductive life wasn't something that had ever crossed my mind until I was living through it. In part that's because so much of the talk about pregnancy and labor focuses on the cascade of interventions. Avoid them, and you'll get the birth you want. The conversation largely ends there. Yet for me, and for many of the mothers I interviewed for this book, C-sections created their own cascade of consequences, shaping our subsequent pregnancies, births, and family size in ways that we couldn't have predicted before the first surgical birth.

"A C-section," Tikvah Azulcir, a PhD candidate in classics, who had an unplanned C-section for her first birth, is "going to tailor your path of your life: your spacing of your children, the number of your children, the method of your birth, the ability to give birth," she told me. "It really changes everything."

For me, it was largely the C-section's trauma that kept me from getting pregnant sooner. Delaying pregnancy following a bad birth is not unusual; a 2018 review of twelve studies that appeared in the *Journal of Advanced Nursing* found that many mothers who'd had a negative childbirth experience delayed future pregnancy, whether they'd birthed vaginally or by C-section.[1] But even if they go well, C-sections shape how a person grows her family, many women I interviewed said. "Once you've had that first C-section . . . it just changes everything. You have so many fewer choices that will be supported by OBs in future pregnancies,"

Justine Richardson, who had her first C-section in 2018, told me. And while some of the data is conflicting about the ways that a C-section shapes a person's future pregnancies and family size, one thing seems clear: a mother who's had a C-section is less likely to have subsequent children than a mother who's had a vaginal birth.[2]

There are many reasons that C-sections are associated with this phenomenon. At the most basic level, simply having a C-section makes it more likely that a mother will have a hysterectomy, the last-line treatment for hemorrhage during the operation, and that makes it impossible to get pregnant again.[3] And while the data is conflicting, there is also some evidence that a previous C-section may make future miscarriage as well as ectopic pregnancy more likely.[4]

A prior C-section also makes it more likely that a mother who gets pregnant again will develop a problem with her placenta, which can endanger mother and baby. The more C-sections she's had, the higher her likelihood of such a problem.[5] These problems include placental abruption, a serious emergency in which the placenta detaches from the uterine wall; placenta previa, when the placenta covers the cervix, necessitating another C-section; and placenta accreta, when the placenta grows too far into the abdominal wall, which makes hemorrhage more likely during birth.[6] And while placenta accreta is unlikely, there is no question that the rising number of cesareans has increased its incidence. From the 1930s to the 1950s, it occurred in fewer than 1 in 30,000 births.[7] By 2016, according to one study, it was occurring in 1 in every 272 births, likely because of the increase in C-sections.[8] As a result, one OB remarked to me, we now have centers of excellence for treating placenta accreta—which we surely need, because the condition increases the risks of severe bleeding and death. Yet, she noted, these institutions exist largely because of problems of our own making.

Perhaps most devastating, though the data don't all agree, is that some research has shown that women who've had C-sections are less likely than women who've had vaginal births to be able to conceive again. Researchers—primarily obstetricians—long assumed that women who'd had a C-section didn't have more babies because they didn't want any. But as Penn State professor emeritus of Public Health Sciences Kristen Kjerulff has shown, by interviewing women before and after their first births for her NIH-funded First Baby Study, women who've had C-sections and women who've had vaginal births are just as likely to report that they want another baby—both before and after they become mothers.[9] The difference is that women who've had a C-section have a harder time getting pregnant the second time around.

It's not for lack of trying. In Kjerulff's study, C-section mothers had even more unprotected sex than women who'd had vaginal births. "They kept trying and trying, month after month," Kjerulff told me. In another study, she found that within eight and a half years of their C-section, 40.2 percent of these mothers didn't have another "live birth," compared with about a third of women who'd had a vaginal birth.[10] Adjusting for age, race, health conditions, and other factors, women who'd had a C-section were still less likely to have another baby—which meant they'd stopped at one child.

Yet in her research, Kjerulff found that most women didn't pursue fertility care when they couldn't get pregnant. "They thought, *Well, that's nature. I'm just not going to have another baby.*" Surely financial considerations play a role here, she pointed out; fertility treatments are expensive, and insurance companies don't always cover as many cycles of IVF as needed to conceive. But she also thinks that mind-set is part of the decision for these mothers to forgo fertility treatments. "A lot of women have unprotected intercourse, thinking, *If I get pregnant I get pregnant, if I don't I don't.* It's an attitude of kind of letting the gods tell you whether or not to have another baby." Yet as her research suggests, to some degree it isn't nature at all, but the unintended consequences of this most routine operation, its impact on what we so often interpret as fate.

There seems to be something so female about this: put your body into control of the medical system, and then fit whatever happens into the framework of destiny. The other possibility is to assume that whatever your body does—or in the case of infertility, doesn't do—is your fault, the result of your own deficiencies. Of the two, leaving it up to the gods seems like a more compassionate way to think.

But the truth is that C-sections, along with many, many other factors—not fate, not destiny—shape how many children a person will have. And we don't adequately respect them for it.

In these ways the operation, this lifesaving and life-changing procedure, is like falling through a trapdoor. It can determine your destiny, the path of your motherhood, even how many children you come to mother. Looking at the history of the operation, and the ways that it coincided with sterilization, shows it has always been thus.

ONE WAY THAT PHYSICIANS MADE the C-section safer in the late nineteenth century was by pairing it with a hysterectomy. With the Porro operation, developed in the late 1870s, removing the woman's uterus after delivering her baby reduced the likelihood of infection or hemorrhage.[11] This is why hysterectomy is a possible, if rare, outcome from a C-section today; it's a last-line treatment if nothing else can staunch uterine bleeding.

Cesarean-hysterectomy had another advantage in the late nineteenth century: it made another pregnancy impossible. As one doctor in 1880 wrote, the Porro technique protected a woman from undergoing "another capital operation."[12] He called this "a boon to her, though she may not be aware of the loss of her womb"—meaning she did not know about the hysterectomy. That might seem patriarchal, or cruel. But given the dangers the operation posed to a mother's life, making another pregnancy impossible could also have been understood as good medicine in an era without reliable birth control.

But there were other, more disturbing instances of C-sections being used during this period to end women's future fertility, even after doctors developed methods of operating that were as safe as the Porro but also preserved women's uteruses. In the late nineteenth and early twentieth centuries, some doctors used C-sections to sterilize disabled women without their knowledge or permission—and they did so because they believed them to be degenerate and thought they should not bear any more children. Obstetricians, like others in medicine, were among the most enthusiastic champions of eugenics in the late nineteenth and early twentieth centuries. And some believed that the very things that made women candidates for C-section—poverty, illness, or physical condition—made them candidates for sterilization, too.

Eugenics, the pseudoscience of perfecting humanity by rooting out "degenerates" and encouraging births among people of "good" stock, dominated medical, legal, and sociological thought in the US at the time.

In his development of Nazi ideology and law, Adolf Hitler would even borrow language from a California law that called for sterilizing the unfit.[13] In the US, of particular concern were the economic and social costs that indigent, criminal, and physically or mentally disabled people posed to society. So, too, were concerns about the ways that immigrants who weren't white or Anglo-Saxon might "degrad[e] the nation's gene pool," writes Adam Cohen in his book *Imbeciles*.[14]

These eugenic ideologies shaped obstetricians' practices. In medical journals, they wrote of the "social and political" imperative to sterilize poor women who needed C-sections because they were "deformed from disease." Not only were such women "not capable of giving that care and attention necessary for the sustenance of their children," they and their children end up "cast upon the public charities for support," wrote one physician, who was then emeritus professor at Bellevue Hospital Center in New York.[15] "Many women that come to cesarean section belong to the depraved and degenerate classes," declared an article in a 1909 edition of the *American Journal of Obstetrics and Diseases of Women and Children*. Because "they and their progeny may become a burden on the State, . . . the continued fertility of these women is therefore undesirable." Another obstetrician, writing in 1911, explained the necessity of sterilizing women during C-section who were "deficiently developed mentally, who should not reproduce their kind and who are likely to be a charge upon the community."[16] These women typically weren't sterilized at state-run institutions, but at the whim of doctors who believed they were doing their best for society and the future of humanity. As for the women, they happened to need a C-section at a time in history when that need could also permanently end their fertility—even as there were other, safe ways of operating that spared a woman's uterus.

Just as in the earlier descriptions of cesareans, in so many of the books and journals about these forcibly sterilized women, the women themselves are largely absent. I saw many drawings of pelvises, uteruses, and sometimes even full skeletons, but rarely encountered descriptions of the mothers, their responses to the operation, what they looked like, or even their names. I didn't realize how accustomed I'd gotten to reading about these silenced, anonymous, and disembodied women—women who'd been reduced from whole people to their malfunctioning or diseased reproductive organs—until the afternoon that I opened a 1911 textbook titled *Operative Obstetrics*. I was alone in a library study room, and when I turned the page to read about techniques of sterilization, so that a "patient may not again be exposed to the dangers of childbirth," I gasped. A photograph of a naked woman stared back.

Turning the page, I saw that she wasn't the only one. The book was full of photographs of expectant new mothers, photographed similarly: naked, hair piled on their heads so to better see their bodies. Some stand with sheets or hospital gowns puddled around their feet, their torsos crossed with surgical tape and sutures. Many are shown from the front and the side, like mug shots. Two are Black; one looks no older than twelve. All were sterilized and delivered in the same operation.

At first I felt excited—the photos seemed to promise that finally, I'd get to see some of the women I'd been reading about. But the women weren't posed in portraits meant to portray their humanity, but to exemplify them as types who "needed" to be sterilized. A few wear towels draped over their heads, perhaps to protect their identities, but in a way that to a contemporary viewer seems only more degrading.

Such was a typical use of photography at the time, as a tool to visualize "normal" and "abnormal," and to categorize ethnicities into hierarchies and types.[17] Daguerreotypes of enslaved people, made some fifty years earlier, had served a similar purpose—and the photographer had posed their subjects in a similar way: naked, full frontal and from the side, sometimes from the back.

It didn't help that, like the women identified only as dwarves in Dr. Robert P. Harris's list of C-sections from the 1800s, these women are also only identified by their disability: flat pelvis; achondroplasia; rachitic pelvis; kyphotic pelvis, rear view; highly flattened pelvis with paresis.

"Vision," feminist scholar Donna Haraway asserts, "is *always* a question of the power to see."[18] My freedom to look at the women put me, most weirdly, among the class of people—physicians, medical students, eugenicists—for whom these women functioned not as humans, but as scientific material. That medicalized gaze narrowed what I could see about them, much as it limits what's visible about C-sections in the public culture.

At the same time, I felt a kinship with these women. We had something in common: we had all met our babies by C-section. I gazed into the eyes of one of the youngest-looking mothers, her large eyes—looking to me, nearly one hundred years after she'd been photographed—mournful. I found myself thinking back to Sabine Hildebrandt's observation: the truth of history permeates our daily living. From that point of view, the shame that attends C-sections today can be traced back to the operation's past, its practice—predominately—on women who, a century ago, were branded the lowest, most degenerate members of their communities, destined to be a lien on the public purse.

DURING THE AGE OF EUGENICS, which lasted in the US from the 1870s until roughly 1942, C-sections were still rare. There were fewer than ten recorded in the US in 1892.[19] At one such operation in 1895 at a hospital in New York, it was so unusual some three hundred physicians observed it.[20] When a hospital performed one for the first time, through the end of the nineteenth century, the operation was so significant as to make the newspaper, the way the first implantation of an artificial heart once did. Nationally, they constituted 2 percent or fewer of births through the 1920s.[21] Soon, though, its comparative safety, and its potential to save the baby, meant that it had become an operation with which an obstetrician would be familiar.[22]

Some C-sections during this period were practiced on the affluent. The *New York Times* ran an article about the cesarean birth of British actress and aristocrat Lady Diana Duff-Cooper in 1929, whose good looks were so well regarded she likely helped to set beauty standards for everyone else.[23] Nevertheless, through the 1930s, the operation's chief subjects disproportionately continued to be drawn from more vulnerable members of society—women who deviated, physically or economically, from feminine and maternal norms. And those very qualities also put them at risk of sterilization.

As a result, even as surgeons developed safe ways to operate that also preserved women's fertility, some doctors continued to do the Porro operation—the technique that permanently removed patients' uteruses—at hospitals with predominantly Black patients. At Johns Hopkins, as medical historian Jacqueline H. Wolf found, Porros consisted of a third of the operations through the 1920s, because "a large number of our patients are colored women of relatively low intelligence in whom we have felt that an unlimited number of repeated Caesarean section was not justifiable," wrote the department's chair, prominent obstetrician John Whitridge Williams.[24]

Other doctors used slightly different procedures, but with the same result of sterilizing their patients. At Charity Hospital in New Orleans, Black women comprised nearly 88 percent of patients. From 1938 through 1959, nonemergency (elective) cesarean-hysterectomy comprised 12 percent of all C-sections.* That means of the 6,609 women who had cesareans over that time period, 800 had their uteruses removed during their C-sections as an elective procedure—not to save their lives. Physicians performed a third of these 800 cesarean-hysterectomies on women because of a "defective uterine scar," though these operations may not have been necessary; according to the study, their uteruses could have been repaired—and preserved. Another third lost their uteruses explicitly for the purpose of sterilization. For all these mothers, it's not clear how much choice they had in the matter. Of the 800 cases of elective cesarean-hysterectomy over those twenty-two years, 45 percent took place on women having their first cesarean section.[25]

In fact, as recently as the 1970s, at the LA County Hospital, doctors seemingly used C-sections as an opportunity to coerce Mexican-born, mostly Spanish-speaking women into hysterectomies at the same time as their children's births—believing that this group of women was having too many children, and that doctors needed to bring their birth rate down.[26] In that way, C-sections were one tool among many that have been used to control and limit fertility—including coerced sterilization and state-funded distribution of long-acting and difficult-to-reverse contraceptives such as Norplant and Depo-Provera—particularly among poor women and women of color.[27]

The cesarean's relationship with sterilization and its impact on family size only amplified the shame and lack of power conferred by the opera-

---

* In an emergency hysterectomy, the physician removes a mother's uterus to stop the bleeding or because of serious infection. In these cases, the hysterectomy is a lifesaving procedure. In a nonemergency hysterectomy, the hysterectomy is medically optional, and done for the purposes of sterilization.

tion in the first place. In such cases, the operation exerted a clear and definite shape on a woman's life. *"Acabo la cancion,"* said one woman sterilized at LA County Hospital in the 1970s. *My song has ended.*[28]

IN ADDITION TO EUGENICS, C-SECTIONS have also long limited family size due to the operation's dangers. Until the 1960s, doctors routinely sterilized women after their third C-section, because the operation's dangers increase with each subsequent section. (Some even sterilized women after their first or second operations.[29]) The widespread belief throughout the twentieth century—which, despite evidence to the contrary, still persists in some corners of the US medical establishment—was "once a cesarean, always a cesarean," meaning if a woman had a C-section, she'd need to have a C-section for all births to follow.[30] And she wouldn't have a choice but to stop at three. Jackie Kennedy's fourth cesarean in 1963 helped to put an end to that practice, by demonstrating—publicly, and on an elite woman—that a woman could have more than three operations.[31]

Yet some doctors still refuse to do more than three C-sections on the same person, a kind of backdoor family planning that people don't typically think about until after they've had the operation. That is because each subsequent cesarean is more dangerous than the last.

But a VBAC after three C-sections is out of the question at nearly any US hospital or birth center because of liability concerns that a woman's uterus will rupture. Which means that women who want another child after three C-sections, like an acquaintance whose doctor refused to do a fourth cesarean, can't have one without defying their doctor's advice and possibly endangering their lives. This is yet another cascade of consequences relating to personal and reproductive autonomy that doesn't become fully visible until after a cesarean's first cut.

At the same time, and though paternalistic, that doctor's refusal to do the C-section is rooted in evidence: compared with a first-time C-section, after four C-sections a mother is nine to thirty times more likely to develop placenta accreta, the condition that puts her at risk for severe bleeding and hysterectomy.[32] She's also more likely to need more than four units of blood transfused (we have only five liters of blood in our bodies) and is at a substantially greater risk of being put on a ventilator after the surgery.[33] What's more, people heal differently. While one person might have a lot of scar tissue after a single C-section, another might have hardly any after several. There is no way to predict this, or even to visualize it, outside of a laparoscopy or a subsequent cesarean.*

According to the authors of a 2006 article on the topic, because the risks of serious harm to mothers increase with each cesarean, parents should take into consideration how many children they intend to have when considering that first or subsequent C-section. But in practice, this kind of counseling is nearly impossible to do. Deciding how many children to have is deeply personal and complex—a decision that, as one mother described it to me, is almost mystical in all of the factors that go into it, some of which are clear and others only vaguely felt. What's more, an unplanned pregnancy can throw off a parent's most rigid plans. And as virtually every obstetrician and midwife I spoke with lamented, a typical prenatal visit is too short to accommodate meaningful education of any kind—to say nothing of extensive education about family planning and future cesareans. For now, C-sections' potential limitations of family size may be best known in groups that value large families—such as Hasidic or Haredi communities—and that as a result are often home to providers with some of the country's lowest C-section rates.

When it comes to decision-making about the risks of each cesarean: Who should get to decide if a woman has had "enough" C-sections? Or who should decide how many C-sections rule out a woman trying for a vaginal birth? It's a question that, most uncomfortably, sits on the same continuum as the arguments that have been deployed by physicians and lawmakers about whether a woman has had enough, or too many, children—from arguments about a woman's incapacity to support her children financially, to natalist discourses from a century ago that (white, middle-class) women must grow the nation.

As Dorothy Roberts, Loretta J. Ross, and other leaders of the reproductive justice movement have demonstrated, such discussions have long

---

* In fact, when I developed abdominal pain while writing this book, multiple providers suggested that it could be from internal adhesions—scar tissue from my section. The only way to know was to look inside. (The pain turned out to be caused by my appendix and an enlarged lymph node.) Seven years had passed since the operation, and it was still coming back to bite me in the ass in ways no one had thought to mention when I had the C-section.

pivoted on race, or race and class. Women of color, and poor women, and most particularly poor women of color, have since slavery's abolition—from the point of view of the state—been having too many children. By contrast, women who wanted to be sterilized—those with the freedom to make this decision, meaning they were more affluent and less vulnerable—couldn't do so if they wished, either. Until 1969, ACOG guidelines established that a woman could only be sterilized if, multiplying her age by number of children, the sum exceeded 120.[34] (As I write this book, aged forty-one, with two children, I still wouldn't have made the cut.*) But the question about C-sections and future fertility is also something obstetricians have been debating since the operation's inception, never quite arriving at an answer—in part because each person heals differently, and in part because they don't have enough data to draw a definitive line.

As my friend Aidan pointed out, even that argument can be sexist; NASA long refused to send women to space because they didn't have data to indicate it was safe. And the reason they didn't have any data is because they hadn't collected any; it didn't seem important enough to. Likewise, the reason we don't know how many C-sections is "too many," or how many C-sections a person can have and then go on to have a safe VBAC, is partly because we've never collected sufficient data on that, either.

The association between C-sections and unfit parents is still ambient. Shortly after my daughter's birth I came across a story about a study in the *Proceedings of the Natural Academy of Sciences* that theorized that cesareans are shaping human evolution.[35] Brain size at birth correlates with body weight and, by extension, good health and survival. But growing a baby with a too-large head will kill its mother, because it becomes impossible to birth vaginally. This is known as the obstetrical dilemma, as popularized in the 1960s by anthropologist Sherwood Washburn; we evolved to grow babies with large brains, but we also developed narrow pelvises,

---

* Before my appendectomy, which I had while writing this book, my trusted midwife, Lena, suggested that I choose to have my fallopian tubes cut during the same operation, to lower my future risk of developing ovarian cancer and for permanent pregnancy control. I didn't; I wasn't ready. As the history of the "Mississippi appendectomy" shows—operations when women of color were sterilized without their consent, and sometimes without their knowledge, under the guise of this other operation—so many other women in my position would not have had the autonomy to say no.

necessary to walk on two legs. The mismatch of baby and mother size is ill-designed for reproductive success, and emblematic of the medical model's definition of birth as inherently dangerous. And it doesn't make sense evolutionarily, according to the study's authors: "It is puzzling why the pelvic canal has not evolved to be wider to reduce rates of obstructed labor." Because women whose pelvises are too narrow for their large babies, write the authors, "[fall] beyond 'the fitness edge,'" their bodies are not fit" from an evolutionary perspective.

Thanks to C-sections, the authors explain, such women survive birth. In turn, we pass on our pelvic proportions, and propensity to grow babies with large heads, to our children, who pass them on to their children, and on, and on. As a result, the authors predict, C-sections are changing bodies: babies are getting bigger; pelvises aren't. But none of this is because of evolution; it's the intervention of an unnatural operation that's changing human bodies.

Reading the paper now, I can see how an evolutionary biologist might conceive this idea. But when I read it shortly after my daughter's birth, it felt like an insult. The thesis, I thought, was that people like me—if not me in particular—should by all evolutionary logic have gone extinct. I overlooked one fundamental aspect of the paper: that the operation is lifesaving. I focused instead on the stigma: that my body, and the bodies of other women who have C-sections, are aberrant. Beyond the "edge of fitness." Not natural. Not meant to be mothers.

TRAUMA WASN'T THE ONLY REASON I waited so long to have another baby. Another big factor, as I ambled into what's charmingly known as "advanced maternal age," was my husband's commute to the city. After years of freelancing he'd landed a full-time job as staff photographer for a lifestyle website. We finally had enough money, but now he was never home: up at five, out the door by six, home thirteen hours later, three or four days a week.

As a consequence, I found myself solo parenting, dawn to dusk, while holding my own job and inching toward tenure. I remember days when I'd run—literally—from day-care drop-off to my office to teaching to a meeting to therapy and then back to teaching. And that was the warm-up.

After my last class, I raced to pick up my daughter from day care—they charged you $1 per minute if you were late—drove us home, cooked dinner, and got her ready for bed. Only after she was asleep, or sometimes just before, I'd hear my husband's key in the door. The sound triggered physical relief. Finally, backup. But it also triggered anger: it wasn't his fault, but I was often furious that I was doing so much parenting alone.

These days were so packed that adding to my responsibilities by having another baby seemed crazy if not irresponsible. So as much as I felt scared by the idea of another birth, when I tried to contemplate how it might go differently, I had trouble getting there; I was too tied up by the exigencies of my everyday reality.

Still, thanks to therapy, I knew that I did want to have another baby. I had no idea how that would work, but I'd located my desire, which felt important. And I didn't want fear from the past C-section to set my future.

I remember broaching the possibility of another baby with my mother for the first time. We were sitting in her living room in New York City. I knew what I wanted, but I also wanted her approval. Some kind of assurance that I was better, enough.

"Do you think I should have another baby?" I asked. She didn't respond right away. We gazed at my daughter, who was playing on the thick blue carpet at our feet.

My mother told me that children take a lot of chi, meaning energy. "That's why they're called children," she said. She was responding to how burned out I seemed, how close to the edge I was living; she was speaking from a place of concern for me, her baby. But I took it to mean that I wasn't handling motherhood, that perhaps I wasn't fated to have another baby—an example of how trauma can distort reality, how my C-section seemed to be shaping my relationships in ways I'd never imagined and couldn't even see at the time.

UNLIKE THE WOMEN PHOTOGRAPHED FOR *Operative Obstetrics* who'd had their uteruses removed, my C-section didn't end my fertility. But it did shape my life, like a boulder that falls into a stream and changes its course. If I hadn't had such a bad first birth, I wouldn't have waited four and a half years to get pregnant again. So even though I went on to have another baby—a boy—I also believe that I would have had a baby sooner, after my daughter and before my son. That I would have had three children, not two.

This very personal aspect of C-sections' cascade of consequences is what made this chapter the most difficult to write. For while I wasn't sterilized after my C-section—my organs were intact, and I got pregnant again, easily—I identified with the women whose C-sections meant they had fewer children than they may have wanted. For all the reasons going into family planning—time, money, space, career, the physical impact of pregnancy—my C-section is the single biggest reason I will only have two children.

Putting my children to bed one night, the darkness in the room felt velvety, thick. As I held my children in my daughter's bed, I felt the presence of a third child—a baby. I could feel this baby's weight on my body. This, I realized, was the feeling that my friend Diana had described: a person on the other side of the wall. And while I could have, theoretically, tried for that third child, I didn't feel confident that I could throw the dice again and win. I'd gotten lucky, twice; I'd birthed two healthy children; I survived. Instead of increasing my confidence, my son's birth had humbled it. I wasn't sure I'd get that lucky again.

NOT ALL OF THE CONSEQUENCES that the C-section set into motion in my life were bad. I highly doubt that I'd have written this book were it not for my C-section; before it, as an assistant professor of journalism at a teaching-focused university, I was writing an academic book about how photographs in the media help us to remember some parts of the past, while enabling us to forget others. One day in the shower, I had a realization: my C-section was the dividing line in my life, possibly one of the most important things that would ever happen to me. That's what I had to write about. It sounds almost too neat, but I put the academic book in a drawer that morning and began working on this book the next day.

In that way, the surgery sent my life in an unexpected but fruitful direction. A writing professor in college, Michael Koch, had once told me I was like a thoroughbred looking for the race I wanted to run. Possibly he was referring to my impatience to do something big, like a horse pawing the ground at the starting block. But I took it to mean I hadn't found the right project for my energy. Deciding to write a book about C-sections, I remembered his comment; I felt as though I'd finally found the race. What a gift, perversely, the surgery had given me.

The surgery gave me something else, too: in the days after my daughter's birth, I wondered what would have happened to us if C-sections hadn't been invented. I knew little about obstetric history and assumed we'd both have died. I developed an image of this, the two of us during the labor, under a black sky dotted with stars. The image felt so real, so close and palpable, it's as if it happened, and it's nothing like the fantasies of a "natural" birth I'd entertained. I see it now as the truth of birth, the most honest understanding of it I could reach: alone, one body, two people. Sundered from the plane of regular life, together we touched eternity. Never again will we work this way together, in such unison, at a single, most primal task. The image feels untroubled, almost beautiful, even as it's born from fear of death. It's only thinking about my C-section that brought me this weird gift. I wasn't otherwise able to process or hold this feeling of suspension—something I hadn't felt before—during the labor or birth.

5

THE AMERICAN (MEDICAL) WAY TO BIRTH

OVER THE COURSE OF ABOUT HALF A CENTURY IN THE US, BIRTH moved from the home, where women midwives attended it, to the hospital, where male physicians managed it. Profound medical and social transformations hastened these changes, including urbanization, blood banking, the adoption of antisepsis techniques, and the discovery of antibiotics. Today, the vast majority of US births take place in a hospital, where they're overseen by an OB. The medical model of birth has triumphed.

In that way, the medicalization of birth is key to understanding how we've arrived at the current C-section rate—despite consensus among the medical community that the US does too many cesareans. Because while the increased safety of C-sections made the surgery more practicable, birth first had to transform into a medical event—one that discounts the value of spiritual care, personal relationships, and human touch—for cesareans to become as widely accepted as they are today. Aspects of most every birth now resemble a medical procedure, which makes birthing a baby surgically not unusual or miraculous or even remarkable.

Crucially, the medicalization of birth also devalued the practice of midwifery, whose definition means "with woman," and whose basic principles assert that "human presence" is essential to care. That's evident in the decimation of the midwifery workforce—something that sets the US apart from its peer countries, where midwifery is far more integrated into health systems and where larger percentages of the population birth with a midwife. It's also demonstrated by the now-dominant logic of obstetrics, which has historically valued tools and intervention over patient-centered care and human touch, and continues to do so.

To be sure, not all midwives hew to the importance of the human presence. The midwives from my first pregnancy and birth did not; those midwives seemed absent not only physically but in spirit, as well. Nor is personal support always possible, because the medical model of birth values and rewards technology, speed, volume, and efficiency—ideals that promote C-sections and technological intervention—rather than vaginal birth. But it is the way that midwives like Helena A. Grant practice when they attend mothers in the hospital. As we'll see, it's how midwife Jamarah Amani practices, whether at a birth center or in someone's home. I'd also find out that this is the way that Lena approaches pregnancy and birth—the midwife who had taken care of me when I'd recovered enough to get pregnant again.

WHAT'S HARD TO IMAGINE, FROM our contemporary stance, is that before birth moved into the hospital, people saw it not as a medical event but as a normal, regular part of life. Partly that's because the average woman had so many children: eight, for white women, during the 1800s. More if you count pregnancies that ended in miscarriage or stillbirth. As a result, the typical woman spent most of her adult life, from her twenties to her forties, pregnant or nursing.[1] Women with similarly large families surrounded her: her sisters, her friends, her neighbors. These pregnancies must have felt as if they created their own seasons, circumscribed how women kept time. They shaped when, how, and where a woman traveled; "what she planted in her spring garden," writes historian Janet Carlisle Bogdan, "and harvested in the fall"; the clothes she sewed.[2] As historian Laurel Thatcher Ulrich writes, they determined when she hefted "a heavy wash kettle," whether she rode horseback to the city, or stayed "at home" to "brew beer."[3] The vestiges of this, the palimpsests of such timekeeping, still mark people's experiences of pregnancy, but only as it intersects with and is dominated by the demands of late-stage capitalism: when best to move, start a new job, go on leave, take a babymoon. Largely these are individual questions, concerns that a couple sorts out together, without the support of a larger community.

Before the nineteenth century, in the colonies and then in the US, pregnancy and birth belonged nearly exclusively to women.[4] A pregnant woman depended on her community for support and knowledgeable care throughout her pregnancy. She wrote to and received letters from her mother, sisters, and friends, asking for advice and commiseration. "I seem to fatten all over," one mother wrote to her friend in 1837. "My feet and legs swell considerably and heartburn and acid continue, otherwise I feel pretty well." Another wrote to her sister about whether "the birth of a baby is as bad as having all your teeth drawn at a sitting."[5] Caring for her other children while pregnant, another woman wrote to a friend, is a "dog of an occupation."[6]

But in the era of community birth—when it took place within a web of social relationships—and before birth became medicalized, it wasn't only one's own pregnancy that shaped a mother's experience of time; other women's births exerted a pull. When a woman's labor started, her community of women came to her home to encourage her, share expertise, cook, wash clothes, and watch her older children. Alongside her midwife, they kept her company through labor. Archives from the 1600s and 1700s in the American colonies show anywhere from as many as seven to a dozen to all of the married women in a given settlement attending a woman's birth.[7] Albrecht Dürer's sixteenth-century woodcut *The Birth of the Virgin* shows an example of one such scene: in the background, the new mother rests in her bed; an exhausted midwife leans beside her. In the foreground—Dürer's real subject—eight women sprawl on benches, drinking and talking. One woman washes the new baby. Another holds a child to her lap. For most of human history, these scenes were private and thus largely out of view. They were also common, and part of women's domestic responsibilities—not the domain of experts.

When labor first got going, it "probably took on something of the character of a party," writes historian Laurel Thatcher Ulrich. The expecting mother provided food and drink for her attendants, including "groaning beer" and "groaning cakes"—probably consumed during the labor. Her attendants, she knew. These were women who'd been through birth before (though it's not clear if newly married women or young girls could attend), and who'd probably been to or personally experienced dozens of births.[8] The laboring mother ate, too—light foods like eggs, broth, and bread dipped in wine.[9]

As labor progressed, the women gathered around the laboring woman and quite literally held her. "A mother might give birth held in another woman's lap or leaning against her attendants as she squatted on the low, open-seated 'midwife's stool,'" Ulrich writes. In that way, a laboring woman was surrounded by and cared for people who knew her, who were also the experts on childbirth—gleaned from knowledge passed down through generations and gained from enduring and watching birth.

This combination of personal and experiential knowledge is hard to imagine in contemporary, twenty-first-century life, given the emphasis on specializing in distinct, even esoteric skills and separating the personal from the professional. In my own life, the only equivalent I can think of is the day of my wedding. I was thirty-one, in graduate school, and had come home to New York to be married. In my hotel room in Manhattan, my mother, closest friends, and future sister-in-law hung out. I vibrated with fear and excitement as we had our hair and makeup done. Most of my friends were already married; Rebecca G and Rebecca W were already mothers, and still nursing; both sat against the wall at various points, close to an outlet, as their Medela pumps pulled milk from their breasts. Female friends who weren't in the wedding party also came by to visit, hug, and reassure me. In my nervous haze I repeatedly misplaced envelopes containing cash to pay the makeup person, the band. Meanwhile, at the venue some blocks away, friends from Syracuse, where we were living, built the chuppah and decorated the tables.

A wedding isn't a grueling, embodied experience, but it is a liminal one, a transformation that many of these friends had been through but that I hadn't. (I'd "learned" that I could get ready for my wedding in this way by doing the same kind of prep before friends' weddings.) And because they knew me, how I acted when I was scared, these women knew how best to steady me—emotionally, but also physically: I remember gripping their hands, being so nervous I could barely walk on my way to the aisle.

I was off to a new life, which ended the life I'd had before. For that reason we have such ceremonies to begin with. And the security my community brought with me to this phase communicated two essential things: I was about to do something spiritually and personally important, and no matter how the marriage went, I wasn't alone.

BEFORE THE EIGHTEENTH CENTURY, WHEN labor started, virtually all midwives—Black, Indigenous, white, enslaved, or free—attended birth in people's homes or, for some Indigenous people, in a shelter made from brush.[10] On plantations, enslaved and free Black midwives attended everyone: other Black women and white women. Their skills made them so indispensable, some earned the honorific "doctor woman."[11] Men weren't permitted in the birth room, and physicians were called for only during exceptionally difficult labors.

The particulars of how a woman labored varied based on her culture. Puritan women were supposed to bear their labors quietly, as a way of demonstrating their piety and resignation to "God's will."[12] By contrast, in fifteenth-century Italy, women were encouraged to scream as loud as they could "even if it does not hurt you so much:" that way, "your husband and the others in the home, feeling sorry for you, try to put down such great fire with capons, sugared almonds and good wines."[13] In some African communities, women gave birth quietly, because prevailing cultural beliefs considered it "shameful to express suffering," and that doing so "damages their babies."[14] European colonialists' observations of these African women, along with their expectation that women "shout very loudly, so that the whole village may hear her!" shaped the expectation that Indigenous and Black women have easy labors, the stereotype that turned up in Dick-Read's *Natural Childbirth.*

Throughout these groups midwives brought special knowledge to bear: they steamed decoctions for women to sit over, prepared syrups to rub on the baby's head and shoulders to try to keep the woman's perineum from tearing, and brewed teas from "amber, saffron, ground cumin seed, sage, and comfrey" to move labor along.[15] They gave mint syrup for nausea. During labor, women moved around a lot: they squatted, held ladders or straps suspended from the ceiling, sat on birthing stools. Some kneeled and reclined into the arms of another woman. Others labored on their sides.[16]

Midwives also steeped teas to address problems like the delayed birth of the placenta or to control postpartum bleeding. They massaged mothers' bellies and helped the laboring woman into different positions to guide babies who'd folded themselves up in ways that make them difficult to birth: sunny-side up, or head cocked, or breech. After the baby's birth, in the colonies at least, a friend or neighbor probably nursed the baby first, because the new mother's milk was believed to be "impure."[17]

From a twenty-first-century perspective, it is easy—too easy—to dismiss these practices as belonging to the past, from before there was "real" medicine, or to diminish this as "folk" tales, not real knowledge. But these skills worked "in many instances in healthy birthing outcomes," Linda Janet Holmes, the author of two books about historical midwifery practices, told me in an interview.[18]

Midwives also took responsibility for their spiritual charge bringing mothers through birth. Black midwives in the southern US, and in Africa, for instance, sang, hummed, and invoked God, Holmes writes in *Safe in a Midwife's Hands: Birthing Traditions from Africa to the American South*.[19] They practiced these rituals after the birth, too: not sweeping out the ashes from the fire for the first few weeks. Fox Indian midwives encircled the shelter where a woman was laboring and sang to get stalled labor going.[20] Many cultures still practice traditions that blend care for the new mother's body and for her spirit: the Chinese tradition of "sitting the month," for example, in which the new mother doesn't leave her home for the first thirty days postpartum while her family cares for her. But it's important to point out that midwifery practiced here, in the US and in precolonial times, included rituals intended solely to care for the mother's spiritual and emotional well-being.

This volume of knowledge can be hard to conceive. Midwife Jamarah Amani told me about the Black and Indigenous grand midwives who are now at the ends of their lives, who learned the art and craft of birth attendance from their elders, and who over many decades—longer than she or I have been alive—have been keeping the practice of midwifery going: "You know the saying: when an older person dies, it's like a library burns down. An entire university."

Medical science has fenced off the knowledge these midwives developed, deeming it irrelevant. It has discarded the knowledge that women who weren't midwives inherited as well. To our peril. Recognizing the value of these practices isn't romantic nostalgia for the illusion of a more authentic past. The value of these practices demonstrates what we routinely neglect: birth—as anyone who has been through it can tell you—is as much about the safe passage of the body as it is about the soul.

DESPITE BEING SEEN AS A regular and normal part of life, childbirth in the 1800s was undeniably dangerous. Historian Judith Walzer Leavitt estimates the risk of dying during childbirth in the nineteenth century, over the course of a woman's life, at one in thirty.[21] This isn't because each birth was very dangerous, but because women had so many children—enslaved women, used to breed slaves, all the more—they were exposed to the dangers repeatedly over the course of their lives. The risks of long-term disability were higher still, and may have been more common among enslaved and lower-class women, for whom birth injuries—perineal tears, incontinence, infection—could be amplified by "hard physical labor," as the historian Nora Doyle writes.[22] Yet even white, middle-class, healthy women feared for their lives during pregnancy. Thus, on learning she was pregnant, a woman prepared her will.

In part because of these dangers, and believing physicians' new tools to be superior to midwives, wealthy women in the US began inviting male physicians into their birth room early in the 1800s. To some extent, physicians did appear to have better tools; they used forceps to assist with difficult births and, after 1845, administered ether and, later, chloroform to numb women from the pain of labor.[23] Women's interest in pain relief seems particularly relatable. Even today, the promise of the epidural is one reason among many that home and birth-center births aren't more popular.

But even as physicians attended them, women still birthed at home, amid their communities of women. The nation didn't have many hospitals or obstetricians, particularly in rural areas. Even in large cities, only a "small proportion" of medical care occurred in hospitals, writes historian Charles E. Rosenberg. Typically, only impoverished or single women birthed in the hospital, and only because they lacked community support—so great were the taboos about birth out of wedlock—or could not afford a midwife.

At the time, hospitals in the US and Europe were the last place you'd want to have a baby. They were, in one writer's description, "cesspools of infection": overcrowded, awash with dirty linen and used bandages.[24] Hospitals were so filthy that women who birthed on the streets of Vienna were less likely to die than ones who birthed in the hospital.[25] Women died from infection at such great rates at hospitals that in at least one European hospital they "were buried two in a coffin" to conceal how many were actually dying.[26] For these reasons, even C-sections were thought to be safer if conducted at people's homes than at hospitals, and some twentieth-century obstetrics textbooks include directions for how to prepare a home for the operation.

In addition to the dangers they faced, the unfortunate women who had no choice but to birth in a hospital often served as raw material on which physicians and medical students practiced, much as enslaved Black women once had. In fact, until the end of the nineteenth century, physicians would collect money from medical students to pay pregnant women to give birth in front of a class; such payment—bribery, really—is how she'd be enticed to submit to such a practice.

And while physicians' tools meant they could ease pain and bring down babies stuck in labor, as we learned in chapter 2, these interventions created new problems: Ether and chloroform could cause babies to asphyxiate. Forceps could maim or kill mothers and babies if applied inexpertly.[27] These tools also spread infection, further imperiling mothers. Handwashing was not regular practice, and physicians spread infection by, for example, moving from conducting autopsies to the labor ward, where they unwittingly spread germs via their hands from mother to mother.

While some leading physicians cautioned about the overuse of interventions, the "do something" approach to obstetrics would ultimately win out. Interventions also gave physicians justification for charging more than midwives did. Such interferences came to define the boundaries of the profession: "By surgical flamboyance the obstetrician set himself apart from the midwife and justified his fees," writes British physician and medical historian Irvine Loudon in his landmark book *Death in Childbirth*, published in 1992.[28]

In a lesson we still haven't learned, these interventions didn't necessarily mean better outcomes. As one nineteenth-century physician noted,

"Perhaps the best way to manage normal labor is to let it alone, but you cannot hold down a job and do that."[29] So while medicine "may have improved comfort levels and may have rescued some women from complicated labors," Leavitt writes, it "did not, on the whole, increase women's chances of survival in the nineteenth century."[30] But the conflation between interventions and safety would remain; indeed, it is still a fundamental delusion of our time.

By the start of the twentieth century, male physicians in the US were attending about half of the nation's births. Midwives attended the other half.[31] To move the needle still further—to demonstrate the need to fully transfer birth to physicians—required reimagining birth itself.

DR. JOSEPH B. DELEE, KNOWN to his family as Dr. Joe, was "often described in the American lay press as 'No. 1 obstetrician, U.S.A.,'" the *British Medical Journal* noted in his 1942 obituary.[32] In fact, the journal declared, "he was actually the world's foremost obstetrician."

DeLee, the son of Jewish immigrants from Poland and Prussia, is associated with the excesses of medicalized interventions during labor: pain relief, episiotomies, and forceps. He helped promulgate the idea that pregnancy and birth are not normal, regular parts of life, but rather pathological and states of illness. Instead of relying on "a medical student, a midwife, or even a neighbor," DeLee wrote, mothers needed highly trained obstetricians to see them through.[33]

DeLee believed that labor endangered mothers and babies: uterine contractions were akin to slamming a baby's head in a door; a baby that passed, unassisted, through the cervix and vagina damaged mothers' perineums as if they'd fallen on a pitchfork. The trauma of labor, DeLee argued, caused long-term physical impairments from prolapsed uteruses to infant brain hemorrhage. (*Tristram Shandy*, the eighteenth-century novel, has a similar passage; though it's a satirical novel, maybe that's where DeLee got the idea.) DeLee had worked at a so-called baby farm during medical school, which also may have shaped his ideas about the potential harms of labor. At baby farms, which existed throughout the United States and were reviled by the press, working and often unwed mothers paid other women, who were also poor, to care for their infants. (In that regard they aren't that different from US daycares today, notes at least one historian, which are also typically staffed by low-paid women, and sometimes derided as a necessary evil so that mothers can work outside the home.) Sometimes baby farms were also a repository for unwanted or illegitimate babies. These babies, who could be as young as a few hours old when they arrived, often did not fare well or live long, and DeLee believed that the brain aneurysms he saw among some of them were the results of injuries they'd sustained during birth.[34]

All told, DeLee's concern about the perils of labor led to what, by contemporary standards, read as outrageous comments, such as his oft-quoted observation that, if they were so frequently hurt by the processes of childbirth, it was a wonder women didn't simply die after birth—like salmon. His concerns also inspired him to raise the standard obstetric care for all mothers, which he sought to do through a rigorous commitment to antiseptic techniques—critical for preventing maternal mortality in the era before antibiotics—and by medicalizing birth. To that end, in addition to the many textbooks and journal articles he authored, and the students he taught, DeLee founded the Chicago Lying-In Hospital, a hospital dedicated only to pregnant and laboring women.

At the same time, DeLee's home-birth dispensary for indigent women, the Chicago Maternity Center (CMC), promoted birth with few interventions and championed the necessity of antisepsis techniques. In so doing, it achieved some of the best outcomes for mothers and babies in the world, in an era when a woman in childbirth was more likely to die than "her father or brother in taking part in the bloodiest battle of the Civil War," as another leading obstetrician put it. In these ways, DeLee is emblematic of the tension of obstetrics—intervene or wait, operate or tolerate—that the profession is still trying to work out.

It is not entirely clear why DeLee practiced in such a contradictory manner. Judith Walzer Leavitt argues that DeLee wanted to raise the standard obstetric care for all mothers by expanding the ranks of well-trained medical providers and replacing midwives. The best obstetric care, DeLee believed, was available in a hospital. But poor and working-class women couldn't afford that. DeLee's home-birth dispensary, Leavitt argues, helped to both replace midwives and train physicians to practice sound obstetrics—particularly through unstinting antiseptic techniques. By contrast, historian Carolyn Herbst Lewis argues that his tendency toward intervention came toward the end of his career, when obstetrics had turned in that direction anyway, and he was trying to keep up with the times. Regardless, DeLee is best remembered for the type of medicalized intervention that inevitably and ineluctably creates harm. Yet he is often overlooked for his meticulous adoption and championing of antiseptic techniques, in both "prophylactic" intervention and in his home-birth dispensary—which remain essential to preventing maternal death.

Methodical and perfectionistic, DeLee, who never married, reviewed patient records late into the night. He scribbled "R.O."—rotten obstetrics—on records where he identified physicians' mistakes, including his own. He often read while eating, his menus rigid and fixed: lamb on Mondays, fish on Tuesdays. In his study he kept a sign that said IN CASE OF FIRE, SAVE MY BOOKS. He was fine-boned and slim with a serious look, and for decades suffered from chronic sore throats and stomach problems, enduring surgeries including gallstone removal and an appendectomy. On multiple occasions in his diary he lamented that if it weren't for his throat pain, he could work three times as hard; he wished he could work all night. His siblings—he had eleven of them, though not all survived to adulthood—repeatedly urged him to rest, relax, lest he drive himself into an "early grave."[35]

Because of his reputation, I was primed to dislike DeLee. But the more I learned about him, the more I identified with this ambitious, work-obsessed, perfectionistic son of Jewish immigrants, trained as a young adult in traditional Orthodox law (his father, who'd gotten his start peddling clothes up and down the Hudson River, not far from where I live, had wanted him to become a rabbi). Like DeLee seems to have behaved, I, too, spent much of my life plowing on as if I didn't really have a body, just a brain. Or, as if my body didn't matter for its own sake, only to the extent that it got in the way of the work. The birth trauma I suffered disabused me of this idea. The wrongs done to my body had transformed into a problem in my head, which then showed up in my body when I was scared. I got hot all over; my heart sped up; I shook. My blood felt bubbly, carbonated. Only once I worked to reintegrate my body and my mind did I see how much I'd behaved as if the two were distinct—a Cartesian view at the core of much contemporary medicine, and one that undergirds the medical model's approach to birth.

FROM A CONTEMPORARY PERSPECTIVE, IT'S easy to dismiss DeLee's notions of pregnancy and birth as artifacts of the patriarchy. But it's also important to recognize that when he entered medical school in 1888, birth and pregnancy were the leading causes of women's death because of infection, eclampsia, and hemorrhage.[36] Infection was so horrifying it would sometimes sweep entire hospital wards, killing mothers and babies, as physicians moved from patient to patient without washing their hands. Antibiotics hadn't yet been invented, so for these infections, there was no cure; "doctoring in that pre-antibiotic era," physician and writer Abraham Verghese observed in the *New York Times*, "was mostly about observation and hope." For that reason, DeLee desired to open a hospital only for birthing women, which he believed would protect them from other patients' pathogens. (To underscore the severity and danger of these infections, it's important to note that even today, postpartum infection causes about 10 to 15 percent of maternal deaths worldwide; in the US, it's responsible for 12.5 percent of deaths, according to the CDC.[37])

Data from the turn of the twentieth century attests to birth's danger. In 1915, six women died in every one thousand live births; infant mortality was about 10 percent.[38] For nonwhite people, those figures effectively doubled.[39] As is the case today, at the turn of the twentieth century, the US lagged behind much of Western Europe, the Nordic countries, Japan, and Australia when it came to keeping mothers and babies alive.[40] Reading the literature from the era is depressingly familiar.

Leading public-health reformers, and physicians like DeLee, conceived of the country's abysmal rates of maternal and infant mortality as issues of great national concern. Improving obstetric training was one important front. But, they argued, bringing maternal mortality under control also necessitated cracking down on another class of workers: midwives.[41]

For centuries, midwives had been suspect, associated with witchcraft in Europe and in the American colonies. Margaret Jones, a midwife convicted of witchcraft, became "the first person executed in the Massachusetts

Bay Colony."[42] Now, at the turn of the twentieth century, virtually all midwives found themselves under attack, assailed as "dirty, ignorant and totally unfit to discharge the duties which [they] assum[e]," wrote Thomas Darlington, a New York City commissioner of health.[43] The *Public Health Nurse*, a professional journal, engaged such descriptions for decades, deriding midwives as "the more ignorant class of people" who were "teachable and imitative," but who could not be thoroughly educated.[44] As they once were in medieval Europe, midwives were especially vilified for doing abortions; in 1907, nurse F. Elisabeth Crowell wrote, in an investigation of midwives, "some go so far as to say that the two terms 'midwife' and 'abortionist' are synonymous."[45] Their perceived lack of qualifications has stuck around; while I was working on this project, one person, a mother of two, asked me—with a hint of disdain—"Do midwives even go to college?" (The answer is not necessarily, depending on whether she's a CNM, which means she holds a master's degree, or a CPM, for which she doesn't need a baccalaureate.)

In the early twentieth century, the nation's anti-midwife rhetoric also took on classist and racist edges. "Foreign" midwives faced rancor for engaging in "age-old, unclean practices." Black midwives attracted racialized scorn, like the one critic who described them as "a cross between a superstitious hag and a meddlesome old biddy," which Alicia D. Bonaparte, the Pitzer sociology professor, notes is "an attack against the very bodies and ages of Black women."[46] Felix J. Underwood, who for thirty-four years served as director of the Mississippi State Board of Health, lamented midwives as "filthy and ignorant, and not far removed from the jungles of Africa, laden with its atmosphere of weird superstition and voodooism,"[47] while magazines ran stories of Italian and Russian Jewish midwives attending the births of "deformed babies."[48] Turning birth over to physicians, public-health workers in several states argued, would improve neonatal outcomes—though in fact it did not.[49] And because midwives were competition for physicians, physicians had another reason to push for medicalizing birth—doing so justified their existence.

Though physicians and public-health reformers largely reviled midwives, immigrant and Black women relied on them. They had reason to: midwives were more affordable. They spoke the same languages. They offered the traditions that immigrant and Black women would have expected, comforts and knowledge that we now describe with the anodyne phrase "culturally congruent care." What's more, in some communities, seeing male doctors was inappropriate. In other communities—especially in the South—Black women couldn't afford or access an OB, or even receive treatment at a white hospital.

Reformers first attempted to drive midwives from the profession by passing new regulations and licensing requirements. Massachusetts, for instance, outlawed midwives altogether.[50] But that didn't do much to keep midwives from practicing. More regulations followed, including mandatory classes, supervision by doctors, literacy tests, white uniforms, and the requirement that midwives "be of good moral character and clean person." Such broadness left much open to interpretation; in Georgia, for instance, midwives could not practice if they had a venereal disease.[51] At the federal level, the Sheppard-Towner Maternity and Infancy Act of 1921, which provided $1 million a year in federal money for establishing clinics that provided care for children and pregnant women, further regulated midwives by putting them under physicians' and public-health nurses' supervision.[52]

At the same time, beginning in the 1920s, nurse-midwifery began to emerge as a new type of midwifery originating from the ranks of public-health nurses focused on maternity. These midwives tended to be white, whereas traditional midwives were not. They received their training in school; traditional, or lay, midwives learned through apprenticeship or through their grandmothers and mothers. CNMs aligned themselves with obstetricians to "eliminate the traditional midwife," and to supervise her, CNM and historian Katy Dawley writes.[53] In time, states would grow to recognize nurse-midwives, while also refusing (or making it difficult) to grant licenses to traditional midwives, thereby pushing Black, Indigenous, and immigrant women out of the profession.

Importantly, of the 7,950 CNMs in the US today, the vast majority are white; only 7.3 percent of CNMs or certified midwives, who hold a similar degree, identify as Black.[54] This isn't an accident; registered nurses are also overwhelmingly white, despite nursing's diverse history, and certified nurse-midwives come out of nursing.[55] And while they still often operate at the bottom of the medical hierarchy, nurse-midwives have achieved greater acceptance. The profession has taken on the cloak of professionalization of medicine, even as it's still illegible, as Helena A. Grant pointed out; when I call to make an appointment with my midwife, the schedulers refer to her as "doctor," even if I pointedly say, *midwife*.

As discussed in chapter 2, there can be much antipathy between these two kinds of midwives, who have different types of qualifications and scopes of care. The disagreements among these groups, and their relationships with physicians, are far from the public eye. What matters about this puzzle of regulations and licensure is the end result: mothers in the US have fewer choices about who can attend their births, even as the United Nations has recognized that midwives with both types of training can safely attend birth.

Both types of midwives also operate in an environment in which the obstetric outlook on pregnancy and birth—that it isn't normal, but pathological; that it's a risky state of preventable disaster—continues to define obstetrics' professional ideology. As obstetrician Dr. Nicole Calloway Rankins, who posts on Instagram and hosts a pregnancy and birth podcast, described it to me, "obstetrics is generally set up to expect that every single pregnancy, every single delivery, is going to be a disaster. And we have to be prepared . . . to act immediately to avert disaster." That dominant, medicalized logic makes it difficult for midwives to practice their profession, no matter their path to midwifery.

WHILE THE EARLY TWENTIETH CENTURY featured widespread contempt for the old world, and for Blackness, in many ways the societal mood was poised to embrace contemporary modern medicine and extend its faith in science and doctors. In the 1920s, scientists developed a vaccine for diphtheria, a common and often fatal childhood malady.[56] They discovered how to prevent scurvy and rickets. The cultivation of penicillin, sulfa drugs, and streptomycin over this same period gave doctors the capacity to treat and cure TB, pneumonia, syphilis, and childbed fever (postpartum infection), thereby saving the lives of an estimated 150,000 Americans between 1936 and 1952.[57] Other public-health initiatives, most notably clean water technologies such as filtration, chlorination, and sewage systems, are also credited with extending human life and curbing infectious disease. By one estimate, between 1900 and 1940, mortality rates fell an average 1 percent per year. A person born in 1940 could expect to live to sixty-three, sixteen years longer than someone born in 1900.[58]

At the same time, birth shrank from its domination of everyday life. The average white, married American woman in 1900 had fewer than four children, less than half of her predecessor from a century earlier.[59] Public-health reformers and physicians campaigned to persuade women that when they did become pregnant, they deserved the best, most modern care they could find. And that care came from physicians at a hospital, not at home with a midwife or with her community of women.

Within this science and health-obsessed national mood, fears about germs and infection were also substantial. Germ theory of disease, only recently understood, held that invisible germs lurking in air, soil, and water could only be eliminated with proper cleaning, chemicals, and hot water, transforming housework into a moral and hygienic imperative. Achieving proper hygiene for home birth seemed dubious—but it was exactly what a sanitary, modern hospital could offer.

As people moved to cities and left behind traditional networks, urbanization complemented and reinforced this focus on scientific expertise. Because of large numbers of people on the move, mothers could no longer rely on women in their communities to take care of them—and their older children—during birth. By contrast, the hospital freed women from their duties at home—with the added bonus of being cared for by medical experts, and the promise of accessing pain relief during labor. Little wonder that women in the 1920s and 1930s believed that by going to the hospital, they were making the safer and saner choice.

In a society that "had come to embrace the model of disinterested, professionalized science," writes scholar Charlotte G. Borst, midwives, largely seen as possessing "traditional, artisanal skills, ceased to be valued."[60] By contrast, "physicians and hospitals became definitive symbols of safety, sanitation and cleanliness," concludes sociologist Keisha L. Goode.[61] In fact, we now know that moving birth into the hospital didn't make it any safer. Some evidence even suggests that between 1920 and 1930, as more women began to birth in the hospital, birth became more dangerous still.[62]

By the end of the 1950s, what we now think of as normal birth was born. Birth had become anesthetized, routinized, anonymized—

one doctor described women lined up to birth as if in a factory—and nearly all US women birthed in the hospital with a physician, alone.[63] Efforts to eradicate midwives worked stupendously well; presently, only about 10 percent of all births in the US, at home and in the hospital combined, are midwife attended. The ranks of midwives of color, and Indigenous midwives, were decimated, and midwifery in the US became a predominantly—though not entirely, as midwife Jamarah Amani points out—white profession. And birth's transformation into a scientific, medical event that takes place in the hospital, primarily attended by a physician, has not changed since.

THE HOSPITAL WHERE I HAD my daughter was once a pioneer of an institution that promoted a mother-centered approach to labor and birth. To some degree, when I toured it in late fall 2015, it resembled a wannabe birth center—a freestanding, homelike facility that is not a hospital, whose birth rooms are usually furnished with real, queen-sized beds and bathtubs or showers, and that provides care for low-risk pregnant people according to the midwifery model. The hospital where I birthed had large labor rooms with patterned wallpaper, which my husband likened to a nursing home for its kind of institutional, impersonal efforts at affecting a caring aesthetic.

I hated it, I told my husband when we left. Even the town felt like a bad fit: an upscale community I'd otherwise have little reason to visit, populated by retirees and second homeowners. But the practice I'd switched to only delivered babies at this hospital. So, though I didn't like it, and because a home birth was out of the question—too expensive, too far from the hospital—there wasn't anything to be done.* Even now, I think that having a baby not at home was the right choice for me, though in retrospect I wish I'd had the option of a real birth center.

Still, researching this chapter I found it difficult to read about community birth. Because even before the operation, when labor went off the

---

* Despite their different reputations as being more or less medicalized or mother-centered, and though I didn't know it at the time, the hospitals near where I lived all had around the same C-section rate of 30 percent.

rails, I felt alienated and frightened, my body a problem no one seemed to know how to solve. My labor was nothing like the books I had read. I was in so much pain in my back that I kept picturing the frazzled frowny face that was the image the doula had used in our birth class to describe the pain of transition, when a person dilates from seven to ten centimeters. But when I got to the hospital, at about two in the afternoon, the midwife who checked me in—someone I'd never met before—told me I was only a centimeter dilated.

The general consensus of hers, and the doula's, seemed to be that I was worked up, possibly exaggerating, scared. And I *was* scared. Because the pain was so intense I couldn't think. My body seemed scared, too, set on pushing her out as quickly as possible, but to no avail, like a trapped animal throwing itself at a door. The contractions dominated me, stacking one top of another without rest, but I didn't dilate.

What went unsaid: if you think this is pain, honey, you're in for some seriously deep shit. What was happening: I was having back labor, which nobody seemed to notice—or if they did, no one explained it. Instead they suggested I get into the birth tub, where I waited for the anesthesiologist to arrive so I could get an epidural. Only once he'd arrived and started the epidural, and I was hooked up to the monitor, did anyone countenance what I'd been feeling for hours: the contractions were so big, one nurse described them as "monster" contractions. One after another after another. Me, the nurse, my husband, the midwife, the doula: we all stared at the machine. The dial reached to the very edge of what it could measure. The contractions were literally beyond its scope. "Wow," someone said. "Look at that."

There are many reasons why no one really registered my pain when I described it. I'm a woman, in labor, which has an exponential expectation of hysteria. Also, I didn't scream, or cry, but went quiet and internal— somewhere deep inside the ocean of my person. But no one in that room, besides my husband, knew me. They didn't know what that quiet meant.

By dinnertime I'd still barely dilated. The doula and midwife told me they were stepping out, that I needed to "rest." They'd check me when they got back. I remember them leaving the room. It was dark. I pictured them shrugging at each other, all out of ideas. I lay in the hospital bed, certain I was going to have a C-section. When they returned,

I'd dilated to ten centimeters. The room got really busy. Lights came back on. Someone turned on the baby warmer. Lots of people crowded my bed. I had a dark sense of foreboding. Things only got worse from there.

Set against such a scene, it's easy to romanticize community birth. It's especially enticing because the love and ferocity my mother and friends would have proffered, I wanted to believe, would have protected me from the carelessness of what felt like being discarded by my birth attendants and, surely, from the pain that came next. I can imagine my five-foot-four-inch, salt-and-pepper-haired, then-seventy-two-year-old mother snarling, and in her deepest, most fearsome voice, telling the midwife, the doula, the obstetrician, *You leave my daughter ALONE.* I can see Rebecca G, my best friend from high school, a nurse by training, opening the door to the hospital room and telling them, calmly and terrifyingly, *Out. Get out.* It is simultaneously easy and almost heartbreaking to imagine this. Rebecca W, who'd have flown in from LA, would have sat on my bed, looked me deep in the eye, and in the no-nonsense voice of the litigator she is, told me, *You can do this. You? Somerstein? Come on. You can do it.* Those words—*you can do it*—I don't think anyone said them to me during any part of that birth. Heartfelt or not, I needed to hear them. I needed to be with people who knew that I could get through it, who'd supported me through the pregnancy, who'd known me since I was a teenager, and who had been through childbirth themselves.

And while it's just as easy to dismiss community birth as fantasy—work, family, and geography might have made such a gathering of women impossible—that misses the point: How can I know if these women could or would have arranged their schedules, navigated around their own families, to show up for me? I am such a product of my culture, of the individualistic white American way of birth, that I never even thought to ask if they could.

WITHIN THE MEDICAL FRAMEWORK, WHICH reified the role of doctor, hospital, and science, C-sections—even if they were exceptional—came to be accepted and began to appear as triumphs of medicine and modernity. In part that's because they became safer: by 1950, the American

College of Surgeons boasted that "only one woman in [one hundred] now died after a Caesarean operation," compared with one in ten in 1920.

That's thanks to blood banking and effective asepsis, implemented in the 1930s and 1940s, which made it possible to treat hemorrhage and discourage infection.[64] The low-transverse incision—for which the surgeon opens the lower part of the uterus, the most common technique used today—also improved the operation's safety. DeLee's legacy is evident here, too, because it's an approach that he promoted.[65]

It's also possible that C-sections' reputation improved because they were associated with doctors, who at midcentury commanded widespread authority and prestige. And, by the 1930s and 1940s, the operation began to be practiced because of fetal, not only maternal, need—not only because a mother could not birth vaginally. Doing C-sections because of fetal distress or because a baby was in the breech position, for example, may have further loosened the operation's association with othered and impoverished women.[66]

Soon, and even as they were relatively rare, C-sections also became associated with some of the most advanced medicine that a doctor could offer. In 1953, the capacity of medicine to override vaginal birth could deliver almost magical achievements: Lucille Ball had her son delivered by C-section on the same day her TV show, *I Love Lucy*, ran an episode about the fictional Lucy's birth.[67] By 1960, when Jackie Kennedy, the incoming First Lady, was going to have a C-section for her second birth, the *New York Times* quoted a "Washington physician" as saying that "the risk involved in a Caesarean delivery was 'practically infinitesimal.'"[68] He was right; between 1950 and 1965, the risk of dying from C-sections at leading hospitals in the United States was less than 1 percent.[69] And in 1967, a doctor eager to make history—to ensure that the baby he delivered by C-section would be the nation's two hundred millionth person—intentionally delivered the baby at 11:00 a.m. on the dot,[70] the time when President Johnson had said that person would be born. (The baby's time of birth was technically 11:03 a.m., but the doctor still met his goal.)

This ambition is both magnificent and hubristic, an emblem of C-sections' hypermodernity. And it's of a piece with the US's embrace of an aggressive, interventionist approach toward health and disease, which as journalist Lynn Payer argues in her book *Medicine and Culture*, has endured since colonial times. Could there be any greater example of a doctor's power over nature, which bespeaks American dominance over land and body, than timing birth for such a milestone?

WHAT'S CRITICAL TO SEE, RISING in the background of these changes to birth, is the development of what sociologist Barbara Katz Rothman calls biomedical imperialism. Just as land gets colonized, she says, so does knowledge. By laying claim to birth, medicine established boundaries about who has authority to attend it. Knowledge accrued over generations, or belonging to a midwife who'd attended births without the supervision of a doctor, no longer counted. That manifested through standards that prohibited midwives from practicing not because of lack of skill, but because of country of origin, class, lack of formal credentials, or willingness to practice abortion.

Rothman, a professor of sociology at CUNY, has been studying birth since the 1970s when, as she puts it, women were handcuffing themselves to their husbands so that they wouldn't have to labor in a hospital alone. Now in her midseventies, with a streak of purple in her gray hair, Rothman is a legend in the world of women and gender studies. Our hour-long conversation feels like a master class in birth politics, and I find myself imagining what it would have been like to have studied with her.

Right away, Rothman tells me that C-sections save lives: her grandmother had one with her mother. This is important ground to stake out early, because Rothman wants to be clear that medical imperialism has done a lot of good; we have it to thank for our contact lenses, antibiotics, and pacemakers. Yet what territory the medical establishment colonizes means that it claims some knowledge as real, trustworthy, and legible, while also excluding and deauthorizing other knowledge as unreliable, untrustworthy, or not real knowledge. And by fencing off some knowledge as illegitimate, it loses a lot. In the context of birth, midwives' knowledge that wasn't colonized was dismissed or rendered illegal, no matter how good or bad it might have been.

The ideology of medical imperialism, which flared during the 1920s and again after World War II, is critical to understand not only the rise in C-sections in particular, but the framework in which we birth: a depersonalized process controlled and administered by medical specialists, where other kinds of (nonmedical) knowledge is dismissed. That's one reason no one besides the laboring woman was permitted in the hospital until the 1960s, says Rothman. In such an environment—where medicine reigns supreme—these relationships, and the knowledge they might bring, do not matter. Once husbands were allowed in, says Rothman, "it wasn't, 'You can bring who you need'—[it was] 'You can bring the father of the baby,'" which is more about the father's rights as a man, than a laboring woman's desires. "For some women, [the father] is the person you want. But for other people, 'My big sister, who's gotten me through everything I've ever done. Can she please come with me?'" says Rothman. "But no. It's not about you. It's about the baby." And about the man.

Dismissing these other relationships clearly makes birth harder and lonelier for people who would prefer to be surrounded by community. But it also has implications for the kind of care that providers can offer. "If you've been with somebody when she's had an orgasm, when she's dropped a book on her toe, when she's gotten horrible news—you know her face," says Rothman. A stranger, or someone you've only met a handful of times at fifteen-minute visits in an institutional setting, won't have that knowledge.

Rothman gives another example: "I have two daughters. When one of them says, 'I can't, I can't, it hurts,' I say, 'Come on, let's, you can.' When the other says that, I say, 'Okay, I'll call an ambulance.' They're different people. But if I didn't know them, and somebody falls on the ground and says, 'I can't, I can't, I'm hurting, I'm hurting'—I just call the ambulance. This kind of anonymization of the patient" frequently describes hospital birth today—where a person's labor is monitored remotely from a nurse's station outside the room. In such a setting, she says, "You can't give real care." You don't know what a person really means from what they say or how they look, because you don't know them.

I confess to Rothman that I had a birth like that, and that it never even occurred to me to ask anyone besides my husband to accompany me. It's almost embarrassing to reveal to her how thoroughly and unthinkingly I complied with the individualistic American medical model.

I feel relieved, almost forgiven, when she says, "Why would you? It's essentially a medical procedure. You don't invite your friends in. You say,

'Afterwards, I'll need some care.'" If you were having your gallbladder removed, you wouldn't tell your friends, "'What I'd really like is five of you with me to get me through this.' . . . Once birth is categorized as a medical procedure, that's the way it goes."

In fact, at some hospitals, if mothers bring their community to their births—a tradition particularly common among some Indigenous communities—they're castigated for it. "I've heard people say, 'Oh, they have such a big family," says Rebekah Dunlap, a doula, birth worker and member of Fond du Lac Band of Lake Superior. "'Why do they have to bring so many people all the time?'"

IN THE LATE 1990S, CANADIAN researchers initiated a large, international study comparing the safety, for the breech baby, of C-section and vaginal birth. They recruited more than two thousand women from twenty-six countries pregnant with breech babies and randomly assigned them to birth by C-section or vaginally. The results showed vaginal birth to be considerably more dangerous for the infants, so much so that researchers recommended that all breech babies be scheduled for C-sections. The impact on obstetric practice was immediate and profound: "Rarely in medical history have the results of a single research project so profoundly and so ubiquitously changed medical practice as in the case of this publication," one obstetrician reflected.[71]

Within five years, in eighty institutions across twenty-three countries, nearly all had "completely abandoned planned vaginal breech delivery in favor of" C-sections. It's for this reason that people like Lindsay Quella, who lives in Vermont, couldn't find a provider in her state who would attend a vaginal breech birth when she was pregnant for the first time. "I wasn't, like, thrilled with a C-section, but I also felt like unless I wanted to do something more rogue, I didn't really know what my options were," she says. If she wanted to birth in a hospital—which she did—she didn't really have any.

"Anything that shows a safety or better outcome for the fetus is really quickly adopted—with good intention. If you harm the baby, that's a whole lifetime full of harm," says Dr. Elizabeth Langen, an associate professor of obstetrics and gynecology at the University of Michigan and a specialist in cardiovascular disease and pregnancy. So in addition to recommending women with a breech baby plan a C-section, or an external cephalic version, a procedure used to try to turn a baby's position so that it's head down, most obstetricians have stopped training to do vaginal breech deliveries—meaning they can't offer that to women who'd prefer to deliver that way. Although doctors practice on simulators, and occasionally attend a surprise breech birth, people seeking to birth vaginally—"who might want to accept that risk for their baby," says Langen—often don't have that option, "because people aren't trained." This approach to vaginal breech is emblematic of medical imperialism: though well-intentioned, defaulting to a C-section dismisses the skills needed to attend vaginal breech birth as well as the reasons a mother might choose it.

At the same time, it's worth noting the moral injury that a provider might feel in response to a bad outcome. Dr. Nicola Pemberton, an obstetrician who runs the Birth Center of New Jersey, notes that "everybody's experiencing trauma—from the doctor to the nurse to the patient—when an outcome doesn't go in the way you hope it to go. I think everybody processes those traumas differently." Some practitioners, she says, in processing that kind of trauma, "may say, 'Never again. I'm never—that's never going to happen to me ever again.'"

MEDICAL IMPERIALISM'S DISMISSAL OF OTHER, more routine labor-management skills also shapes the births of NTSV babies—term, head-down, single babies, their mothers' first. When I was in labor, not once did the midwife or doula suggest I turn on my side, massage my back, or use a peanut ball to open my pelvis—all standard interventions that can happen even if you're hooked up to a monitor. Instead, when neither the tub nor the epidural helped me to dilate, the midwife asked if I'd had any operations on my cervix, as if my body had to be the problem. I'd had a colposcopy in college, basically a cervical scraping, which was in my medical records; I hadn't hidden it from the OBs or midwives. I remember thinking, *How are we only talking about this now?* I also see now that this moment shows how completely underprepared I was to cope with labor, too; I had no plan, and no knowledge, other than to see how it went.

Writ large, the loss of labor-management skills matters because stalled labor—not progressing to full dilation—is the number one reason for C-sections in the US.

"There's a midwife that I work with that if someone's labor is progressing slowly, I'm like, *Oh, great. She's on.* Because she will be able to help this woman be in different positions and push in different ways, and she will get this baby delivered vaginally," says Langen. "There's always someone on the team who we all know can help someone deliver vaginally. And I think what we haven't figured out is how do we take that expertise that these folks clearly have and disseminate it among all the nurses, all the midwives, all the doctors," she says. "Recognizing the importance of normal labor and how it looks and how to help manage it is something that in really busy OB-GYN residencies sometimes doesn't get prioritized."

Rebecca R. S. Clark, an assistant professor at the University of Pennsylvania School of Nursing, makes a similar observation. "Physicians especially don't have tools, if a labor isn't progressing," to move it along. "A lot of nurses might not have those tools, either," she says—such as how to help someone change positions, or do a side-lying release, or use a rebozo—a large piece of fabric that's wrapped around a woman's belly and hips and used to gently help a baby rotate or to relax a mother's pelvis. Certifications in obstetric nursing, she points out, tend to focus on electronic fetal monitoring as opposed to skills to address the baby being hung up at a given point, and deciding what's next.

I've gone back and forth about whether my C-section was necessary, not least because the midwife told my husband after the fact that the baby might have slid out on her own. She said this with a voice of deep regret; perhaps she wished it were true but didn't actually believe it. After the section, the OB told my husband that my daughter's head was turned to the side. (It wasn't clear if anyone knew this was her position when I was in labor, or if they only saw it once she was born.) Still, with a midwife, nurse, or OB who knew how to turn a baby with a sideways head— someone like the kind of midwife or nurse Langen describes—I don't believe I would have needed that operation. But I also don't believe that my daughter would have slid out without help. She was in a bad position.

In that hospital, that night, with that staff, there wasn't anything else they knew how to do. For a more complicated labor like mine, the only tool they had was a hammer—or in their case, a scalpel. If I'd been some-where else, with staff with different training and other outlooks, perhaps I wouldn't have needed a C-section. I'd get confirmation of this belief with my next baby, who positioned himself seemingly identically—from the back labor to the slightly cocked head.

I could blame myself for my C-section: I should have done more re-search. I should have made better choices. But this is so clearly the result not only of multiple systemic failures, but of medical imperialism's di-minishment of the value of personal relationships and the kind of labor support Rothman calls "hand skills."

I was sitting on the sofa talking with my husband when I under-stood this. It was late; the kids were in bed. Though we've gone over the birth many times, I felt such urgency as we talked about it that night in light of medical imperialism. My husband, a sociology major in college, a systems-thinking kind of guy, seemed to get it before I did. And then it was almost as if, for the first time, I saw what had happened: no one there understood the situation well enough to deliver my baby vaginally. This insight felt almost like physical relief. There was nothing that I, or even anyone in that room, could have done to prevent that C-section. But the conditions that led to these circumstances were not inevitable. And they needn't continue to be.

BY THE MIDTWENTIETH CENTURY, THE public had largely accepted the medical model of birth, by virtue of the fact that most people birthed in the hospital. But scientific and medical advancements around birth, and even around pregnancy, came at a price. Thalidomide, a sedative and anti-nausea compound once "marketed as freely as aspirin," caused birth defects in babies born to mothers who'd taken it to combat morning sick-ness early in their pregnancies.[72] The drug's British packaging read, "No known toxicity and free from untoward side effects." In fact, it hadn't done "the standard testing."

While Thalidomide affected an estimated 147,000 babies worldwide, only 24,600 lived to their births. Those who did had shortened or mis-shaped legs, arms, and internal organs, and crooked spines.[73] (Notably, Thalidomide hurt fewer people in the US than elsewhere, because the

FDA never formally approved the drug for marketing or distribution.) While the scandal led to new drug-testing regiments, and distrust of pharmaceutical companies, it also became twisted in such a way as to emphasize individual women's responsibilities to manage risk during pregnancy. As one cardiologist concluded, "Married women of childbearing age should avoid drugs as much as possible, particularly new ones."[74]

During this same period, birth advocates also publicly voiced concern about doctors' overuse of interventions. "That Mothers May Live," a story about maternal mortality in the November 1939 issue of *Ladies' Home Journal*, promoted medicalized childbirth by focusing on physicians and the necessity of prenatal clinics. But the writer also critiqued "the abuse of interference with labor—reliance on labor-hastening drugs, forceps delivery, Caesarean sections instead of the old doctor's maxim: *Here I sit and twirl my thumbs / And catch the baby when it comes*."[75]

Yet regulations that made it difficult for midwives to practice only continued in the decades since. In states such as Mississippi, for example, where Black midwives had continued to attend Black women's births through midcentury, the state required midwives to renew their midwifery permits yearly. In order to do so, they needed a physician to assert that a given county still needed her services, writes historian Yulonda Eadie Sano.[76] If she could not secure this recommendation, then she could not renew her permit and would have to retire.

Many of the women lay midwives saw in the South were very poor. It wasn't uncommon for a midwife to go unpaid for her work, or to receive food instead of cash. As one midwife recalled, "If I'd a stopped 'cause they didn't pay me, I'd a stopped a long time ago."[77] And while the introduction of Medicaid in 1965 covered these mothers' births, it did not cover births midwives attended—and so had the result of further medicalizing birth. (Private insurance plans such as Blue Shield did not cover midwife-attended births, either.) These are but two ways that we socialized women to have births in the hospital, and also made doing so an economic necessity, as Helena A. Grant pointed out.

Who Made the Lamb (1964), writer Charlotte Painter's chronicle of her pregnancy and birth, expressed the emotional and psychic costs of an excessively medicalized model of childbirth. Recuperating from her cesarean, her bed "no more than two feet" from a man "moaning horribly," Painter's obstetrician comes in to check on her. "I thought: I am receiving the best of all possible modern medical care. But what I said betrayed an ungracious turn of mind: 'This place must be the latest thing in snake pits.'"[78]

In the decades since, we've kept childbirth in the hospital, where it is most often overseen by OBs. New technologies, like electronic fetal monitoring, have further squeezed out labor support, personal relationships, and even human touch. But because birth takes place in a hospital, with a constantly monitoring set of machines, that lost knowledge can be hard to see. Like Painter, we are the recipients of the most modern medical care—but not necessarily the kind of care that's needed most.

When my daughter was six months old, we held a baby naming for her in our backyard, a Jewish ritual to welcome her into the community. It was a warm day in October. My father led me through a recitation of Birkat ha-gomel, a blessing traditionally said after surviving danger, such as having crossed a desert, recovered from a serious illness, or given birth. The *bracha* translates, roughly, to mean: *Blessed are you, God, for bestowing good to me, despite my being undeserving.* A person says the blessing in front of a minyan, or group of (traditionally) ten men, and then receives an answer from the community: May God bless you with good forever.

When I said this *bracha*, I wasn't yet able to speak about what had happened to me. The blessing was as close as I could get, and I could barely finish saying it, I was so moved. My father responded to me, a recognition I took to mean, *Yes, I see you. In fact, all of us gathered here see you. The danger you endured did happen.*

There's not a word in the blessing about the dangerous journey having been worthwhile; the point is the danger that you survived. The communal recognition of having survived a perilous journey serves as an antithesis to the comment, *At least your baby is healthy.* It is said in front of a community who sees both your trial and your presence. It recognizes that the mother has a soul, fears, and other emotions besides joy and delight. It is an example of how such a form of collective spiritual support can help to keep you alive. It is almost like being witnessed into being.

After my son was born, in June 2020, Lena, my midwife for my second birth, did something similar. Because of COVID, no one could come to see us, not even my daughter. No one could send flowers or meals. We weren't even permitted to leave our room to walk the halls. But she came to see me, drew a chair close to mine. It was a Wednesday afternoon; she wore scrubs; she had other places to be. Her visit was a surprise. "How are you?" she asked. She leaned forward, elbows on her knees, and smiled, ready to listen.

6

"HISTORY IS SHOWING THEM HOW TO TREAT US"

VICTORIA WILLIAMS STARTED SEEING HER OBSTETRICIAN EVEN BEFORE she got pregnant. She already had one daughter, Saniya, born in 2005, during Victoria's first year of undergrad. Her pregnancy had gone well. It had also gone long. At forty-one weeks pregnant, though she and her baby were doing okay, Victoria's doctor induced her. During labor, Saniya's heart rate plummeted, and Victoria had a cesarean. "What I know now is of course that [induction] caused me to have the style birth I had, because of the Pitocin—because it stressed [my daughter] out," she says.

But almost a decade had passed since that birth. And Victoria's life had changed a lot during those ten years: she'd graduated college; moved with her daughter to New Orleans; earned an MSW from Tulane; met and married her husband; made a career working in nonprofits. In that way this next pregnancy was a bit of a "redemption" from her first, Victoria says. At the same time, "I still felt that single baby momma syndrome," she says. "Those are wounds I'd never dealt with or healed. I still felt that shame of a nineteen-year-old girl in another state."

Still, as with any mother who's had a C-section, especially with her first birth, Victoria's decade-old C-section initiated a cascade of consequences, such as whether Victoria should try for a VBAC or schedule a repeat cesarean. But for Victoria, who's Black, racism would further shape the ways her future births played out. In essence, this is what is meant by "intersectionality," the term that scholar Kimberlé Crenshaw conceived.

In her pioneering work on Black women and work, and later, on Black women and violence perpetrated against them, Crenshaw theorized that "race and gender interact to shape the multiple dimensions" of discrimination, subjugation, and vulnerability.[1]

In other words, a C-section sends a mother down the chute of consequences no matter her race or class. But a Black, white, Hispanic/Latinx, Indigenous, or Asian woman comes to that C-section—and to motherhood writ large—through specifically raced and gendered experiences. And the path of C-section mothers' subsequent reproductive lives— whether they want to have more children or don't, seek contraception or abortion, want to VBAC or schedule repeat cesareans—is constricted and textured by virtue of the ways that gender and race interact to create, foreclose, or shunt someone along different paths, narrowing their choices.

At first, Victoria liked her new doctor, a white woman. When she told her that she wanted to try for a VBAC, her doctor seemed enthusiastic. Looking over Victoria's records, "She was like, 'Yes, you can do this, and [the first C-section] technically doesn't really count. It was nine years ago. Your scar tissue should be fine and not a big deal.'" (Some obstetricians caution against trying for a VBAC any earlier than two years after a C-section, because of concerns that the uterus hasn't had enough time to heal and to safely sustain the pressure of labor.)

When Victoria became pregnant, she had a good full-time job with a "great company." But during her pregnancy, Victoria was laid off. She lost her health insurance as a result and needed to apply for Medicaid. Going from a "private payer" to a person with public insurance seemed to change how her doctor thought of and treated her. "I looked a certain way, and then boom, I lost my job and I became this different person to her."

At a prenatal appointment at the beginning of Victoria's third trimester—at around twenty-six weeks pregnant—her doctor said, "Time to schedule."

"Schedule what?" Victoria asked.

"You have to have a C-section."

"No, I'm not. I thought we had talked about this."

Victoria tried to switch to a different provider. She went to the Alternative Birthing Center at Ochsner Baptist, a birth center staffed by midwives and located within the New Orleans hospital. It resembles freestanding birth centers both in practice—"We believe labor and birth are normal events," it declares on its web page—and its treatment of laboring mothers, who aren't hooked up to electronic fetal monitoring, can wear their own clothes, and can eat and drink during labor.

But the staff told Victoria that they couldn't take her, that they don't accept new patients after twenty-four weeks. Victoria was frustrated. She was just past the cutoff. She explained, "I'm having this situation. I just found out about you guys. This information was not offered to me when I got here."

No, they told her. They weren't accepting new patients.

Being on Medicaid hampered Victoria's choices further. Not all doctors take Medicaid. Some advertise that they do, but when you call, it turns out they aren't accepting patients with that type of insurance. Nor could Victoria afford to hire a midwife and pay out of pocket. Her doctor, she said, had "box[ed] me in at the right time." She was stuck.

Over the coming weeks, Victoria's doctor emphasized the risks of VBAC. "There's 1 percent chance of this, 1 percent chance of that," Victoria recalls her saying. At first, Victoria was thinking, *Okay, those are risks, but I'm healthy.* Nothing was going on clinically, like diabetes or hypertension, to make a C-section more likely. But at her prenatal appointments, her doctor kept emphasizing the bad things that might happen if she had a VBAC, without sharing the risks of a repeat cesarean.

Although she didn't know it at the time, Victoria now thinks that her doctor may have used a race-based formula to determine her likelihood of having a VBAC. The VBAC calculator uses a person's age, hypertensive status, reason for prior cesarean, and whether she's ever had a prior vaginal birth to create a likelihood of VBAC success. Until 2021, this calculator also asked about and factored in a person's ethnicity.[2] It automatically gave a lower score to Hispanic/Latinx and Black women seeking VBACs compared to white women with identical risk factors, because— statistically speaking—those groups are less likely to have a VBAC. In that way, it functioned as one among other racist tools that, Victoria says, shape the "trajectories of how you give birth."

Ultimately, Victoria scheduled the C-section. "I let the angst of the situation get to me," she says. But even scheduling it was a struggle. Her doctor wanted her to give birth before forty weeks; Victoria refused. She told her doctor that her first birth went beyond forty weeks and, moreover, that "that's normal. That's okay. Why do I have to tell you, OB lady? This is stuff that you should know." But her physician didn't listen to her. "Even to the day of my birth she wasn't listening."

Victoria's C-section was scheduled for noon. The morning before, her doctor called and said, "We have to move your time to five a.m."

"No," Victoria told her. She already had it lined up: she'd bring her daughter to school in the morning; go in for the birth; her husband would pick her daughter up from school at three o'clock. Moving up the operation to 5:00 a.m.—with less than a day's notice—meant Victoria would have to find someone to care for her older daughter.

"That's the only time I have available," the doctor told her.

"Okay," she said. "Give me another day."

"An extra day isn't going to give you a baby," her doctor responded, showing how much she knew Victoria wanted a VBAC.

Victoria was furious when she hung up the phone. She tried to get labor started at home, holistically—eating lots of pineapple, which is said to kick-start labor. But ultimately, she says, "I [didn't] have another option. I wasn't immersed in the birthing environment that I am now. I succumbed. I so [wish] I'd [gone into labor and] showed up with a baby."

"The history has been written for Black women," Victoria tells me. "They are the people who have been experimented on. History has already told [doctors], 'They have a high pain threshold. They have high blood pressure. They don't eat well. They're already stressed out. They don't have social support.' History is showing them how to treat us."

IN THE UNITED STATES, BLACK, Hispanic/Latinx, and Asian women are disproportionately more likely than whites to have C-sections. Rates among Black women are highest. In Louisiana, where two hundred years ago François-Marie Prevost used enslaved people to experiment with cesareans, the patterns are the same, but worse. Today, the state commands the second-highest C-section rate in the country, behind only Mississippi. More than a third (37.9 percent) of Black mothers there have C-sections, according to the March of Dimes.[3] Even initiatives in other states that have successfully brought down the C-section rate—like the California

Maternal Quality Care Collaborative—have seen these racial inequities persist.

Since the pandemic, C-section rates have gone up for mothers in all ethnic groups, to 22.4 percent of all births in 2021, from 21.6 percent in 2019.[4] That may be because mothers with COVID, whether they had a severe case or not, were counseled to have a cesarean to be able to better treat COVID, which can be serious in pregnancy and even cause stillbirth. It's also possible that providers "lowered the threshold" for C-sections in order to "reduc[e] inpatient maternal stays, cross-infection and the use of protective equipment," write obstetricians Wissam Arab and David Atallah in a 2021 letter to the editor of the *European Journal of Midwifery*.[5]

But C-sections increased most for mothers who are Black, Hispanic/Latinx, and Native Hawaiian or Other Pacific Islanders (NHOPI). So while primary C-sections increased 2.8 percent over that period for white mothers, they increased by 4.4 percent for Black and 14 percent for non-Hispanic/Latinx NHOPI mothers.[6]

There are a number of reasons for these inequitable rates, and racism—from the structural to the individual level—lies at the center of them. Perhaps most telling that it's racism, not race, as Dr. Joia Crear-Perry of the National Birth Equity Collaborative put it, is that low-risk Black women are more likely than low-risk white women to have a primary cesarean. At the individual level, "pressure and coercion and discrimination in the patient-provider interactions contribute to these high rates," says Dr. Nicholas Rubashkin, an associate professor of obstetrics, gynecology, and reproductive services at University of California–San Francisco. Rubashkin has a PhD in global health and has studied the VBAC calculator's racist design.

Discrimination and coercion take place between people in a private setting, so they can be hard to track. And while mothers of all backgrounds are pushed into interventions they don't want, according to a 2019 study in *Reproductive Health*, women of color are more likely than whites to say that they have been pressed to accept an unwanted intervention, and to have been scolded or yelled at, or refused help when they asked for it.[7] In another study, from 2013, 13 percent of Black mothers and 19 percent of Hispanic/Latinx mothers said that during childbirth they had been discriminated against based on their race, ethnicity, culture, or the language they spoke.[8] This discrimination often reflects racist and classist stereotypes, as Lisa Keyser, a mother who lives just outside DC, experienced. A former Division III swimmer, Keyser, who is Caribbean American, became pregnant in her twenties. Though she came straight from work in blouses and pencil skirts, and had gotten pregnant at a healthy weight, at her prenatal visits her doctor told her to stop drinking soda and to walk faster at the mall.

Such discrimination is also borne out in hospital-level data. About half of hospitals in the US have C-section rates that differ for Black and white patients—with Black women's rates being higher. This isn't inevitable; the other half have C-section rates that are the same regardless of the patient's ethnicity.

There's also evidence that hospitals treat Black and white mothers differently, particularly when they decline an intervention. A white woman who does so may be perceived as "well-educated and decisive," write scholars Laura B. Attanasio and Rachel R. Hardeman in their study on the topic.[9] But a Black woman may be treated "as non-compliant, aggressive or as the 'angry Black woman.'" That's what may have happened during Victoria's second pregnancy. She refused a C-section, only for her doctor to pressure her further, using scare tactics. Then, when Victoria could not accommodate her doctor's last-minute change of the time for her cesarean, the interaction grew even more hostile, with the doctor's cutting remark that one more day wouldn't get Victoria a baby.

Dr. Karen A. Scott, an obstetrician who created the PREM-OB Scale to measure and visualize obstetric racism—a metric that quality improvement surveys for hospitals and physician practices don't otherwise track—saw this in her practice.[10] There's "such grace," she says, extended to "white reproductive labor and bodies not given to Black women and their babies. White women will sometimes just demand, 'Get out of my room. Don't touch me anymore. I fire you!'" she says. But when a Black woman says something similar, it's, "'Let's call security. Let's call the police. Put her in restraints.' There is a threat of a Black woman who asserts herself and her authority, and God forbid if the Black male partner is just as, if not more, protective," says Scott, who recently departed the University of California San Francisco to focus full-time on her work improving birth outcomes and measuring obstetric racism.

Denise Bolds, a licensed social worker and doula who runs Black Women Do VBAC, an organization that trains doulas to support Black women who've had a cesarean and want a vaginal birth, and that trains doulas to support women preparing for surgical birth as well, also notes that many of the Black mothers she's cared for were pressured into C-sections by providers who cautioned, "You don't want your baby to die, do you?" That line is so profoundly coercive, she says: "I did all this work and now you're going to tell me I'm going to go home and lose her?" It's also effective, she points out, because it taps into the legacy of Black mothers who historically were separated from their babies when they were enslaved. Black "babies have always been the Gross National Product—Black women have always been the gross national product of this country," says Bolds. "The woman has come from ancestors where baby" was separated from its mother. "It's a traumatic trigger for Black women. You're saying that to me—my ancestors went through this. I'm not going to. I'll let you cut me.'"

That hospital staff treat Black mothers differently from mothers of other races is also evident in the results of a randomized clinical trial on induction. In the study, led by University of Pennsylvania obstetrician Rebecca Hamm and published in 2020, researchers enrolled expectant mothers into two groups: one induced according to their providers' preferences, the other according to a standard protocol.[11] The researchers found that C-section rates dropped dramatically among Black women whose doctors followed the standardized process. In that group, Black women had a C-section rate of 25.7 percent. But among women whose doctors induced them however they saw fit, Black women had a C-section rate of 34.2 percent. And that's not all: in the standardized group, Black infants also benefited. They were born healthier, needed shorter stays in the NICU, and were less likely to need supplemental oxygen. Notably, the protocol did not change the C-section rate among non-Black women, or the health of their babies—demonstrating that the physicians, knowingly or not, treat Black women differently than whites. (Similarly, standardizing protocols for how to treat hemorrhage has also been shown to make birth safer for Black women; as with the study about induction, the standard protocol did not have any effect on white women's outcomes.)

Even the reasons that Black and white mothers have C-sections differ. Black mothers are more likely than whites to have a C-section for nonreassuring fetal heart tones—whose interpretation is highly subjective, which we discuss in chapter 8. White women are more likely to have a C-section for stalled labor. "Those are really different reasons," says Rebecca R. S. Clark, the assistant professor at Penn. "There's a lot of provider subjectivity in both of them." When it comes to nonreassuring fetal heart tones, are Black women "having their labors intervened with more frequently, more aggressively?" asks Clark. This can stress babies, and such stresses can make a baby less tolerant of labor, which happened in Victoria's first birth. Or, asks Clark, "Do [the mothers] not feel safe? Likely, in the situation. So therefore, they don't respond well, therefore, their fetus doesn't respond well. Your blood pressure is up, you don't feel safe—[mother and baby] are connected at this point."

Rei Shimizu, an assistant professor of social work at the University of Alaska–Anchorage and the author of a 2022 report on inequitable maternal outcomes in Alaska, sees a blanket distrust of women's bodies at the core of such discrepancies. There's an "assumption in the health system, and particularly in [OB-GYN] health systems, that nonwhite female bodies cannot give birth safely without intervention, when in fact BIPOC people have given birth safely for centuries without Western medicine," she says. To some extent, given how institutionalized medicalized birth has become, that assumption may shape many women's births, no matter their race. But thinking intersectionally—looking at why and under what conditions Black women in particular have C-sections, and at the ways that history has shaped these conditions—suggests that Victoria's race and gender shaped her pregnancies and births, whether her doctor was conscious of that assumption or not.

YOU ARE TREATED WITH LESS COURTESY than other people are.

You are treated with less respect than other people are.

People act as if they're better than you are.

You are threatened or harassed.[12]

These statements, writes Linda Villarosa in her book *Under the Skin*, get at the "steady, soul-crushing experience of everyday racism."[13] But it wasn't until the Black Women's Health Study, which launched in 1995,[14] that researchers developed and used these queries to assess how everyday racism affects people's physical health. Until then, Villarosa observes, the bulk of US studies that look at health over the long haul had enrolled almost exclusively white participants.

The researchers found that the accumulation of discrimination stresses Black women throughout their lives. Like a toxin that the body can't flush away, such accumulated stress wears on—and wears away—health. In a series of academic articles she published beginning in 1992, Arline Geronimus, a professor at the University of Michigan School of Public Health, termed this accumulated stress "weathering."[15]

At the time, convention had it that babies born to teen mothers had worse outcomes than those born to women later in life. But when Geronimus looked at the data, she found the opposite to be true for Black mothers: the older a Black mother at the time of her baby's birth, the less likely her baby was to survive. Geronimus hypothesized that "weathering" on people's bodies, caused by "social inequality," compounds over time—such that a Black fifteen-year-old has had less stress on her body than a Black woman at twenty-five. Over time, Black women accumulate more "insults to health," through racism in all its forms—systemic to interpersonal—insults from which white women are comparatively protected. The reason that Black babies born to Black women in their twenties and older were dying at higher rates than whites, she theorized, was because their mothers were in worse health than white women of the same age. "That prolonged, effortful, active coping with social injustice may, itself, exact a physical price," she wrote.[16]

Researchers have identified how chronic stress harms a person's health. When a person is stressed, her immune system is distracted from defending the body from infection. Stress also activates cortisol, and aldosterone, secreted by the adrenal glands, which cause inflammation throughout the body—initiating physiological changes that can be harmful, from elevated blood pressure to an increase in visceral fat, which is more damaging to inner organs than fat stored elsewhere on the body. Chronic, unpredictable, and negative stressors are believed to add to a person's allostatic load: the "wear and tear" on a person's body. Where some kinds of stress are important and physiologically useful, too much stress, or "allostatic overload," writes Bruce McEwen, a neuroscientist who studied the effects of stress on the brain, "serves no useful purpose and predisposes the individual to disease."[17]

Physiological evidence for weathering may also be apparent in our telomeres, a sequence of repetitive DNA. The job of telomeres is to protect chromosomes, like a buffer. During the process of cell division, telomeres shorten. What this means is that our telomeres invariably shorten as we age. When they are too short, the cells that they're part of either die, or if they survive, they can't create new cells.[18] "If they erode completely, then the DNA sequences at the ends of the chromosomes degrade, which can cause a host of diseases seen in premature aging," explains Meghan Blair Turner, a PhD student in pharmacology at the University of Kentucky who studies the metabolic impacts of stress from early in life.

Prolonged exposure to stress, especially in early life, is believed to shorten telomeres prematurely. Emerging research suggests that, between birth and adulthood, Black people experience telomere shortening at a much faster rate than whites—likely because of exposure to racism, not because of any inherent physiological traits. At the same time, it is important to point out that the rate of telomere shortening can also be slowed down over the course of a person's life. They aren't static—shortening, and shortening, and shortening until you die. (There is also a mechanism for rebuilding telomeres, but it isn't well understood.) Still, telomeres are a biomarker for how much stress a person is under at the time that they're measured.

Taken together, researchers postulate, the accumulated stresses from weathering cause Black women to be at a physiological disadvantage when they become pregnant. This is partly why having more education, or more money, doesn't protect Black mothers or their babies from poor birth outcomes the way that such advantages protect whites. As researcher Fleda Mask Jackson found, the stresses of racism among college-educated Black women are pivotal—particularly regarding their "sense of obligation to protect children from racism," as well as racism they face at work.[19] "These are professional women," says Victoria. "These are doctors and lawyers who mentally have made it. But then you try to do this grand accomplishment of having a baby, and you die. Or you have some major complication."

The physiological effects of chronic stress may also create biological conditions that make for a poorer environment for babies in utero. Compared with whites, Black women are twice as likely to have babies born prematurely and at lower birth weights. Frankie Robertson, who runs her own firm in Lafayette, Louisiana, consulting on the social inequities of health for Black birthing people, needed an emergency cesarean at twenty-eight weeks. Though she can't prove it, Frankie believes that the stress she experienced before and during her pregnancy—stress caused by racism, and her fight against it—led to her hypertension, the early C-section, and her daughter's fifty-six days in the NICU. "My issue was an abnormal amount of stress and trauma," she says now.

Frankie, who was forty-one at the time and living in New Orleans, had already had a baby—a boy born after a healthy pregnancy. But with her daughter, she began experiencing heart palpitations midway through her pregnancy that would not stop. She didn't fully connect the dots about how the activism she'd been engaged with, regarding police violence against Black people, or the work she was doing in her community around health and structural racism, might shape her pregnancy. Not because she was doing something wrong, but because of the seeming ubiquity of structural racism she was encountering in so many corners of her life. Frankie developed pregnancy-induced hypertension, and a spike in her blood pressure just after she started her third trimester sent her to the hospital. While her own health stabilized, her daughter wasn't doing well, and doctors told her the baby had to be born.

At the time Frankie wasn't aware of weathering and initially blamed herself: "Did I do this wrong, was I too active, should I have turned the news off because all these things are stressing me out?" she says. "These societal issues, these larger structures—they do chip away at us," she says. "That's the essence of weathering, whether you know it or not."

JAMARAH AMANI, A LICENSED MIDWIFE and the founder of the National Black Midwives Alliance, is based in Miami, where the C-section rate is over 45 percent.[20] Amani, a mother of four, found midwifery during her first pregnancy when her OB—seeing her "list of ten questions"—told her, "You know, there's a midwife down the hall.'" Amani laughs. "That was the best thing that could have happened to me as a young mother," she says now. The relationship she formed with her midwife was much more reciprocal. She wasn't only open to Amani's questions, a receptiveness symbolized by the couch in her office, but her midwife asked Amani questions, too—how the pregnancy felt, what it meant to her.

When Amani and I spoke on Zoom, she wore big earrings, a nose ring, her hair wrapped back in a scarf. What brought Amani to midwifery as a profession were the gaps she saw in the reproductive justice movement, to which she'd committed herself in her early twenties. She saw the movement's strengths defending the right to abortion and had worked to make access to abortion and emergency contraception more available. At the same time, she believed that the movement needed to focus more on birth. So she began training as a midwife. In 2011, she became the executive director of the Southern Birth Justice Network, a grassroots organization training midwives, doing policy work, and advocating for Black maternal health. Several years later, in 2018, she started the National Black Midwives Alliance, encouraged by Black grand midwives, her mentors, who've been practicing for half a century or more—the midwives public-health departments intentionally drove from the profession.

Amani says that it's important not to underestimate or downplay "the impact of interpersonal racism on how the white majority of providers deliver care to birthing people of color." Yet, she cautions, interpersonal racism is "not the only type of racism. We have to address not just who's in the room, those two individuals, but this entire system that is based on white supremacy." I ask if she can think of an example in which white supremacy is codified in the practice of healthcare. She answers immediately: BMI.

TAKE YOUR HEIGHT IN CENTIMETERS. Convert your weight to kilograms. Divide weight by height, and that's your BMI.

Developed in the 1830s and popularized in the 1970s, BMI purports to assess body fat as a proxy for a person's health. It categorizes people into underweight, ideal, overweight, and obese categories. Researchers developed these groupings using the heights and weights of about seven thousand white, middle-aged men—hardly a diverse population. Today in the

US, Black and Hispanic/Latinx women are disproportionately likely to fall into the overweight or obese categories.

BMI continues to be used in research on populations because it's a "quick and dirty" way of assessing health, one researcher explained to me. But it provides far less insight into a singular person's health. About a third of people with a "normal" BMI have metabolic syndrome, meaning they're prediabetic. They may be a "normal" weight, but they aren't healthy. BMI also fails to assess where a person holds fat. If it's predominantly on their belly, they're at a higher risk for metabolic and cardiac disease, even if they're at a normal BMI. In that way it misses people who appear "normal" but are in fact at risk of disease.

At her first meeting with an expectant mother, Amani must assess her BMI and assign her a risk number between 1 and 3. That she does so is written into Florida law. But it's more than that: if a person has a BMI over a certain number, then Amani must determine that their pregnancy is a 2 (medium-risk) or a 3 (high-risk).

Because Black and Hispanic/Latinx women are more likely to be categorized as obese, they are more likely to automatically fall into those higher-risk categories. But being classed as higher-risk can increase the interventions in a person's pregnancy, labor, and birth—including the likelihood of a C-section. "Wait, so you're telling me that I could end up with a C-section because of my weight," says Amani. "But the reason that I would end up with a C-section is because you're deciding that I'm high-risk because of my weight. So you created the narrative, and you're creating the procedure to address your narratives, but neither are really based on the truth. And your narrative is leading to this very unnecessary procedure," she says.

Some data suggests that this is exactly what occurs. Because while high BMI is associated with higher rates of C-sections, it isn't clear whether fatness causes C-sections or is merely associated with them. A 2011 study of nearly twelve thousand mothers found that providers are more likely to use Pitocin and epidurals during labor when treating fatter patients, and less likely to use forceps or vacuums (to assist with vaginal birth). They're also more likely to call a C-section earlier in labor than for slimmer people.[21] In that way, BMI may function similarly to race. And while a higher BMI may make it harder to have a vaginal birth—many of the obstetricians I spoke with said that it does—it may also inspire physicians to treat mothers differently.

To be clear, the physicians I spoke with were divided about the potential impacts of inequitable treatment. Some believed that higher BMI makes it harder to birth vaginally, period. Rebecca Hamm, the obstetrician who led the study about induction of Black and white mothers, told me that she ran a similar study on induction and BMI—to see if standardizing protocols made a difference in C-section rates. It didn't. (It's important to point out that not all C-sections result because of failed induction.) Other physicians noted that the association between BMI and higher C-section rates might result from a mixture of implicit bias and physiology: a higher BMI does make vaginal birth more difficult, and some physicians may treat fat patients differently than thin ones.

What's uncontested is that C-sections for obese mothers can be risky. The overall operation takes longer than operations on slimmer mothers. And the time between incision and the baby's birth is also longer, according to a 2014 study—even accounting for previous C-sections.[22]

High BMI also casts a shadow that is profoundly stigmatized beyond obstetrics. Obesity is often framed as a public-health crisis, one for which individuals are held personally responsible—even though access to nutritious food, safe places to exercise, and genetic disposition play key roles in a person's weight. Yet in media and public-health messaging, obese people "are figured as a heavy burden on self, family, and society," writes Sabrina Strings, an associate professor of sociology at University of California–Irvine. "In other words, they are endangering not only their own health with their high-risk practices but the health of their families and the public health."[23]

The medical literature framed the impoverished and disabled women in the late nineteenth and early twentieth centuries, on whom C-sections were developed, as similarly degenerate. Moreover, their bodies' capacity to reproduce was a threat—their children a future financial and social burden to society. Sterilizing these women, physicians and eugenicists argued, was essential, which is why some used cesarean sections as an opportunity to do so.

I'm not suggesting that physicians are sterilizing mothers with high BMIs against their will. But it strikes me that perhaps we've created another class of people who are treated as though they are ineligible for and incapable of vaginal birth. People for whom, given the value and shame placed on their bodies, surgery becomes the right answer. Physiological processes may only compound that treatment, if obesity does make it harder to birth vaginally.

But BMI is so frequently used because it is easy, fast, and inexpensive to assess. The better and more holistic ways of assessing a person's health that Amani named take more time and money: glucose levels, cholesterol, and blood pressure. Notably, about a year after we spoke, the American Medical Association announced a new policy in response to BMI's limitations—the ones about which Amani had expressed frustration. Rather than use BMI as a stand-alone metric, in a clinical setting, the AMA advised providers to employ "other valid measures" such as "visceral fat . . . waist circumference, [and] genetic or metabolic factors" to assess a person's health.[24]

It is easy to see how, in a system that prioritizes efficiency and speed—at the expense of personal relationships between doctor and patient—clinical use of BMI would have become so widespread. "People have care providers that don't see them in their fullness of their humanity," Amani said. "They see them as their race, their BMI, their blood work."

On the obstetric side, that's exacerbated by how short prenatal appointments tend to be, says Victoria. Doctors don't get to know you. That was likely another component in the dynamic with her doctor—another reason why, after Victoria lost her job, her doctor seemed to treat her with less respect. She didn't know Victoria was a self-described "academia-type person," always reading a book or listening to a podcast. She didn't know that Victoria loves school so much that she recently completed an accelerated doctoral program in healthcare administration in fourteen months with no breaks—a sprint of a marathon for which, because she works full-time and has young children, she'd study at two or three in the morning.

It's striking, I said to Victoria, that after you lost your job, your doctor treated you as if you weren't trustworthy or responsible, instead of responding with compassion. As if losing your job and health insurance during pregnancy wasn't hard enough, I said.

Yes, Victoria agreed. But she didn't sound surprised.

OVER THE PAST FIVE YEARS or so, the mass media has focused on the elevated risk that Black and Indigenous mothers face of dying during pregnancy and birth. These deaths include ones that happen during pregnancy and within a year postpartum. And the majority of these deaths—four out of five, according to the CDC—are preventable.[25]

The leading cause of pregnancy-related deaths in the United States is mental health–related: overdoses and suicide. But such stories don't make the headlines, says former Woodhull nurse-midwife Helena A. Grant, or fit with the conception that practitioners are the only ones responsible for the country's maternal health emergency, not a wider societal responsibility. "It's deplorable, despicable, for Black and Brown women—for all women," she says. "And we have an expectation that Black women are going to fare worse—the ones who get the short end of the stick in all. It's built into the historical essence of this country," she says.

To make a real dent in the crisis, she said, we must change the system: for instance, offer paid family leave to mothers and their partners. And, she points out, that leave must begin when a person is still pregnant. One outcome that emerged from COVID is that when communities locked down, rates of preeclampsia and preterm birth decreased, says Grant. There's even evidence that lockdowns decreased total allostatic load. "Why are we not making that [data] usable? Why are we playing these games?" she asks. "We need to be thinking more holistically." (To be fair, some OBs I talked to suggested that the rates of preeclampsia did not actually decrease—they simply went under-reported. Studies on preterm birth during the lockdown period are uneven; some found a reduction in preterm birth, while others haven't. What does seem clear is that preterm birth because of cesareans and inductions fell during lockdown—possibly, according to authors of a 2022 study in *Pediatrics*, because people weren't seeing their obstetricians as often, and fewer "indications for delivery" were identified. Or, in other words, because people were left alone to go into spontaneous labor.[26])

Keisha Goode, the assistant professor of sociology at SUNY Old Westbury, pointed out that focusing on individuals' deaths "removes responsibility [from] big-picture structural issues" that shape a person's health long before and long after they become a parent. The insurance a person has—or doesn't have. The birth centers where they can get an appointment—or can't. These inequitable systems, structures, and investments profoundly shape the communities where a person is born, grows up, lives, raises her family, goes to school, works, and grows old.[27] They influence a community's potential for wealth and economic stability, the quality and availability of its schools and healthcare, how safe or violent it is, its degree of environmental degradation, whether there are parks or paths to walk or ride a bike.

Such social determinants of health, researchers have found, play a far larger role in a person's health than the sum of her personal choices. Yet in the US we tend to focus on individual health markers, like a person's weight, or BMI, and to overlook how social determinants of health play a larger role in shaping those metrics. An efficiency-driven health system may be one reason for that. But when it comes to birth, this focus on individual and quantifiable metrics is also reflective of the medical model of birth.

By comparison, midwifery is philosophically grounded in a more comprehensive understanding of health, one that, according to the International Confederation of Midwives, encompasses "the social, emotional, cultural, spiritual, psychological and physical experiences of women." As a consequence, midwifery stresses more holistic questions about a person's health, says Holly Smith, a certified nurse-midwife and consultant on the executive committee of the California Maternal Quality Care Collaborative. These questions get at some of the social determinants of health, like your living situation, where you work, how you get to work. Yet one of the sad consequences of social determinants of health is that Black women in the US have disproportionately less access to midwifery care, which may also contribute to their elevated likelihood of having a cesarean. It's for these reasons that midwives like Jennie Joseph, whose Commonsense School of Midwifery is based in Florida, are seeking to train a new generation of midwives of color.

Focusing mostly on death or near-misses is also problematic, says Pitzer sociologist Alicia Bonaparte, because it "obscures that there are Black birthing parents that are able to birth their children." And it plays on a long history of pathologizing Black mothers as unfit and aberrant, and that pathologizes pregnancy as well. "That's very familiar to people, right?" says Bonaparte. "'Look at the horrible things that are happening to these Black women.'

"I'll be honest with you," Bonaparte says. "I'm growing tired of seeing this in the media. . . . I'm more so interested in focusing on the folks that are addressing it." Yet stories tend to focus on the crisis, obscuring the solutions that scholars, midwives, activists, and others are already working to effect. It also obscures that Black mothers do have safe, healthy births every day. And that the goal of birth shouldn't just be about survival—it "should be about joy, pleasure and excitement," says Keisha Goode. "There's such an association with birth and death. . . . We have to shift the conversation a little bit here."

The emphasis on deaths and near-misses presents another problem: it skims over mistreatment that might not end in any quantifiably "bad" outcome. The emotional wounds from everyday racism resonate long after the moment of insult, and not only physiologically. Overlooking this pain is like discounting a person's emotional experience of her birth—like telling a mother who felt traumatized by her C-section, *Well, at least you're both healthy.*

"If somebody walked up and called you a name, or insulted you—like, 'Hey, you're an ugly bitch.' It's going to affect you and you're going to remember that for a long time," Jamarah Amani says. She gives an example of a baby who, after its birth at her birth center, needed to go to the NICU for a higher level of care. The parents were Black Caribbean. When the family arrived at the hospital, she recalls, "The nurse said, in front of the parents, 'This is a dirty baby.'"

The parents were stunned to have been "disrespected in this way," Amani recalls. The insult brought them both to tears during what was an already stressful situation: their baby's needing to be admitted to the hospital. "To have the staff, who was also Black, refer to their baby in that way—it's devastating. It's the thing that they remember most about their hospital experience," she says. "And the white supremacy is so deeply embedded into the system that even people of color are perpetuating it."

Helena A. Grant made a similar point. "A lot of people say, 'culturally concordant care,' or, 'Let's put Black cops in neighborhoods.' When you start aligning with the very system that is very broken, and that energy, and the mentality, you become part of it—you structurally become part of it—you start doing the same damn things that you're seeing done." It takes a "strong person energetically, spiritually, mentally, to be in a system and still say, 'I will not become that. I will not align with that.' But most people—women, men, Black people—when they get in a system, they become that. White supremacy, it's not about white people. It's about characteristics that develop."

In healthcare, Amani says, we let "a lot of things slide because, 'Oh, well, you know, they're saving our lives,'" she says. "I don't even know why we give such a pass to people who are supposed to embody the word 'care.' But care is not calling someone dirty to the face, or their child. That could just not happen in any other setting." Yet these kinds of racist insults "happen all the time," she says. "They don't get addressed. Because of the power dynamic. If I'm that angry parent, especially if I'm Black, I might be the one that has DCF [Department of Children and Families] called on me." In that way, letting what may seem like "minor" hurts go unremarked perpetuates racist systems; there is ample evidence that Black infants are more likely than whites to be removed from their families' care; that Black mothers are more likely to be drug-tested than white mothers; that Black mothers are more likely to be harshly punished if they test positive for drugs.

Amani shares the story of Syesha Mercado, who had her thirteen-month-old removed from her care when she went to a hospital to ask for help feeding him. She was pregnant, and her breast milk had dried up. But her baby—exclusively breastfed—refused other liquids. Mercado, a singer-songwriter, is a minor celebrity; she was on *American Idol*. She's married. Beautiful. And, because her baby was dehydrated—again, the very reason that Mercado brought him to the hospital—the consulting pediatrician called DCF, which removed her son to foster care.

But Mercado's nightmare took a turn for the worse after her second baby's birth. Because she was already flagged by DCF and had a child in the system, authorities seized her baby ten days after she was born. "How can we not relate this to chattel slavery?" Amani asks, referring to the 1662 law, passed in the then-colony of Virginia, that an enslaved woman's children would have the same "status" as their mother. "When these types of situations happen, that's in our minds," Amani says. "Like, 'Let me not be the parent who's angry, who speaks out, and then I walk out here without my baby.'"

Nicole Carr grew up in south Florida and speaks with a mellow twang. Now an assistant professor of English at Texas A&M University–San Antonio, she studies Black motherhood and is working on a scholarly book on the topic, *I Am Not Your Mammy: Black Feminist Mothering in the Twenty-First Century*. When we spoke on Zoom one blisteringly hot day in August, she had just wrapped filming a documentary about Black mothers called *High Risk: Black Mothers Protecting Themselves and Their Babies*. In our meetings she looked at once elegantly and casually put together, in a crimson silk top and sporting petite gold hoops, a gold necklace, and cat-eye glasses, with her twists pulled partly away from her face. Like a Hollywood ideal of an English professor.

Carr, who's Black, was working on her PhD at the University of Miami when she decided to start a family. Her mother, aunt, and grandmother were all birthed by midwives; "it seemed natural" that Carr would do the same. She also disliked hospitals and couldn't imagine birthing in one.

Carr bonded deeply with her midwife, a Cuban American woman from a big family like hers. But the birth, at Carr's home, was unexpectedly difficult. Carr's daughter had shoulder dystocia, which means that, as she was being born, she got stuck behind Carr's pelvis. Carr and her daughter were both admitted to the hospital. Carr's daughter stayed in the NICU for nine days, and during that time, Carr said, "I was very cautious about saying too much and not challenging the doctor too much." Carr grew up in a diverse community that included whites. When her daughter was born, she was living in southern Florida—what she calls "plantation Florida." She says, "That's why I knew to, like, be quiet, not to ask the doctor too many questions, even though it's my child. I knew not to upset them, knew just to be quiet. You want her to come home."

I asked if she'd worried staff would call Child Protective Services. Carr says she didn't think that would happen. But she felt the doctor's distrust. "We felt like when we said something, they would hold her longer" in the NICU, she says.

When the NICU doctor told Carr and her husband that they'd seen her daughter have seizures—there were video monitors filming the babies all the time—Carr and her husband asked to see the footage. They were told, "You don't need to see it"—though this was their baby.

For the rest of her daughter's weeklong stay, she perceived the staff's disrespect. "I absolutely knew that when they admitted me, they're saying, 'A poor Black mother who made the stupid decision to have a midwife.' Even though I was working on my PhD at the time. I knew what they were seeing."

It never occurred to me, until I talked to Nicole, that we had felt no obligation to act deferentially to anyone after my C-section. In fact, a few days after my daughter's birth, a hospital administrator came to my room to see how we were doing. I didn't really understand why she was there at the time. She was tall and blonde, dressed professionally, in heels, no white coat. Now, I think, she wanted to take the temperature on our likelihood to sue. Which is so disappointing, because what we really needed was a counselor, a therapist, someone to talk to. I remember trying to nurse and feeling distracted by the baby, and by my pain. I really wanted her to leave. My husband chased her out. "Get the fuck out of here," he yelled.

My husband is white, over six feet, broad-shouldered. He hadn't slept, showered, or shaved in days. He'd been wearing the same clothes the whole time, including what was probably a dank hoodie; because we weren't planning to have a C-section, neither of us had packed for more than twenty-four hours. The rims of his eyes were inflamed. He probably looked scary and, possibly, dangerous. I'm certain he intimidated the hospital flack, who left her card, fled, and never returned.

What freedom we had, to express rage without worrying about the repercussions, like whether she would call security, or child welfare, or find some other way to punish him or us or our baby for his anger. That's the cloak of whiteness. The "grace" that Dr. Karen A. Scott spoke about.

As for the hospital, it's telling—of our perceived class? Of the degree to which they knew they'd fucked up?—that even in their mistreatment they tried to accommodate us. In a 2018 survey run by the International Cesarean Awareness Network of women who'd had a similar experience—who'd felt unbridled pain during their C-sections—most were ignored. Some were given token apology gifts: one mother received a gift card to Walmart and a water bottle.[28]

And even as some providers sought to blame me for the pain—one person told me my body hadn't metabolized the anesthesia the way "normal" people do—the hospital administration recognized that things had gone wrong. Moreover, and crucially, this wrong mattered, or at least seemed to make them nervous, perhaps because of my race and class.

AFTER BEING PRESSURED INTO HER two C-sections, when Victoria Williams was pregnant with her third baby, she approached the alternative birthing unit at Ochsner Baptist in New Orleans, hoping to avoid another cesarean. The intake coordinator—a midwife—told her that wasn't a problem, and set up an appointment with a midwife.

But at Victoria's first prenatal appointment, the midwife told her that she couldn't continue at the birthing center, as she'd had too many C-sections. Five years later, that still doesn't make sense to Victoria. "I could have seen an OB and a midwife," she says. "I just wanted the care." I thought of something Helena A. Grant had told me in one of our first conversations: every woman deserves the touch of a midwife.

Victoria found a Black OB, then, thinking that might make a difference. "She was one of those doctors that took her time," Victoria remembers; she'd wait forty-five minutes to see the doctor, and then, because she was balancing work and care for two children, she'd run out of time and have to leave in the middle of the appointment.

By this point, Victoria had already lost much of her faith in the obstetric system. She had trouble trusting her doctor. And this doctor, too, pushed her to have a scheduled cesarean. The risks of a VBAC were higher now that she'd had two sections. Her doctor shared these risks with her, the percentages of one or another thing going wrong. Victoria is a determined person; at Birthmark Doula Collective, where she's worked for five years, she's done a lot of direct support of new and expectant mothers. Now, she focuses on crafting and pitching policies to the Louisiana state legislature meant to support mothers so that they don't get "bamboozled." Still, she says, when you're pregnant, it's hard to make sense of the real risks, to unpack them and make the best decisions for yourself and your children. Especially when, like Victoria, you know the risks that Black women face, and especially those like herself: well educated, partnered, knowledgeable about pregnancy and birth. "You're in between a rock and a hard place," she says. "I'm a Black woman. I don't want to freaking die trying to give birth."

As she got closer to her scheduled C-section, her doctor pushed Victoria to have cervical checks, to see if she'd dilated. Each time, Victoria declined. What was the point? "We already knew how far along I was," she said. "I didn't want to keep being prodded." Part of her hoped again that she'd go into spontaneous labor before the cesarean, and she knew that repeated cervical checks would increase her risk of infection.

"Then that's another reason for her to say, 'Oh, you need a C-section,'" she says.

Her doctor gave her pushback about declining the checks, Victoria says. She told her, "'You just want to control everything.' It's like, 'No, I want to get the birth that I want.'"

"This is how you understand it's a system," she says. "It's not individualized care. It's system care. The only thing I got to control" during birth, in that bright OR—another C-section—"was the music."

As is typical in the US, Victoria's postpartum care was practically nonexistent. She had no physical or occupational therapy. No weekly checkups. She would have been given more instructions, she notes, if she'd had knee surgery. In that light, it's "ludicrous," she says, that after each operation, she was cleared for activity at her eight-week postpartum visit.

Still, she says, she's healthy, and always has been. So she healed quickly. "I think," she adds. But maybe it isn't that she healed quickly; maybe she healed slowly, or not entirely, or as quickly as the average person, but had no choice but to act as though she'd healed fast. "Society expects you to just get up and keep rolling and keep moving." Even more so for Black women, she says. In fact, the "glorification of the postpartum period" as one of rest and support—most significantly at luxury postpartum hotels, discussed in chapter 10—isn't available to most Black people, she says. "We can't afford to do that."

On the outside, Victoria looks well healed. She didn't have any major scarring. But her body remembers. She still has severe back pain from the epidurals. And occasionally she has muscle spasms, which feel like pinching and pulling sensations from the bottom of her stomach. Those may be from the scar tissue, she thinks.

And even though her children are now fourteen, seven, and four years old, there's another level of healing she's working on: repairing grief and trauma—from the births, other hardships in her life, even inherited sadness from her mother. Victoria herself was a C-section baby, born while her mother was grieving the loss of her mother. Enveloped in that grief, her mother's body shut down; she had very little amniotic fluid. Growing up, and even as an adult, Victoria reflects, "I felt that innate responsibility to heal my own mother." She wants her children to live with a different narrative, so she has been working with her mother to heal some of this pain: writing letters, putting out photographs of her grandmother. "I want to heal that for my own children."

Victoria's story shows how trauma gets passed down through generations: personally, through a family, but also among whole groups of people—in the ways that "history" is telling physicians how to treat Black women. At the same time, Victoria's story shows how a person can channel that inherited trauma—can aim it in a certain direction. Because even as she's working to heal inherited grief by reaching back into the past, her children are also starting to do their own work with that history, which will shape the future: her eldest daughter, she tells me, is planning to become a midwife.

7

"YOU'D BE NAIVE TO THINK HEALTHCARE ISN'T A BUSINESS"

IF THERE'S AN ARCHETYPE OF THE CASCADE OF INTERVENTIONS AND the medicalized model of birth, Justine Richardson's labor might be it. Justine was thirty-one and living in Charleston, West Virginia, when she went in for a prenatal appointment the day after her due date in February 2021. COVID was raging in Charleston at the time, and neither Justine, who's white, and works in supply chain management for a Fortune 500 company, nor her husband, an attorney, had yet been eligible to receive the vaccine.

Justine had wanted an unmedicated birth. This wasn't a common choice among her friends or family, but it had been important to her. For that reason, she'd planned to birth in a birth center. But the facility, the only accredited birth center in West Virginia, abruptly stopped allowing births when Justine was thirty-two weeks pregnant.

Justine did not have much of a choice about where to have her baby. There are only two hospitals in Charleston that offer maternity care; the next closest, in Huntington, is a one-hour drive away, and doesn't have as advanced a neonatal intensive care unit. Some five hospitals in West Virginia have closed since 2005, in part because they do not generate enough money, their owners say, to keep them open.[1] She also didn't have much time to search for an obstetrician, because she was so far along; she'd been under a midwife's care at the birth center and had to transfer to an obstetrician she found through friends' recommendations. The hospital where he delivered had a 24.7 percent primary C-section rate in 2021, slightly less than the state average that year, but Justine didn't know that at the time.[2]

At a prenatal appointment the day after her due date, Justine's doctor recommended that he induce her. "I did not have high blood pressure, I was not significantly overdue, I was just kind of due," she recalls. He didn't give her information on the risks of induction, and she felt ready to meet her baby, so she agreed.

When she arrived at the hospital that night, monitors showed she was contracting, though she couldn't feel it. But in fact, she was already about two or three centimeters dilated, and had a lot of bloody show. Because she was already in labor, the nurses didn't insert Cervidil or Cytotec, medications that ripen the cervix. Instead, they kept her on the monitors and told her to relax. In retrospect, Justine wishes she'd been sent home; she lives only fifteen minutes away.

At 6:00 a.m., Justine was hooked up to Pitocin to speed up her labor. She moved around the room as much as she could, changing positions, even as she was connected to the IV and the monitors. A few hours later, her doctor recommended breaking her water, to make her labor go faster still. She agreed, thinking how on TV, "that speeds things up."

Although it wasn't evident to Justine at the time, this emphasis on speed is a hallmark not only of the medicalized model of birth, but of the ways that capitalist values—speed, efficiency—have seeped into medicine, and into expectations of childbirth in particular. That's evident, too, in the ways that in some hospitals, providers often depend on technological and medical interventions to move labor along, like Pitocin and epidurals—which can ease pain, and in turn can sometimes help a person to dilate (though they can also slow labor)—rather than less-invasive techniques like using a peanut ball, which opens a mother's pelvis, or other modes of helping a laboring woman into different positions.

That morning, Justine continued to dilate. But her doctor seemed impatient and gave her the impression that he didn't have faith that she'd get to full dilation. She was given cervical checks every hour. Once she'd reached six or seven centimeters, her progress seemed to stall. She started to get scared that she was going to need a C-section, which she had really hoped to avoid. She wondered if her doctor was concerned because there'd been meconium in her water—feces in utero, which can mean a baby is stressed—though the baby wasn't in any distress according to the monitor.

As her labor wore on, Justine began feeling more and more nervous. She thought her fear and anxiety might be stalling her labor and asked a nurse if an epidural would help her to relax and dilate further. The nurse brushed her off—"Uch, maybe," Justine recalls her saying, sounding as if she didn't care what happened to Justine. Desperate to make the vaginal birth work, and without other resources—like encouragement, or suggestions on how she might position herself—Justine elected for the epidural.

Justine held herself very still as the anesthetist placed the epidural in her back. Without waiting until the medication had taken effect, the nurse inserted the Foley catheter into her urethra. "I was not numb when they did that. It was a very painful, humiliating experience," Justine says. "I kind of remember screaming, 'What are you doing? Is this necessary?' And just being ignored."

The epidural meant Justine couldn't move from her bed. In that way it didn't help; what she really needed, she says, was something like a Xanax to take her mind off of the pain. In fact, now that she was stuck in bed, the epidural ended up only increasing her anxiety. (She's not against epidurals, she clarifies—they can help people have the birth they want. But she wishes she'd known more about what getting one meant for lack of mobility.)

A few hours later, Justine's cervix hadn't dilated much more. She'd started to swell a bit, "probably from all these people touching me," she says. But on the monitor the baby looked fine. "Finally, my doctor was like, 'Let's call it and do a C-section.'" She hadn't even been in labor for twenty-four hours. Her water had only been broken for about six. "I was given very little time, especially for a first-time mom," she told me.

"It was horrible," Justine said. She cried all the way to the operating room and remembers yelling, "I want you to know that I tried, I really tried." Her baby was born healthy, weighing eight pounds, twelve ounces. His Apgars, which measure a newborn's well-being by assessing respiration, color, heart rate, reflexes, and muscle tone at one and five minutes after birth, were about as high as they can get: nine and nine.

In her room later that day, Justine texted photos of her baby to family and friends. But then a text arrived that surprised her. It was from her insurance company: they'd received a claim for the epidural she'd had only hours before.

The message caught her off guard, she says. "I think at first I laughed, like, *Wow, that was quick*." But then she "kind of felt like a cog in the machine."

"I already hadn't wanted an epidural and had felt fearmongered to get one. And then to be billed so quickly just kind of hit like, 'I'm just money,'" she says.

That text was the first of many messages about claims that she'd get from her insurance company. In all, the sticker price for Justine's birth— what it would have cost without insurance—totaled about $33,000. Though Justine had private insurance through work, she ended up owing about a third of those costs. She negotiated with individual physicians' offices to reduce the fees. But the hospital, a nonprofit, refused to negotiate; they told her that they discount care only if, by submitting proof of all of their assets, patients can demonstrate that they are destitute.

Justine knew she wouldn't qualify; both she and her husband work. And yet, "we also don't have unlimited money," she says. After talking with the different doctors' offices, she was able to reduce her debt to $10,000, her out-of-pocket max for the year. She paid what she could from a healthcare savings account and the rest she put on rewards credit cards. "Might as well get that five percent cash back," she says ruefully.

"I really hadn't expected to have a C-section. I'd planned on this other method of birthing," she says. The bill for a vaginal birth "probably would have been half" what she paid for the C-section.

"To this day I don't quite understand why I needed one," she says. "It feels like it wasn't necessary. It feels like I was really set up for failure."

CHILDBIRTH IN THE US IS expensive. While rates vary from one hospital to another, even within the same city, the average cost of a C-section in the US is around $17,000; vaginal birth costs an average of $12,000.[3] Insurance typically reimburses hospitals about 50 percent more for a cesarean than for a vaginal birth.[4] And compared with vaginal births, C-sections are more efficient. Particularly if they are scheduled, a hospital can do far more of them than vaginal births in a day. Physicians compensated by services rendered—rather than by salary—also make marginally more from cesareans than from vaginal births (though such fees don't account for how long a provider spends with a mother during labor, for example). On its face, then, it seems simple: do more C-sections, make more money, for institutions and physicians alike.

But the truth is a lot more complicated. And while there's widespread agreement among the doctors, economists, healthcare analysts, and other experts I talked with that economics contributes to the number of medically unnecessary C-sections that we do, there's a lot less agreement about why.[5]

One thing is clear: the US healthcare system is fast turning away from one driven by an imperative to heal and care for patients toward one led, first, by a focus on profit. And while this drive is transforming every medical specialty, from dermatology to radiology, gastroenterology to neurology, for birthing people, the drive to use healthcare as a means to extract profit has profound implications for where, how, and with whom they experience prenatal care, labor, and birth. So while there doesn't appear to be any smoking-gun evidence that hospitals specifically push C-sections as a way to generate profits, the macro-level conditions that favor income also create a culture that promotes surgical, rather than vaginal, birth.

To be sure, when it comes to clinical practice, the CEOs of hospital and health systems will be the first to say, "'I'm not a doctor. I don't make clinical decisions. It's [the doctor's] job,'" says Dr. Vikas Saini, a cardiologist and president and CEO of the Lown Institute, an organization that assesses hospitals. "But it's damn sure certain that the hospital administrators have every reason to look the other way" if doctors are doing more procedures than are clinically necessary, says Saini—from cardiac stents to C-sections.[6]

Americans are accustomed to healthcare being something we pay for, something that isn't free or a human right, something that, by 2022, has landed approximately four in ten adults into medical debt.[7] But over the past several decades, healthcare in the US, along with other aspects of the economy that on their face have little to do with financial services—like housing and education—has been transformed into a financial tool to make money, like stocks or bonds. Importantly, making money by *doing* healthcare—getting paid for doing your job—differs from *using* healthcare as a way to maximize profits. Increasingly, hospitals and healthcare systems, private equity firms, and other private companies are bending the industry toward the latter.

University of Chicago professor of health administration and policy Colleen Grogan traces the ideological seeds of this profit-driven phenomenon, known as financialization, to the 1860s, when government rhetoric began to conceal the consistent, financial commitment it made to public health, and insisted instead on the role of the private market.[8] But the actualization of healthcare financialization began in the 1980s and '90s. As Rosemary Batt and Eileen Appelbaum explain in a paper for the Center for Economic and Policy Research, the process took place from "the inside out": nonprofit hospitals and health systems began to act like for-profit institutions.[9] They adopted "non-healthcare-related financial strategies to survive," such as taking loans from investment banks to buy and leverage assets, participating in the stock market, even launching their own venture capital funds. At the same time, financialization occurred from "the outside in." Private companies and private equity funds that previously weren't in the business of healthcare entered that sector because it appeared to be "a lucrative investment."

Overwhelmingly, evidence shows that financialization of healthcare is bad for patients, whether they're entering the world or getting ready to leave it—or anything in between.[10] That's because organizations use "financial analysis" to assess "whether to invest in a given activity," write Appelbaum and Batt. "Patient care becomes a secondary—not a primary—mission of the organization."[11]

This bears out in the ways organizations cut costs. For instance, some hospitals slash the number of nurses they staff to levels that fall below safety thresholds, even though there is evidence that the more nurses in a hospital, the better the outcomes for patients.[12] Health systems may also steer patients toward physician assistants or nurse practitioners, who are cheaper to employ than doctors. PAs and NPs can end up doing procedures, or making diagnoses, that an MD should, putting patients at risk. Still other financially driven organizations delay or forgo investing in new technology, or keep less medication or fewer supplies on hand, leaving patients vulnerable to emergencies, shortages, inadequate systems, and poorly maintained technology.

Financialization also means that hospitals and health systems organize themselves toward generating income. Overwhelmingly, data shows that patients now pay more for their care, though outcomes haven't improved.[13] Patients may be counseled toward unnecessary tests or procedures, like inductions, which are becoming so common—the rate has tripled since 1990—that one labor and delivery nurse told me the staff cheers when someone comes in who's actually in labor.[14] In medicine writ large, more invasive or technological interventions don't necessarily equate to better care or outcomes. In birth, as the past century has shown us, they're almost always worse.

Hospitals are further incentivized to promote technological responses to childbirth because these are the kinds of care that insurance companies reward. By contrast, so-called high-touch, low-tech labor support is poorly compensated; one nurse-midwife told me that for labor support she can bill about $30 an hour. Similarly, notes Penn's Rebecca R. S. Clark, hospitals and insurance companies may invest in more advanced electronic fetal monitoring, but refuse to recognize, or compensate, nurses with training in Spinning Babies, a movement program in which a nurse or doula guides a mother into various positions to open her pelvis during labor to promote vaginal birth. Labor support is squishy to define: it can mean being in the room with the mother, encouraging her, trying different types of pelvic release. But this care is not only essential to supporting vaginal birth, it also gives labor and birth its texture: the degree to which a provider was present, or (seemingly) not available, helps shape the birth experience. Surely, notes Pitzer College sociologist Alicia D. Bonaparte, we could figure out a better way to code for such support; we've "figured out how to code for tongue depressors," she says dryly.

That's reflected, too, by the fact that insurance companies pay more for a primary cesarean than a vaginal birth. This is backward, according to some physicians. "If it's someone's first birth, you should probably get paid more for a vaginal birth than for a C-section. Because for your first birth, you walk in and I do a C-section, and that takes an hour, and I'm done," says University of Michigan's Dr. Elizabeth Langen. By contrast, "if I have to support you through your labor, that might be twenty-four hours." In this way, insurance companies are a critical part of the system that enables, and rewards, an interventionist, high-tech, and surgical approach to birth.

But C-sections' elevated costs fall onto parents' shoulders. On average, according to the Peterson-KFF Health System Tracker, the cost of maternity care for a person with employer-provided private insurance who's had a C-section is $26,280, of which $3,214 is out of pocket. Vaginal births cost an average of $14,768, with $2,655 out of pocket.[15] And as in other aspects of healthcare, even having insurance doesn't necessarily make birth affordable. Alicea Bahl, who owns an Italian restaurant in Florida, had insurance through Blue Cross Blue Shield when she had her first baby in 2012. She'd planned a home birth but ended up with an unplanned cesarean in the hospital. The hospital billed her insurer $48,000, she says. Blue Cross Blue Shield negotiated that down to $36,000; Alicea had to pay half of that negotiated rate, or $18,000. That far exceeded what she'd prepaid—$2,200—for a vaginal birth.

"When you hear people talk about affordability, you're generally talking about the ability to afford the insurance and not the care once you get the insurance," says Cora Opsahl, director of 32BJ Health, a self-funded plan that provides healthcare to two hundred thousand 32BJ union members and their families in New York. But copays and deductibles can be so high that people can't "necessarily afford" care, as Justine's and Alicea's experiences show. "We're bankrupting parents," says Opsahl.

If insurance covers most of your birth, as it did for me, the costs of a C-section can seem opaque and irrelevant. As Justine put it, claims statements can seem like "fake money."

That's how I felt about my C-section at the time. The sticker price was about $50,000, and while I remember my shock at the sum, I also didn't really care. We must have just come in from a walk; I stood beside a pile of our boots and coats as I stared at the explanation of benefits. *Do I need to keep this piece of paper?* I wondered. When I shared it with my husband, and he became furious—"$50,000 for a botched operation!"—I felt impressed at the depth of his rage. "I know, it's disgusting," I told him. But

I believed it didn't really touch us. It wasn't a bill; we didn't have to pay it. I also couldn't imagine that when my midwife dragged my OB out of bed at 1:00 a.m. to operate, she was thinking of how much more money the hospital would pocket because my birth had turned surgical. In fact, she might not even have known how much the C-section cost; these figures can be opaque for providers as well.

But this attitude, that the financial or systemic costs of C-sections aren't relevant, is problematic because of what it conceals: that the majority of us birth in a system increasingly run by private owners, or profit-driven nonprofits, that prioritize efficiency, speed, and maximum returns at minimal cost. So although I didn't want to think about it, the explanation of benefits I shrugged at was much more important than I'd recognized. It was a trace, an output, of the industries powering the biomedical empire Rothman described.

The profits that hospitals enjoy from medically unnecessary C-sections, as well as other medically unnecessary tests, procedures, and interventions, are one more aspect of the operation to which most people don't know they're consenting. They are unwittingly participating in a system that uses healthcare as an opportunity from which to extract as much profit as possible. To me, this is among the most stomach-turning aspects of contemporary American birth. For if the medical model discards the mother for the baby, the financialized model throws out us both.

ONE OUTCOME OF FINANCIALIZATION THAT hurts patients, and that may result in unnecessary and otherwise preventable C-sections, is scarcity of care. As hospitals consolidate, they tend to close the smaller, more rural, and less profitable hospitals and obstetric units they acquire. It's the opposite of what the nation did in 1946 with the Hill-Burton Act, which devoted $75 million a year for five years to hospital construction around the country, in an attempt to bring healthcare in the United States thoroughly into the modern era.[16] (How modern is debatable, as the program erected segregated hospitals.)

Hospital consolidation began after the 1970s, when federal and state governments cut how much they reimbursed hospitals for Medicare and Medicaid. Many public hospitals quickly ran out of money. Some told patients to bring their own blankets and toilet paper. Around the same time, smaller community hospitals—where you'd go to have a baby or set a broken arm, and which would refer you to specialists at larger hospitals if you needed more advanced care—began to consolidate with other institutions or to close. They also had to look for other ways to make up for the financial shortfalls they were now facing.

Hospitals had incentives to join larger health systems. Consolidated hospital systems can "wield an extraordinary amount of market power and negotiate extremely high prices with commercial payers," meaning private insurance companies, says Zach Levinson, a researcher at Kaiser Family Foundation. They also save money on billing, scheduling, and other back-office duties.

Other hospital systems have saved money by closing obstetric units. They've done so in areas where they say birth volume is too low, particularly in rural areas. In fact, these closures appear to be driven by a commitment to maximize profits: wealthier counties' hospitals are much less likely than poorer counties' hospitals to close. And the smaller private, nonprofit, and for-profit hospitals in these rural areas are three times more likely than public hospitals to close their maternity units.[17] (Public hospitals may be more likely to stay open because, the researchers conclude, they "focus on community needs," even as obstetric care is unprofitable.) These smaller hospitals are especially vulnerable because rarely can they access the other, nonfinancial avenues to drive profits that a large academic medical center can—like starting a venture capital fund or borrowing large sums from an investment bank—that would entice their new owners to keep them open. "From just a straight-up financial return on investment perspective, it makes complete sense, right?" says Colleen Grogan, professor at the University of Chicago. "And that's all they care about."

It's possible that closing smaller hospitals with fewer births could benefit birthing people by shunting them to larger hospitals where providers attend more births and have more opportunities to hone their skills. There's also some evidence that OBs who attend fewer births are more likely to do C-sections. This makes sense because their skills may be rustier. Volume matters for skill development. Attend one thousand births, and you'll probably have seen just about every variation that can happen, my midwife, Lena, told me.

But the paradox of birth is that more equipment and more technology, as can often be found at larger hospitals, don't necessarily result in better outcomes. As Penn's Rebecca R. S. Clark told me, at one well-regarded, highly medicalized hospital where she used to work, she and her colleagues used to joke that it was the right place to have a baby if you were "pregnant with twins, an uncontrolled diabetic, and you [had] a gunshot wound." By contrast, "if you're low-risk, you want to go to a place that cares for women who are low-risk," she says.

Closing obstetric units also creates care deserts, forcing people to travel to birth—much as people must travel if they need an abortion. That in turn creates its own inequities, because white women, who tend to be wealthier, can and will travel further for their care than Black women. Clark gives the example of southwest Philadelphia, a predominantly Black neighborhood. Nonprofit health system Trinity Health Mid-Atlantic ceased in-patient services at the community's Mercy Hospital in 2020. It had been open for over one hundred years.

Now, women in southwest Philly typically travel to the nearest hospital to give birth—often the Hospital of the University of Pennsylvania, says Clark, which is a large academic medical center. Even if they are low-risk, they are birthing in "a place that specializes in intervention," she says. White women were more likely to go to a hospital farther away, with a stronger midwifery presence. In this way, hospital consolidation may contribute to unnecessary C-sections, particularly among Black or other underserved communities.

Closing obstetric units also appears to make birth more dangerous, exacerbating inequities even further. One recent study led by Harvard University's Alecia McGregor found that women who gave birth after the obstetric units nearest them had closed were more likely to have a hysterectomy or to need ventilation or a tracheostomy than women who gave birth when their nearest OB wards were still open.[18] That was the case for all birthing people, and for Black and Hispanic/Latinx birthing people in particular.

Closing obstetric units can also harm any person with a uterus—not only pregnant people. "Maternity care is not just having babies," said Lydia Moorman, a Sharon, Connecticut–based activist who fought to keep the maternity ward at Sharon Hospital open, after its new owner,

Nuvance Health, sought to close it, citing low birth volume. "It's having those physicians around for gynecological care and emergencies."

WHILE HOSPITALS HAVE BEEN CONSOLIDATING with one another over the past several decades, corporate and hospital health systems have been aggressively purchasing physicians' practices. According to the Physicians Advocacy Institute, nearly 74 percent of the nation's physicians are employees of hospitals or corporations. Those figures are even higher for OBs: half are employed by hospitals; another 27 percent are employed by other corporations.[19] Independent practices are very much the minority—less than one in four as of this writing.

Corporate or hospital-owned practices aren't bad by definition. Running a practice can be cost-prohibitive, even fundamentally untenable, because of the significant overhead: office rental, an office manager, equipment, malpractice insurance. Independent practices also can't negotiate reimbursements like a powerful corporation that controls a significant portion of the market. Thus, a corporate-owned practice can likely pay providers higher wages. Larger practices—no matter who owns them—are also better for providers' work-life balance; in a small practice, you're virtually always on call. Even taking a vacation can be difficult.

But corporate and hospital-system owners also exert control over how physicians' offices look and feel. By "streamlining" offices, these owners may require physicians to strip their offices of individuality, so that any one office—and any provider—appears to be interchangeable with any other. One midwife who works at Optum, a corporation that made $14.1 billion in 2022, an increase of "revenue per consumer served" of 29 percent from the year prior,[20] told me that when the company took over from CareMount in 2022, it forbade providers from keeping anything personal in their offices—even plants. It also got rid of telephone lines that ring directly to a specific office. An obstetrician at another large health system in upstate New York, who travels among three different offices, doesn't have her own office. A cardiologist at another large health system in New York City is forbidden from hanging up his diplomas.

Corporate and other private owners also shape how clinicians practice. Journalist Eyal Press observed in a 2023 article in the *New York Times*

Magazine that "despite the esteem associated with their profession," over the past several years "many physicians have found themselves subjected to practices more commonly associated with manual laborers in auto plants and Amazon warehouses, like having their productivity tracked on an hourly basis and being pressured by management to work faster."[21]

These working conditions can be misery-inducing. "There's no way that I can see upwards of thirty patients a day and appropriately take care of my patients and take care of myself," one OB with twenty years of experience told me. With such volume, "you're cutting corners, not following up," she says, then coming home and doing "pajama charting"— catching up on patients' charts until midnight. And, she points out, because volume means short appointments, she cannot do meaningful patient education—for instance, really making sure a person understands the risks and benefits of VBAC compared with a repeat cesarean. This OB works for a large nonprofit corporation. Despite what its owners say is their real goal, their underlying mission is "to have a business that pays non-providers, their board, and shareholders," she says. That, she adds, "is obscene." At the end of our conversation, this OB—a vivacious and brilliant person—joked that the reason hospitals' windows don't open is to keep physicians from jumping out.

The latest private owner to take interest in obstetrics is private equity, which began acquiring OB-GYN practices in 2013 and accelerated rapidly during the pandemic. What's different about private equity from other private owners is that they typically expect to make very high returns on investment in a short timeline—like 20–30 percent over the course of three to five years. Private equity firms also usually take on lots of debt. And once they've made their money, through maximizing profits and slashing costs, they often sell the company they bought. As Laura Katz Olson, distinguished professor of political science at Lehigh University and the author of *Ethically Challenged: Private Equity Storms US Health Care*, points out, these firms begin thinking about selling on day one. It's like buying a house to flip it—you might paint, but you won't fix the foundation.

Joseph Dov Bruch, an assistant professor of public-health sciences at the University Chicago, explained to me that private equity might find obstetrics appealing because, as an industry, it's "very fragmented." Many practices are independent, or owned by hospitals, and PE firms see these as an opportunity to consolidate them "into one big portfolio company." They might plan to streamline admin, overhead, and other costs that are otherwise handled separately by each independent practice. Bruch adds that private equity firms might see that they could "complement traditional [OB-GYN] services" with offerings "like IVF or other fertility services," such as egg-freezing, which typically carries high prices, and net substantial profits. In fact, fertility services are so profitable that they are one of the first medical specialties that private equity companies began to acquire, beginning in the 2010s. "While perhaps [OB-GYN] procedures don't get reimbursed the way a dermatologist's would"—an area of medicine in which private equity has made substantial inroads—PE owners are likely thinking, *We can still make a buck*," Bruch says.

These new owners also have profound implications for how providers practice medicine—and how patients experience it. "Once you sell to private equity, you give up all your control of everything," Dr. Clara Surowitz told me. Surowitz, an obstetrician in New Jersey who now runs Trū Birth Center in Lakewood, was part of a group that sold to one such investor. After the sale, she began receiving emails admonishing physicians not to order what were once routine tests for thyroid function or vitamin D on the prenatal panel, "because it costs too much."

Defenders of capital markets and consolidation point out that when a health system or private equity firm buys such a practice, it wipes away the debt and pays the physicians a salary. Together, this can seem like a godsend—making it possible for a provider to retire, for instance. What's more, because small or solo practices are difficult to sustain, there are fewer individuals or small groups to whom to sell a practice. "A lot of medical providers are looking to retire, earlier and earlier," says Lehigh's Olson. "And they have no place to sell their practices to, because these young guys can't afford it. So they sell them to private equity."

"Our healthcare system is so dysfunctional and has been extremely dysfunctional for a very long time," says Grogan. As a result, we give "an outsized superpower to the financial markets. Because they can come in and say, 'We're your savior. We know you need capital investment . . . and we're willing to give the money.'" When they encounter objections—like eliminating standard prenatal testing, for example—their argument is,

"'Well, look at how bad [finances are] now,'" says Grogan. "It's hard to argue against that." But, she says, "their arguments are hollow—and that gives them power."

BECAUSE OF CONSOLIDATION, WHEN I became pregnant, I could choose from four practices—all large groups—owned by two health systems.

Once I chose a practice, as is the custom, I bounced to a new provider at each appointment. I was told this was so that I'd get a chance to meet everyone, so that the person who attended my birth wouldn't be a stranger. These meetings felt like mismatches, each in a different way. At ten weeks pregnant, one doctor told me to stop riding my bike, lest I fall; at sixteen weeks, another shook my husband's hand, congratulated him, and measured my fundal height without acknowledging me; a third prescribed B_{12} and Unisom, a sleep aid, without telling me why—I suppose now because I had said I felt nauseated. This recommendation for medication I hadn't asked for, and with no explanation as to its purpose, was the final red flag. I switched practices at twenty weeks.

The new practice felt homier, in a rambling old house in Kingston with sumptuous rugs and creaky wooden floors, the toilets and sinks endearingly home-builder-grade, not bulletproof institutional. It was owned by the same corporation as the first practice, but still retained the character of its original owner, Dr. B, who wore low-top sneakers and made blunt and outré comments I took as evidence of his authenticity. Along with the furnishings, these outbursts seemed to confirm that I'd be treated as a person, not just a patient.

This practice was a better fit. But when my doula asked who I hoped would be on call when I went into labor, I thought, *None of them*; I didn't really like any of them. I think back now to what Rothman pointed out about how the biomedical empire dismisses the knowledge wrought by relationships, and how that dismissal shapes care. While I don't know that I would have bonded with any of the OBs or midwives at that second practice, I didn't have much of an opportunity to. I'd cycled through them all and had hardly seen any of them long enough to find out. And ironically, despite having met everyone at the practice, the person who attended my birth in the end was a stranger: a midwife who works per diem.

I also didn't know how important a meaningful relationship with a provider would be until I got pregnant for the second time. I recognized Lena even before I went in for my first prenatal visit. I'd seen her around—in yoga, or walking her dogs in the neighborhood. That familiarity made me feel more trust in her, even before I stepped into her office: she knew I was more than a vagina, as Linda Janet Holmes put it. She also happens to be a remarkable midwife, one committed to the value of a consistent relationship: even though she works for a corporate organization, she communicates with schedulers to make sure her patients don't get bounced around from one provider to another. During that second pregnancy, I only saw two other providers for routine visits over the course of my forty weeks. That was important not only because it enabled me to build a relationship with her, but because it kept me from having to tell the story of my first birth repeatedly, which used to make me really nervous.

The impacts of financialization and consolidation also demonstrate why hiring more midwives without reforming the current system won't necessarily revolutionize care. Midwifery, explains certified nurse-midwife Holly Smith, sees pregnancy and birth "not as a disease to be fixed, nor a thing to be managed, but rather . . . use[s] vigilance and care and person-centered support." As a profession, it values "the therapeutic use of the human presence." But a financialized system that promotes volume and efficiency makes it difficult for midwives to practice that way, to realize the tenets of their profession. "Midwifery can't exist in a place that doesn't support it," says Smith, an executive committee member of the California Maternal Quality Care Collaborative, who with colleagues has worked to design a tool kit for hospitals to lower their C-section rates.

That's particularly the case when a financialized system pivots on a medicalized model of childbirth, which focuses on avoiding all risks and often reduces mothers to a mere "vessel for this baby coming out," says Smith. What such a system does not recognize, Smith says, is the mother's experience. And yet, patient experience matters deeply. How mothers "direct their care, and what they want, is in fact the thing that creates the best outcome."

Not everyone cares to form a relationship with their midwife or obstetrician, and that wasn't a priority for some of the mothers I interviewed.

Some people prefer, or feel neutrally about, large or corporate medical settings. But if those don't make you comfortable, it's increasingly difficult to access more personal or small-scale types of care—unless you can buy yourself out of the system altogether, by seeing a boutique practice that probably doesn't take insurance, or by birthing in a birth center or at home.

The same is true for providers hoping to go into private practice—unless they're independently wealthy, doing so may no longer be a viable option. It's a given that a new doctor will lose money the first year and may not make money until the second or even third year she's practicing. But it's not clear that a new, independent provider can ever get on track in the current climate, because it's extremely difficult for small providers to negotiate meaningful reimbursements from commercial insurance companies. "Over 50 percent, and growing every year, of all physicians are employees," says Lehigh's Olson. New doctors may not expect that—or want it. But "they're out of medical school with this huge debt and don't have a lot of choices."

I see that low compensation rate when I review the explanation of benefits for visits to Dr. K, my children's pediatrician. He is the one solo practitioner in our family's orbit. His urgent line rings to his cell phone. I don't know how he survives, financially; he makes less than $60 per visit, between my co-pay and what my insurance pays him. On his own, he covers rent, an office manager, insurance, supplies, utilities. Perhaps this is the reason he is the last solo pediatrician in our county.

Even over the course of my first pregnancy, the pressure of consolidations became apparent: not even the appearance of the seemingly more authentic practice had lasted. The day I went into labor, the office had completed its move to a headquarters just as sterile, just as anonymous, as the offices housing the practice I'd left behind.

IT ISN'T ONLY PATIENTS WHO stand to benefit from forming relationships with their providers. When it comes to obstetrics, relationships can be beneficial, even protective, for providers, too. Because one of the most consequential factors that predicts whether a person will sue her provider for a bad birth outcome is the quality of their relationship. In a seminal study from 1994, researchers found that obstetricians whose patients felt rushed during visits, and reported visits lasting less than ten minutes, were far more likely to be sued than obstetricians whose patients reported spending more time with their doctors.[22] Patients of the frequently sued doctors also said that they were ignored during labor and birth, and that their physicians did not explain to them what was going on. Still other research shows that poor communication is associated with higher rates of litigation.[23] And though I couldn't find a citation in the academic literature, one midwife I talked with learned, at a seminar on malpractice and litigation, that meeting a patient for the first time is a risk factor for a lawsuit.

My nonexistent relationship with the obstetrician certainly played a role when I was trying to decide if I should sue him, in that I never considered what a lawsuit would have done or meant to him personally or professionally. Instead, I went around and around in my head about whether a settlement would be worth it. On the one hand, I didn't want the money, because what could it do for me? It couldn't restore me to who I'd been before the birth, or give my daughter retroactive access to the mother I could have been in her infancy. It wouldn't take away the fear and anxiety I felt when I went to the doctor or dentist. All it would get me was money. And because I thought of myself as a not-litigious person, as someone mostly not motivated by money, that felt dirty—as if it would violate my identity, my primary values.

"Yeah, okay," my friend Laura said, after hearing me out. "But money is still money. And money can buy you a lot of things. Like college tuition."

It's also tempting to believe that litigation is the way to reform a financialized system. As Laura pointed out, money is the language of corporate medicine. You could argue that if you want to change the culture, people are going to have to sue.

But lawyers have reason to avoid these cases—especially if they revolve around harms to the mother, and particularly if those harms are emotional. That's because such cases are hard to win. "It's like going on the Olympic level against the hospitals, taking on an institution that has endless resources to hire endless lawyers and throw money at it. It's literally David and Goliath," one lawyer told me. It's also difficult to litigate malpractice cases for "downstream" injuries, says Deborah Fisch, a Michigan attorney and vice president of Birth Justice Bar (formerly the Birth Rights Bar Association). These include, for instance, uterine scars from earlier C-sections that lead to placental problems in subsequent pregnancies, which can end in serious outcomes. A patient may choose this future risk if a C-section is medically indicated; but for C-sections that aren't medically necessary, says Fisch, or that are performed without informed consent, patients have no legal recourse against an OB who performed the surgery. And, she adds, far from being responsible for damages, the OB may not even know of these downstream consequences.

What's more, our reliance on this tool comes back to bite all of us by reinscribing the fear of possible financial and professional penalties for a birth gone "bad." Physicians practice defensively; patients seek legal restitution. Yet this cycle has not improved birth for anyone. And because most cases are settled out of court, the terms of these settlements are "usually confidential," and may not even admit any fault, explained Fisch—which means that the judgments do not change the healthcare system whatsoever.

To some extent this partly explains why I didn't try harder to find a lawyer. I didn't want money; it couldn't fix my problems. I wanted to make sure that what had happened to me wouldn't happen again. A lawsuit seemed the only way to get near to that. Helen Lowery, a former products and medical liability lawyer whose first birth, an unplanned cesarean, was riddled with errors, knows she would have had a different experience if she hadn't walked into the hospital as a Black woman, she told me. But what goes wrong in the hospital, and even what went wrong in her first birth—which included numerous errors, and culminated in nurses initially not permitting her to breastfeed her baby, who was in the NICU—"aren't always legal problems. Which means there aren't always legal answers." But the US medical system lacks other ways to "help the person find closure," like mediation. "[Litigation] is the tool, and whether or not the problem calls for a sledgehammer, that's the one we use."

OBSTETRICIAN NH HAS SHOULDER-LENGTH STRAIGHT black hair, a muscular build, and the patience and calm of the camp counselor he once was. It's easy to see how he'd be the type of physician who got dinged for spending "too much time" with his patients, as he tells me. In fact, long-term relationships with patients is one reason that NH, thirty-nine, chose obstetrics. But since graduating from medical school nine years ago, he has not been able to develop those relationships, because he's borne the brunt of the financialization of obstetrics. (And it's because of his concerns about future employers that he asked to use his initials.) His experiences are a cautionary tale of what financialization does to providers—and how that shapes patients' care.

At the end of NH's first contract, he was recruited to join a group in Phoenix. The branch he signed with had just two physicians, one of whom was retiring. It was part of a larger group of practices partly owned by the group he was recruited to, and—though NH didn't know it—an array of private equity owners. His new contract provided him with a salary of $300,000 a year for three years.

Around the time of his hiring, a private equity firm purchased the company he'd joined. NH believed that the new owner would honor the terms of his contract. But seven months into NH's tenure, the CEO called him in for a meeting to look at his numbers.

In the meeting that May, NH says that the CEO told him that NH's numbers were trending up. But, he explained, NH had signed his contract with the company's previous owner. The new owner had not committed to paying his salary and overhead. By September, the company would run out of money to pay his salary.

The CEO proposed changing his contract to production only—meaning he'd be paid whatever income he generated, after expenses, what's known in industry parlance as "eat what you kill." At that time NH was generating enough income to cover his overhead, but not earning anything to live on.

The CEO suggested that NH take out a line of credit to pay himself while he went without a salary, which struck NH as nuts. It wasn't clear how long he'd be going unpaid and racking up debt: "Two months, three months, four months, five months, six months—who knows, right?" NH said. The practice couldn't guarantee anything.

Because he'd refused to amend his contract to production only, in late August 2022, he received an email: he'd been terminated. His patients, who'd just started making relationships with him, were disappointed. His absence would mean that they would need to get to know another physician.

"I just turned thirty-nine," says NH. "I could practice for at least twenty-five years. If [they'd] made a small investment to keep me around, they could have gotten a return on an investment. But they actively decided that, 'Okay, he's been there for seven months. He hasn't made enough money. You've got to let him go.' It doesn't make any sense."

Most upsetting, says NH, is that the decision to change his contract wasn't based on the quality of his work. No one asked how well he was doing for his patients, or whether he was practicing evidence-based medicine. "Make a decision based on that," he says. "And if you say, 'Oh, the patients don't like you, you're just not a good fit'—fine. You say, 'You're not meeting objective guidelines. You're doing too many unnecessary procedures.' Fine, okay. . . . But it's not that. It's, 'We're not going to put in any more money.'"

Recently NH was recruited by an obstetrics practice owned by yet another private equity firm. The physicians who work there told him that they're being reimbursed at higher rates, which means they're making more money. But, NH points out, "it's only been a few years" since the private equity purchase—so who knows what's to come. (He did not end up joining the group.) What's more, those physicians have established practices with plenty of patients. For NH, or any other new physician, it would be different: he'd need to build his practice. And while he would expect it to take two to three years to ramp up a full practice, "private equity probably doesn't understand that. They're going to say, 'Well, you've been there for a year. Why are you making these [numbers]. You need to pick it up.'"

IT WASN'T UNTIL WE RECEIVED a bill for $4,000, a few months after my daughter's birth, that I got upset about the money. The bill came from a nurse who was needed during the surgery, but who was out of my insurance network. I'd never consciously met this person, hadn't agreed to have her treat me. Nevertheless, the bill explained, I was on the hook. This is what's known as a surprise bill, and it's now illegal. Private equity firms lobbied heavily against the "no surprises" act, passed in 2021;[24] issuing them was part of their playbook to extract as much money from patients as possible.

I temporarily lost my mind over this bill. It represented all that I hadn't consented to, and all that had gone wrong. While the nurse herself was not at fault, the bill felt like depravity made real, a painful outcome of the financialized system of birth. Because where the $50,000 explanation of benefits felt passively degrading, an exchange of funds that took place outside of but about my person, the $4,000 bill arrived in my mailbox, directed at me. I Googled her, wondering what would happen if I didn't pay the bill. Which I felt certain I wouldn't do. The birth had already cost me enough.

But it also dug into me in part because it gave me a glimpse into what I didn't know about my daughter's birth. Learning of this nurse's existence would become the first of many clues I'd try to gather, over the coming years, of what it must have been like in that surgical suite, during the hour or so that I became a mother. I used to believe that if I looked hard enough, I would be able to reconstruct what I didn't remember, as if by compiling enough detail I could summon the missing tape.

So I Googled her again. I found her address; she lived in a turn-of-the-century home beside a swell in a river, fifteen minutes from my home, on the same road where I'd later pick up a plastic basketball hoop for my toddler. But I couldn't find much else, like when and where she'd gone to nursing school or how old she was. In the strange intimacy of this era of Google Maps, I knew what her house looked like, how much she'd paid in taxes for it over the past decade. But the listing through the healthcare system for which she worked, likely on a contract basis, showed only a featureless icon.

I understand now that in a financialized system, a featureless icon of a provider is effectively the point. She could be anyone, and so could I; we're both interchangeable. The only relationship I had with her, that I knew of, was a financial one. We two had been reduced to a transaction; me, and my birth, to an ATM.

In her book *The Biomedical Empire: Lessons Learned from the COVID-19 Pandemic*, Barbara Katz Rothman writes that the "highly standardized, industrialized hospital system" performs well for acute problems, like an accident or sudden disease. In those cases, "whoever's on duty at which-ever station—intake to X-ray to overnight linen changes—the bureau-cratized, standardized response is pretty much going to be the same and work the same." Though we may wish for some "touch . . . of the per-sonal," writes Rothman, "we usually pretty willingly sacrifice individual-ity for the gown, the bed, the food, whatever the hospital serves up, in trade for the services."[25]

But birth, and death, aren't "procedures, something for which the existentially constant you suits up, deals, and comes through the other end. They are definitionally transformative. You will never be the same. The one of you will be two. Or none."

I came through; my one, or my not-one-but-not-two, became two. The operation, and the birth, ended one part of my life and opened a new one. But, by design, I could not ask this nurse what she thought about what had happened during my operation or who may have been at fault. I could not ask her what my face looked like when the doctor held my baby to me, whether I'd been able to smile at my baby daughter, or if my eyes had even been open. I could not ask her if she'd ever seen anything like this before, or whether she had a hard time sleeping that night. All I could do was send her a check.

8

TECHNOLOGY AND TOUCH

SHORTLY AFTER SHE BECAME PREGNANT IN 2007, JULIE CANTOR HIRED a certified nurse-midwife. Not only to care for her during pregnancy, but to safeguard her autonomy in the hospital. "I wasn't messing around," she says. That she felt the need to do so is striking. Cantor earned a JD from Berkeley Law and an MD from Yale. A native Californian, she speaks with a powerful cadence and a no-bullshit manner, the kind of verbal seriousness sometimes trained out of even the most accomplished women. She was dressed in black when I met her on Zoom, her dark hair pulled into a bun; it's easy to see how she would command the courtroom as a litigator, or the classroom as a lecturer; for years she taught a course on reproductive healthcare and law at UCLA's law school.

But Cantor had seen during her medical residency, and through her own research, how medicalized birth can prioritize physician prefer-ence, even physician convenience, at the expense of mothers' autonomy. She knew mothers whose physicians did episiotomies, vacuum extrac-tion, or C-sections without gaining their full consent, or even despite the mothers' saying no. And she recognized the role that American faith in technology played in these experiences—the ways that it collided with misogyny, and patriarchy, to abet physicians' decisions to override patients' wishes.

At a visit with the midwife when she was six weeks pregnant, Cantor met the OB who backed her up. This doctor had a reputation for being a sort of cowboy obstetrician, sweating it out at labors of VBACs, or twins, that today fewer obstetricians in the US take on for convenience, fear of liability, or both. He pitched Cantor and her husband, a practicing litigator who also has an MD, on choosing him as the primary caregiver instead of the midwife for Cantor's pregnancy and birth.

Then the OB suggested that they do an ultrasound.

Cantor wasn't sure. Did they really need to?

He said they should, to make sure the pregnancy was viable.

"All right, let's do it," Cantor said, thinking, "I'm a doctor. Right? So it's like, 'We're among friends, we're in the club.'"

On the ultrasound, the pregnancy looked fine. Cantor remembers the doctor telling her, "You're exactly X days pregnant, so you got pregnant on September first."

"I didn't. I got pregnant on September fourth or fifth," Cantor responded. "I know exactly what I was doing. I know exactly how babies are made."

"The machine is telling me you got pregnant September first."

"The machine must be wrong, because I was there," Cantor told him.

On its face, a few days' difference in conception date isn't especially high stakes. Based on the ultrasound, it is unlikely that ACOG guidelines would have recommended that the physician change Cantor's due date.* But their conflict is emblematic of what often happens in the American medical system: "objective" data provided by a computer outweighs a woman's "subjective" knowledge—like when a person who's had an epidural tells a provider she still feels pain, and the provider responds that the epidural "should be working."

These interactions can be read to reveal how little a woman's voice matters at so many crucial junctures of labor and birth. But these interactions also demonstrate a particularly American ideology: technology—not the patient, and sometimes not even the provider—must be right. And what's more, technology is exhaustive in the data it supplies. Increasingly, in the medicalized model of birth, we treat the reams of information relayed by machines as so authoritative, so trustworthy, and so omniscient, it is as if they convey all there is to know.

---

* If there's a discrepancy between the date of a person's last menstrual period, and the "age" of the pregnancy on an early (prior to nine weeks) ultrasound, ACOG recommends changing a person's due date to accord with the ultrasound imagery.

THE SUPREMACY OF TECHNOLOGY, CULTURAL critic Neil Postman writes, has changed the way that physicians practice. It shapes how they look for and detect illness; the ways they interact with their patients; how they conceive of their own training and knowledge. For pregnant people, these changes are most evident in the uses and consequences of electronic fetal monitoring (EFM), a technology so thoroughly integrated throughout obstetric wards, OB Neel Shah told me, that wherever there's an outlet, there's a monitor.

As this chapter explores, EFM helped catapult the US C-section rate from less than 5 percent when it was introduced in 1968 to more than 30 percent today. It changed how people labor: where a mother in the hospital once had nurses or her physician at her side, now she can be left alone for longer, while a nurse watches an electronic chart of her contractions on a computer down the hall.

But EFM is notoriously unreliable. And though it has increased the C-section rate exponentially, it has not made birth safer for babies, as measured by rates of cerebral palsy or oxygen-deprived brain injuries. To understand why such an unreliable technology continues to be so widely used, it's essential to look at the medical history that came before it. These technological and ideological shifts developed to intercede between doctors and patients and put technology on a pedestal. They also reduced the apparent pertinence and value of information that a provider can gain from touching or simply being with a laboring person—embodied knowledge that a machine can't possibly know.

VISIT A DOCTOR TODAY, AND the moment she puts a stethoscope on your chest may feel like the most intimate part of the appointment. But the stethoscope's invention in 1816, by a French physician named René Laënnec, marked the beginning of a new distance between doctor and patient. Before Laënnec's invention, doctors listened to a patient's heart by tapping her chest. Or they put a handkerchief on her chest, then placed an ear against it, to hear the heart's rhythm. They also relied heavily on patients' narratives of their symptoms, and on visual observations of their bodies, to detect and identify illness.

One day, in Laënnec's attempt to listen to the heart of a young patient with "plumpness of figure," tapping didn't work.[1] Yet he believed that putting his ear close to the breasts of this young, busty patient—repeatedly described in subsequent literature as the more pejorative "obese"—would be unseemly. So he rolled up a wad of papers to create a tube—the better for sound to travel, something he knew as a flautist—and put one end to his patient's chest, the other to his ear.[2] "Mediated auscultation," he called it.[3] In lay terms: indirect careful listening. A definition that sounds like a contradiction.

It would take a generation before stethoscopes became widespread; "established" physicians rejected them. They criticized the distance the stethoscope created between doctor and patient. Others expressed concern that relying on technology, instead of visual observation and listening to patients' symptoms, would lead to incorrect diagnoses.

Despite these misgivings, including mockery in the form of an epic poem by Oliver Wendell Holmes Sr., father of the famous jurist, medicine adopted the stethoscope.* As Western medicine evolved, it continued in Laënnec's direction. Rather than "rely primarily on the patient's descriptions of his or her symptoms," tools developed to equip physicians to make an "objective diagnosis."[4] Today, these technologies are integral to Western medicine: X-rays, CT scans, MRIs, biopsies, and blood tests home in on organs, bones, and cells to assess the presence or absence of disease.[5]

But a reliance on what technology can identify, the stories it can tell, is problematic. The most advanced technology cannot always perfectly visualize each person's unique anatomy. An ovary may be hidden by a segment of bowel, obscuring cysts in a pelvic ultrasound, for instance. Ultrasound technology is less accurate on expecting mothers who are fat.[6] Still other conditions are notoriously difficult to visualize with a machine alone. The only way to make a definitive diagnosis of endometriosis, for instance, is to look directly inside a patient's pelvis, through a laparoscopic surgery. Likewise, blood tests on people with chronic illness, particularly

---

* His poem, about a young doctor who mistakes the sound of buzzing flies for a patient's heart problem, concludes,
  Now use your ears, all you that can,
  But don't forget to mind your eyes,
  Or you may be cheated, like this young man,
  By a couple of silly, abnormal flies.

autoimmune disorders, don't necessarily reveal visible and quantifiable measures of illness—even if a person is sick.

This approach to the body as a disconnected series of parts is a product of modern medicine. By contrast, says P. Mimi Niles, assistant professor of nursing at NYU and a certified nurse-midwife, the medicine of antiquity saw the body as a whole, much as traditional Chinese medicine or Vedic medicine continue to do. The emergence of specialties that focus only on a single system (cardiology, neurology) in isolation from others further inscribed this fractured conception of the body, one that leaves out mental health altogether—though the brain is part of the body, and despite evidence that loneliness, anxiety, depression, and stress can harm a person's health, even shorten her life.

The evolution of this fractured, objective-seeming approach is evident in medical texts' illustrations, and in their depiction of human reproduction in particular. *The Compleat Midwife's Companion* (1724), like other books from its time period and before, included drawings of a woman's entire body—with a more detailed view of the fetus and the woman's reproductive organs. But by the mid-1800s, with men's entry into childbirth, and the introduction of the stethoscope, illustrations in midwifery texts and general anatomical books changed to show only a woman's pelvis, reproductive organs, or the fetus, without the context of the rest of the mother's body. (At the time, this was a gendered shift; showing parts, not the whole, did not occur in medical illustrations of men's reproductive organs.[7]) It's another reason that I found the photographs of women from that early twentieth-century obstetrics textbook so surprising—they were rare because they showed women as a whole.

These drawings of disembodied reproductive organs read as objective representations of anatomy. But they had a crucial consequence, concludes historian Nora Doyle: they "dissociated childbirth from the body of the mother."[8] In that sense, these illustrations are emblematic of how childbirth evolved to become a mechanical, scientific, and medical process that, above all, is about the expulsion, or extraction, of the fetus. Quite literally, these drawings communicate that birth is disconnected from a woman's body or spirit, and from the relationship she has with the fetus within her—the subjective stuff of birth that makes it so awe-inspiring, so difficult to describe with known language. They also represent the medical-legal perspective that's still shaping reproduction, whether a person wants to keep her pregnancy or wishes to terminate: the uterus, and the fetus within, are very much their own independent things.

THE IDEA OF THE FETUS as a separate being from its mother has a long history; as explored in chapter 3, and most intensively through the eighteenth century, the Catholic Church once pushed for C-sections on women who'd died because it conceived of the fetus as an independent soul that needed to be baptized. But what makes this idea of the fetus especially persuasive today are the dazzling technologies that undergird it, such as prenatal testing, gene editing, 4-D ultrasounds, surgeries in utero, and external fetal monitoring. They provide scientific, visible, and seemingly objective evidence that the fetus is an independent being. And once a fetus is established as separate it can, according to some schools of thought, lay claim to personhood.[9]

At the same time, and though it seems contradictory, medicine and law recognize the fundamental physiological connections between mother and fetus. For instance, mothers have been prosecuted for harming themselves, and thereby harming their fetuses, while pregnant.[10] While recognizing the interconnectedness of mother and fetus isn't new—centuries of maternal impressions theory, popularized by Aristotle, held that women's experiences, encounters, and even desires during pregnancy literally manifested on their babies' bodies, as birthmarks or other traits—in the West, this connection has been conceived and legislated "as a point of competition between mother and fetus," writes legal scholar Isabel Karpin.[11] In this light, "connections are recast as vulnerabilities," pitting the mother's "body against [the] fetus." In such a conception, a mother and a fetus's interests cannot be aligned: it's me or you. There is no such thing as not-one-but-not-two.

The adversarial relationship between mother and fetus, and the notion that they are separate entities, manifests most acutely in arguments about abortion: how, if, and under what circumstances a person has the right to terminate a pregnancy. But these ideas also almost certainly play into the nation's C-section rate, and are buttressed by EFM, a technology that appears to give objective, trustworthy, and authoritative information about how a baby is tolerating labor.

The scientific and empirical information that technology can convey also displaces—and replaces—pregnant people's subjective knowledge about their own bodies. For instance, I knew that my second child was going to be a boy, just like I knew my first would be a girl; I could feel it; I heard their energy with my body. Of course a cynic could point out I had a 50 percent chance of being right. But it wasn't a guess; it was real knowledge. I'd even dreamt of my daughter after meeting my husband, long before I was pregnant: we'd have a daughter with gray eyes. (And we did.) Yet with both pregnancies, I felt the need to confirm my children's sex with technology. Where in 2015 I had to wait until the twenty-week anatomy scan to find out definitively that I was having a girl, when I became pregnant in 2019, a blood test at ten weeks confirmed I was having a boy. That we could know his sex so early and with certainty blew my mind, as did the means by which it was possible: the blood test detected his cells mixed among my own. Yet, on reflection, the blood test revealed what I already knew: my body and my son's body together had made a new person, one both female and male (you're growing a penis, a friend told me, approvingly).

When my son turned two, he wasn't that verbal. What would he want to eat to celebrate? I tried to channel him, to figure out what he'd like on his birthday menu. The answer came through clearly, like an epiphany: chicken for the entree. Brownies for dessert. When I served this food, I felt chuffed, but not surprised, at the intensity of his delight. In fact, part of me felt his delight in my own body. I reflected that the blood-test technology, the whole field of maternal chimera, confirms what I've known since my first pregnancy, and what to some degree feminist legal scholars have also asserted: that to be pregnant is to be neither one nor two people. Or, to put it poetically, that there are parts of my children residing in my "inmost self where the unknown gods abide," as Edith Wharton wrote.[12] And yet, even after I'd already become a mother—and even though technology had failed to keep me safe in my first birth—I still trusted technology over myself.

What women know is often dismissed as "instinct," Rothman told me—the subjective realm that can't compete with objective knowledge.

What men know is praised as wisdom, sagacity, insight, brilliance. The truth, she said, is that you can't always explain how you know what you know.

WHEN NICOLE CARR, THE ASSISTANT professor at the University of Texas–San Antonio, became pregnant with her son in 2016, she felt pressured—by her family, by her then husband, by society—to see an obstetrician, not a midwife, and to birth in a hospital. Carr didn't want to—she preferred to keep seeing her midwife, who she described as "emotionally in tune." But she acquiesced, because her first birth, at Carr's home, was unexpectedly difficult and resulted in shoulder dystocia. (Her daughter largely recovered; she has mild cerebral palsy today.)

Carr began seeing a Black female obstetrician in a two-person practice. "I explained to her what happened with my first child," she remembers. "She kind of was like, 'Well, that's because you had a home birth. What do you expect?'"

At the time, Carr was under intense stress. Her marriage was crumbling; she was finishing her dissertation; she was looking for an academic job. She was open with her OB about what was going on. "Several times I told her, 'I'm really under some stress.'" Her doctor assured her, "No, it's fine, everything's fine." She continued to dismiss her, even after Carr fainted while walking her daughter to the park.

But Carr's sense that there was something wrong mounted. "I had this continuous sense of doom," she told me. She spoke openly about her feelings with her mother, husband, and friends. At one point Carr's mother even suggested that, in order to get examined, she should go to the hospital and say that she was in pain.

During her brisk prenatal appointments, Carr tried to persuade her doctor that she needed extra monitoring. "I had done some research on the language, so I was like, 'I think I should be high-risk. Some women have babies and it's really easy and simple, and I don't think I'm one of those women.'" But Carr's doctor was adamant that her pregnancy was okay. Nothing in routine screening had turned up any issues. Eventually, Carr says, "I think I just gave up. I should have just changed doctors."

That spring, Carr and her husband divorced. In late July she moved to upstate New York, to start a job as an assistant professor of English at SUNY New Paltz (where we were briefly colleagues). Her mother and sisters came with her. At a doctor's visit to establish care with a new practice—Carr was about thirty-three weeks pregnant—the doctor tried to measure the fetal heart rate. She couldn't find the heartbeat and sent Carr downstairs for an ultrasound. Carr knew there was something wrong.

In the dark, the sonographer pressed the transducer to Carr's belly. "You could see on the ultrasound he was not moving. He was the baby who had moved more than his sister." Carr didn't want to look at the monitor. "That's when they told me." Carr's baby had died.

Though she wasn't able to get more regular fetal monitoring, Carr had still had far more testing than with her first baby, for which she hadn't even had an ultrasound. So when Carr heard that her son had died, she almost laughed with disbelief. "Every week and we're running all these tests," she says. "And he *died*?"

"A part of it is these doctors are so removed from their patients," she says now. "You don't come to their homes. You don't see how they live. You just see them as a patient for fifteen to twenty minutes. If there's not anything major presenting to them," then there isn't anything that doctors do. So although Carr told her doctor repeatedly that she believed her son wasn't safe inside of her own body—because of her stress and her sense that something was wrong—there was no test result, no objective diagnosis, that her doctor could act on. She listened to what the technology said, which, in a system that prizes efficiency, we believe tells us all that we need to hear.

After she learned that her son had died, physicians sent Carr to the hospital. She needed to birth him.

There, the attending doctor was "extremely compassionate," says Carr. He was a white man, she says, and told her that he and his wife had lost a child, too. He asked Carr if she had other children, and she said yes. "'She [Carr's daughter] is going to need help. She's going to need therapy,'" he told her. He was also angry, says Carr. He called her pregnancy high-risk. "He told me, 'You should have been on bed rest. You should have been monitored. Because of what happened with your first child, there's no way—I would have had you on bed rest every day.' He had that kind of insight, because he'd lost a child, but he essentially confirmed what I was trying to tell the first doctor—there's something wrong."*

Carr could have been induced to birth vaginally. But the doctor told her that it might take a while, because her cervix wasn't ready. She elected for a C-section under general anesthesia. Part of her hoped she wouldn't wake up after the operation. She wanted to be with her son, whom she'd named Harlem.

Carr's mother held Harlem until Carr came out of the anesthesia. Then Carr took him in her arms. Her ex-husband, who'd flown up, held him, too. "He was a perfect baby," Carr says. The nurses took pictures of him and put him in a cute outfit. They inked his feet and made footprints. When Carr left the hospital without Harlem, she had these mementos that bore his touch, which still means so much to her; she can hold them.

It's not clear why Harlem died. There was no infection. The state of his body at birth suggested he'd only been dead for a day or two. To the best that anyone could tell, her doctor told her, it was an umbilical cord accident. It appeared to be wrapped very tightly around his neck.

"Obstetric racism is about white doctors being racist, but it's also about doctors, white, Black, whatever, that when you're expressing your concerns, they just don't listen," says Carr. "It's the system that makes it so that when you go in and talk about your concerns, it's almost like you're not an expert in your own body." As such, a doctor's race doesn't necessarily indicate whether they will provide adequate care because they're operating in a fundamentally inadequate system.

I asked Carr how she'd worked through her grief. She hadn't cried during the conversation, even as her feelings were right there on the surface.

"I felt shame for a long time," she says. If people asked how many children she had, "I wouldn't have said, 'I'm a mother to a living child and a dead child.'" But once she started speaking about her son, "the conversations changed. Even in my family." She learned that her mother had had a stillborn brother, and that she had aunts who'd lost children. "We don't talk about this side of pregnancy and birth or death. But the more

---

* Shoulder dystocia itself isn't an indicator that a subsequent pregnancy will be high-risk, but it does make shoulder dystocia much more likely in a subsequent birth.

I talked about it, the more people were like, 'I went through something like that.'"

How had she learned to be able to speak about it? I was asking, I said, because for years after I'd had my C-section, I couldn't speak about what had happened to me.

"One thing that helped was to not do that guilt thing that mothers do," she said. "You say, 'Well, it's my fault.' Even though I'm a Black feminist," a scholar of gender, and know "a woman's body is not just meant to reproduce. But when mine couldn't get the baby here, there was that sense that, 'You're a failure. Somehow your body didn't do what it was supposed to do. And you failed your son.' I went through all of that. And I went through moments where I couldn't speak, like you said, after your C-section," she said.

"Now I want to speak. And I want to help people. And I want to at least, with my story, be like, this is a testimony. That you know your body better than anybody else does. You don't have to give in to what society says you have to do." She paused. "If I can speak about it, then I can be better."

WHEN DR. EDWARD HON INTRODUCED the first electronic fetal monitor in 1968, most midwives and doctors used a special stethoscope, called a fetoscope, to monitor infants' hearts during labor.[13] Typically, they listened every fifteen minutes during active labor, and every five minutes during pushing. They didn't listen all the time. Only intermittently.

Hon believed an electronic, continual monitor would help doctors in high-risk labors to be more certain about when to intervene and when to let labor continue. In that way he believed that monitoring would *reduce* unnecessary C-sections, while also making birth safer for babies. (The nation's C-section rate at the time was around 4.5 percent.[14])

Hon's first model was internal and invasive. It screwed to the baby's head and measured a mother's contractions and the baby's heartbeat. Once the external EFM was invented, a few years later, obstetricians and hospitals quickly embraced it.

At its core EFM is a very advanced stethoscope. Its purpose is to listen continually, indirectly, for what are said to be objective and reliable signs of the fetal heart during labor, a proxy for how a baby is faring. Its design, to listen continuously, evinces the ideology of obstetrics: the expectation that during labor, everything can go terribly wrong at any moment.

In 1976, when the first randomized, controlled study appeared that compared EFM to intermittent auscultation, it found no difference between intermittent listening with a fetoscope and EFM.[15] No difference in rates of newborn death, injury, or Apgar scores. The only difference the study found was that the C-sections "markedly increased" among the women monitored with EFM, at 16.5 percent versus 6.8 percent.[16] Yet by this point, half of the hospitals in the United States had already adopted the technology. When used on mothers who have not previously had a cesarean, EFM, according to one study, makes a person up to 81 percent more likely to have a C-section than mothers monitored intermittently.[17] But the technology hasn't reduced rates of infant death or cerebral palsy or intellectual disability, once thought to be caused by oxygen deprivation during labor. And currently in the US, one in four C-sections is due to nonreassuring fetal heart rate.[18]

Despite its flaws, EFM is now ubiquitous. Most mothers who birth in the hospital are familiar with the two belts that strap around the laboring mother's belly. Among mothers who are monitored continuously—which is not uncommon—the belts keep them pretty much tied to the bed, though some units are adopting wireless monitoring now. When a mother moves, the belts slip. This can cause tremendous stress; one mother who was attempting a VBAC told me, about her son, "They kept losing him on the heart monitors," even though her baby was okay. As a consequence, some mothers try to move less to keep the monitors happy, which isn't good for labor. Mentally, EFM can also take its toll: Madeline, who had an unplanned primary cesarean with her daughter, told me that despite being low-risk she was monitored almost continually once she got to the hospital. She was told early in her labor that she couldn't get up to take a walk or shower because she had to stay hooked up to the monitor. "I don't think that made anyone feel any safer," she said. "It certainly didn't inspire confidence."

The heart tracings produced by EFM fall into three categories. Category I heart tracings are clearly okay—the baby is doing terrific.

Category III tracings are seriously dangerous and tell the provider that birth—likely by C-section—is immediately necessary. These tracings are also extremely rare.[19] One study of more than forty-eight thousand people from ten hospitals showed that category III tracings occurred only .0004 percent of the time over the course of labor.[20]

Category II tracings are far more common, occurring at some point during labor in upward of three out of four patients. They are also, in their way, more troublesome, because they are more subject to interpretation; what they communicate is not so clear-cut. These tracings may suggest a stressed baby, but they may not. They may suggest that the mother needs to shift position, or that she needs oxygen, or that other interventions that providers call (rather disturbingly to a layperson) "intrauterine resuscitation" are necessary. In fact, 99.8 percent of category II tracings are false positives for cerebral palsy, meaning they look as if something may be wrong, when the baby is actually doing okay.[21]

I met Chris Verilli, who's worked as an obstetric nurse for fifty years, at a cafe near my house. She is slim, wears glasses, and wore scrubs to our meeting; afterward, she was going to teach her first in-person childbirth class since COVID. Verilli has practiced at the same hospital for the duration of her career. She started before EFM's introduction and remembered learning to use a fetoscope on a mother in labor. "I was shaking like a leaf," she told me. She was so nervous that she wasn't sure if she was hearing the baby's heartbeat or her own pulse, pounding in her ears.

When her hospital adopted EFM, Verilli remembered, "Sometimes you'd listen too long and you'd hear things that were such a minute period of time that really didn't mean there was distress," she explained. "Just like if we held our breath, our heart rate would drop down. That doesn't mean I've stopped breathing."

But interpreting the tracings on EFM strips is highly subjective. There's a wealth of studies that raise troubling issues regarding the clinical usefulness of the strips. The printouts feel like objective data, says Cantor, the lawyer and MD, but they are subject to interpretation. Obstetricians have raised concerns, both in the medical literature and with Cantor, about the ubiquity and near worship of these paper strips. "People who are in the field, if they're honest, will tell you there is no way to read much of what is on those strips with any degree of certainty or replicability," says Cantor. "It's almost like finding meaning in the noise." As cultural critic Postman pointed out in his 1992 book *Technopoly*, we have long believed that cultures may suffer from inadequate information. Only now is it becoming evident that cultures may "suffer grievously from information glut, [and] information without meaning."

For this reason, researchers have tried using artificial intelligence or algorithms to read the strips. But these don't tend to work. No surprise— the algorithms are designed by humans, and thus subject to bias. That we believe we can design a technology to solve problems created by technology further attests to the degree to which medicine has lost its way.

And yet, talking with Susie, another labor and delivery nurse, I imagined how those concerning strips could make it difficult not to act. We were walking on a trail in New Paltz on a warmish day in December, the wind blowing down on us from the ridge. She told me that when you hear a deceleration—when the fetal heart rate goes from *boop boop boop boop boop* to *boop . . . boop . . . boop*—it's "not a good sound." Naturally, everyone in the room who's on the medical side knows that decelerations can be a normal part of labor. Still, she said, the baby nurse standing by is sometimes "twitching," white-knuckling it, until the baby is born. I imagined myself in such a nurse's shoes. Then in a doctor or midwife's position. I thought I might not be able to tolerate that sound, either. Not even because of fear of litigation, but because of the potential to make a wrong call that changes—or ends—someone's life. More than one person's life: the parents' lives, too. For a provider who's had a previous bad outcome, it would be especially difficult, I imagined, to abide these moments.

Which perhaps is a reason not to use EFM, but to return to intermittent auscultation instead. Indeed, the evidence against EFM is so very damning. "The obstetric societies of the United States, Canada, Australia, and New Zealand acknowledge that electronic monitoring provides no long-term benefit for children," concludes a study from 2016.[22] Another notes, "Alas, EFM use continues unabated today as if it were actually efficacious."[23] As many as thirty years ago, the United States Preventive Services Task Force (USPSTF) assessed "electronic fetal monitoring as grade D, the lowest grade possible," declaring, "routine electronic fetal monitoring for low-risk women in labor is not recommended."[24] (As of 2014, the USPSTF considered this recommendation "inactive," because it's either "outside its scope of work," "no longer clinically relevant," or "because it has limited potential to influence public-health burden or clinical practice.")

"We're the only country that does continuous monitoring of infants in labor," New York obstetrician Aliye Runyan tells me. "We see everything that's going on, and not everything that's going on that looks negative is necessarily going to be negative. It all depends on the timing—how far the mom is from delivering. A lot of [intervention] has to do with [how] we know more. We're monitoring more things and try to intervene earlier and prevent bad outcomes for mom and baby."

That imperative can't be disentangled from fear of litigation, she said. In New York, where she practices, parents can sue an obstetrician, on behalf of their child, up to ten years after the birth for an injury sustained during birth. And when a person turns eighteen—the year she is legally permitted to file a personal-injury lawsuit—she has another two and a half years to file a claim for her own birth injury. Though New York's is among the longest lookback periods in the country, it's not the only state that has one. Dr. Elizabeth Lucal, an obstetrician in the Hudson Valley, gets blood gasses from every placenta at birth. She does so to gauge the baby's health. It also serves as evidence for how a baby was doing at birth, should a family come back seeking to litigate.

Barbara Norton, a midwife who runs the Geneva Woods Birth Center in Anchorage, became a nurse right before EFM's introduction—but just barely, she told me. We spent three hours talking at a picnic table in the parking lot of her birth center during summer 2022, as COVID raged across Anchorage. Once EFM was adopted, Norton remembers, "you could just see, we ran back for all these C-sections for fetal distress and the baby came out" perfectly fine. "And that is what you still see. We still don't know how to use that technology."

Norton also saw how the technology transformed labor nurses' tasks. "It allows the nurses to not be at the bedside. They have to be there out at the desk looking at all the screens," she told me. "When I was trained to be a labor and delivery nurse in 1978, I was at the bedside the whole time. I was there supporting and listening and doing my job. . . . But the monitoring took the nurses out of the bed, out of the room."

In that way, hospitals have an incentive to value EFM: it makes it possible to rely on a skeleton nursing crew, to maintain nurse staffing ratios that would have been infeasible before EFM's introduction. Thanks to the advent of central monitoring at nurses' stations, "You can watch two patients instead of one," Norton told me. This may not have been the kind of care intended in fetal monitoring's initial design. But set the tool in an industry increasingly led by financially motivated owners—where it is difficult to staff nurses because of a labor shortage and burnout that's hastened by troubling nurse-to-patient ratios—and to some degree, it's become an electronic babysitter, its beeps and streams of data a substitute for personal, and human, observation and physical support.

Technology and intervention are also the kinds of care our culture rewards. "I don't think we value high-touch, low-tech care when it's appropriate," says Penn's Rebecca R. S. Clark. That is reflected in what kinds of care and knowledge insurance companies recognize and reimburse, as discussed in chapter 7. "We're starting to think about reimbursing for doulas," Clark says. But most of "what we recognize and what we pay for are our medical interventions." Nor do labor and delivery nurses study such high-touch interventions as a matter of course—but they do receive training in how to read and use EFM.

While reporting this book, I remember thinking how clearly eliminating EFM would "solve" the C-section problem. After all, fetal heart tones are the second-most-common reason for C-sections in the US. But I hadn't considered how deeply ingrained technology is in the medical model—to say nothing of our culture overall. In a way, that's reflected even in Nicole Carr's requests for more monitoring, when perhaps what she really wanted was the kind of time and personal care she'd received during her pregnancy from her midwife.

And although there are some initiatives to train providers to use a fetoscope, like the University of Michigan's Obstetrics Initiative, many of the obstetricians I spoke to didn't think that we'd get rid of EFM anytime soon. "Unfortunately, we're well aware that [EFM] increases our C-section rate," Lucal, the Hudson Valley obstetrician, told me. And while the technology might improve—in fact, she's aware of advances that are underway, such as wireless monitors—"It is never going to go away," she says. "You have to incorporate it into your practice, so that everybody has the least negative impact, and you can get the best out that it can offer."

Runyan, the New York City OB, made a similar observation. "EFM has become the star of the show," Runyan told me. "We don't do anything without a monitor." I thought of Julie Cantor's experience—how the ultrasound became the star of her show, how her provider believed it communicated more truthfully than she could. It's not a surprise; I see this in how some of my students think about AI and ChatGPT, and how useful these tools are for "writing," for coming up with ideas, sourcing facts—even though the software is often wrong, its sourcing almost impossible to trace. What's depressing is when they use these tools not because they've run out of time to do the assignment but because they've grown up believing that a computer knows more than they possibly could.

IT'S IMPORTANT TO POINT OUT that Laënnec developed the stethoscope in part because of his disgust with or sexualization of a woman's youthful body. Those qualities forbade or discouraged Laënnec from touching her. Some of Laënnec's peers expressed similar constraints. One doctor who wanted to study circulation wrote that doctors should do so "by placing their hands directly on the heart," but regretted that "our delicate morals prevent us from doing so especially in the case of women." But medicine did not have to evolve in this way. Other physicians at the time critiqued such "false modesty" and "excessive restraint," as Foucault points out in his book *The Birth of the Clinic*.[25] "This exploration, which is carried out very precisely above the chemise, may take place with all possible decency," wrote one doctor in France in 1811.[26]

Male physicians' potential sexualization of, or shame or disgust with, the female body shaped birth, too, in such a way as to put space between doctor and patient—at the patient's peril. (French philosopher and pornographer Georges Bataille "reflected on the 'impossibility' of looking at genitals—like looking at the Sun and the death," Andrea Mubi Brighenti writes.[27]) The drawings of women's reproductive organs separate from their bodies, which coincided with men's entries into the birth room, definitively showed that these men weren't looking at women sexually. But as discussed, these illustrations contributed to a new conception of birth as a disembodied process. Similarly, nineteenth-century birthing stools had skirts around them, ostensibly to maintain women's modesty. But these skirts harbored bacteria that spread infection, making birth more dangerous. The disgust attending women's bodies is also partly why, when birth initially moved to the hospital, obstetricians had women confined to bed and swaddled under sheets.

It would be a mistake to suggest that physicians and nurses rely on technology such as continuous fetal monitoring because they're disgusted or shamed or enticed by women's bodies. But this kind of technology stands in for, and indeed gets in the way of, human touch. It also obviates the need of asking for consent the way a doctor or nurse should ask before touching you with her hands.

EFM is also of a piece with other shifts in medicine that have increased the distance between doctor and patient, and these shifts attest to how the powerful juggernaut of corporate medicine doesn't value personal relationships or human touch. "Nobody tells me to take my clothes off anymore," commented my father-in-law, who's in his seventies. Verilli, the labor and delivery nurse, pointed out that some doctors don't even sit down when they come into the exam room—they have too many people to see in that same fifteen-minute slot. Such distancing diminishes the human character of the provider, too. "Dr. Lucal, if you'd only bring your laptop into the exam room with you, you'd be much more efficient"— that's one of the critiques obstetrician Elizabeth Lucal hears from her supervisors. She counters, "But if I brought the laptop in, I wouldn't look at the patient."

Even the transition from handwritten to digital charting has introduced distance between patient and provider. Where providers once wrote notes, "Now we have boxes to check," Verilli told me. For how contractions feel, "there's strong, moderate, mild, not. That . . . does describe it, but in writing it, you are a little more descriptive. You get a better picture." And while the software allows providers to leave a narrative note, doing so is laborious. At a certain point, given how voluminous charting is, you just don't do it, she told me. So while electronic charts generate reams of data, their quality of information is sparse. By contrast, Susie, the obstetric nurse, told me about the chart from her own birth in England in 1971. It fit on a single index card and spoke to the human scale of birth: the nurse recorded Susie's "lusty cry."

In a sense, electronic charting functions like electronic fetal monitoring:

a near-continuous stream of data, a purportedly objective computerized gaze that, despite its seeming completeness, leaves out the nuance and the context that gives it meaning. It's a similar logic that undergirds our use of closed-circuit television, or Ring devices that record the front door, or even police officers' body cameras—which, despite their promise, haven't been shown to reduce police use of force. We assume that the constantly recording device captures everything, and therefore anything of significance. We believe this visual omniscience will fix the problem. And we discard or forget that events take place outside of the frame, including what subjective, embodied knowledge can reveal.

Yet when it comes to birth, what's outside the frame matters a lot.

Perhaps electronic charting is narrative-less by design, because it is in the best interests of the hospital. Such spare, seemingly objective reporting is advantageous in a highly litigious environment. "I guess, in a court of law, less is better," Verilli muses. "Because then it's 'he said, she said.'"

TRADITIONALLY, PAYOUTS FOR MEDICAL MALPRACTICE during childbirth are for sustained physical harm to the baby. And while Americans have a reputation for litigiousness, "birth injury" lawsuits win substantial awards in the UK and Australia, too. The most common such lawsuits allege that babies deprived of oxygen during labor develop "hypoxic ischemic encephalopathy," or HIE, a brain injury that lawyers argue can cause cerebral palsy or otherwise delay development.[28] The average payout for these lawsuits is about $524,000, but awards for a baby found to be injured during labor or birth can be in the millions.[29]

In a lawsuit, the record produced by EFM makes it possible for a lawyer to point to a heart-rate deceleration and say, *Here is where the baby was damaged*—a claim nearly impossible to verify or, because of the authority we vest in technology, refute.[30]

The majority of obstetricians in the US (about 80 percent) have been sued; lawsuits for HIE account for a large degree of such lawsuits.[31] Hence the bumper-sticker aphorism of birth: you don't get sued for the C-section you did; you get sued for the C-section you didn't do.

But the imperative to avoid a lawsuit for a harmed baby effectively means overlooking the costs of the C-section—or whatever other intervention—on the mother. "Even the [practitioners] I've spoken to who are really liberal and understand it, there's still this pressure, and this fear, that God forbid I have a bad baby case," Julie Cantor told me. "You're better off having a woman who's been violated, [or had] a bad birth outcome, or trauma, than a harmed baby—or, God forbid, a dead baby. Because you know what's going to cost you in this lawsuit? The baby."

A legal emphasis exclusively on harms to the baby also reflects the position of mothers in our society. Cantor points to the case of Kimberly Turbin, a California mother. Turbin's video of her episiotomy, which a doctor performed even though Turbin repeatedly said no, went viral.

"Nobody would take her case," says Cantor. "Either because they didn't think it was illegal. Or they thought, *Well, doctors know best.* Or, *No harm, no foul. I mean, it's just a woman.* Or they thought, *Childbirth is dangerous.* Or they thought, *Even if it was illegal, and even if it shouldn't happen, how much money is it really worth? How much is a harmed woman really worth in this society?*" Cantor and I spoke in March 2022, three months before the Dobbs decision. "We're coming up on overturning *Roe. Roe*, don't look at it like abortion. Look at it as the right to control your body. Guess who doesn't have that right? Pregnant people. And you know who's mostly pregnant people? Women. And you know how women are treated in this society? Not well." (Dawn Thompson, who works as an advocate and doula through Improving Birth and Birthify, ultimately helped Turbin find representation, and Turbin settled the case. As part of the settlement, the obstetrician, who was already at the end of his career, gave up his California medical license.)

But a birth doesn't have to go to court for mothers to know the value their bodies command. One mother in a social media group I belonged to included, in her VBAC plan, "No matter what happens, I am the No. 1 priority." It's telling that she felt she needed to include this directive. And it demonstrates the extent to which mother and baby are separate, and competitors, in the realm of birth.

IN 1994, ARTIST MONA HATOUM had doctors film the interior of her body by feeding an endoscope into her mouth, esophagus, and her vagina. For her piece *Corps étranger* (*Strange body*), she installed the resultant video in a dark, womb-like space. The piece is disorienting; sometimes it is difficult to know what part of the body you're looking at. But that strangeness is the point. Despite the surveillant capabilities of technology, despite all the disease that it can pinpoint—this is the problem, right here!—our inner bodies are largely strangers to us, the people hauling them around.

And in spite of the very deep investigation that technology permits of our selves (and cells), doctors and nurses touch patients' bodies far less now than they once did. In a sense, one could argue that now, all touch is subject to investigation, a consequence of #MeToo. And it's evident that the diminishment of touch, even the fear of it, is also powerfully felt throughout our culture. Young people have a lot less sex than they used to; we spend more time in the virtual world than touching each other. Verilli, the veteran L&D nurse, joked, "Sometimes I don't even know how people get pregnant."

"When a baby is born, a mother is also born," writes Ashley Montagu in his book *Touching*, a bestseller when it first came out in 1971. "There is considerable evidence that at this time, and for months thereafter, her needs for contact exceed those of the infant."

Yet most of the discussion around touch and birth focuses on what touch can do for the baby. The "golden hour" helps the baby during her first hour of life, because touching an infant regulates her breathing and temperature. Over time, it also helps her to develop emotional regulation. In a way, that emphasizes what medical technology has been designed to do: to overlook and bury the mother, the person, the body, the story she's brought to the birth.

As we're talking, Verilli reaches across the table and squeezes my wrist. Her touch is a surprise, but it's nice. For some, touch can be deeply comforting, she says. And for others, touch can be uncomfortable, if touch has been used to abuse or violate. In that way, touch can also offer midwives and doctors important diagnostic information—a story that the body tells, if a practitioner knows how to listen, that technology cannot identify. Labor, says Verilli, and pushing especially, can trigger people who've been abused or sexually assaulted. But labor isn't the time to figure out if this is part of a mother's history. In fact, it couldn't be worse, because of the opportunities for missteps—for the wrong kind of touching. In that instance, a mother "could have had a nice delivery," Verilli says.

"Instead, she's all freaked out." A system based more on touch, rather than technology, could help providers understand that part of a patient's life early on.

When I struggled to nurse my daughter, my mother paid for a lactation consultant to come to my home to help me. My nipples were raw and bleeding from the bad latch. The LC, Jenn Sullivan, with a streak both blunt and empathic, attended me without judgment or horror about what had happened during my birth. I can see now that Jenn was probably less concerned with making sure that nursing "succeeded" than with listening to how I was doing and trying to find a way to reduce my pain. My daughter had a suck like a vacuum, which I understood as her ferocious clutch on life. In the words of psychologist D. W. Winnicott, I had introduced too much of the world, too quickly. She knew with her body how frightening the outside could be. Too much of the bad kind of touch, and all at once.

Jenn helped me to position the baby on my lap and watched me try to latch. Then she helped me to do so, gently bringing my daughter's chin to my breast.

Do lots and lots of skin-to-skin, she counseled me. She wasn't telling me this so that I'd increase my milk or to turn me into a round-the-clock nursing machine. This touch wasn't for the baby. That wasn't the story she was most concerned with. She said, "The baby is medicine for you."

9

PAIN

It is as difficult to think about pain as about love. Both are charged with associations going back to early life, and with cultural attitudes wrought into language itself.[1]

Adrienne Rich, Of Woman Born

THERE'S A REASON THAT NINETEENTH-CENTURY WOMEN WROTE ONE another letters inquiring whether birth hurts as much as having all of your teeth pulled in one go. It's because birth is painful. That's why women invited male doctors into the birth room to begin with: they had chloroform, and then ether, which promised to take away some of the pain.

To a woman of one hundred years ago, the array of pharmacological pain relievers at laboring women's disposal today might seem magical, divine: epidurals, laughing gas, opioids, spinal anesthesia. Sterile water boluses injected into the sacrum. Even nonpharmacological offerings might seem miraculous, like baths, showers, and massagers that emit continuous and never-ending hot water. Amid such a surfeit of coping mechanisms, the support that other women can provide—simply through their presence and encouragement—may not seem important or particularly useful.

While we have solved many of the technological and medical challenges of diminishing childbirth pain safely, though, there's still no way to have a baby entirely without pain, during labor or after birth. That pain can be terrifying, empowering, both, or neither. But it is most certainly normal. Unfortunately, because birth has been medicalized, it can be hard to expect—or accept—this reality. Medicine, delivered in a hospital, is supposed to make pain go away. With childbirth, it can't. Not entirely.

What's important about pain during birth, research into birth experiences shows, isn't only the pain *itself*. It's the way that other people respond to the pain. Pain that's diminished or dismissed causes damage that lasts.

For a long time, the consequences of my obstetrician's dismissal of my pain kept me from seeing how that happens in many other people's births, if in circumstances less extreme. But once I started reporting this book, I started to see these instances everywhere, even if I didn't go looking for them; it was as if I could see new spectrums of light. My friend Danielle told me one such story, unprompted, over dinner. She'd been induced with Pitocin for her second baby and was dilated to three centimeters when she arrived at the hospital. An hour into receiving the Pit, which was dialed to a six (the highest dose is twenty), Danielle—a former competitive swimmer who describes herself as having a very high pain tolerance—asked for an epidural. In fact, she now thinks she waited too long to ask, because by the time she did, the pain was so intense she was having trouble breathing. The midwife, whom Danielle describes as "cold," seemed to think Danielle was exaggerating, and told her to calm down.

It took the anesthesiologist an hour and a half to arrive. When he got there, no one checked Danielle again to see how dilated she was. But a nurse told him, "She's at a three." Danielle was in too much pain to speak up and demand to be checked. The anesthesiologist suggested that Danielle relax, that she had a long way to go. And though he appeared to insert the epidural, it didn't work. The minutes passed, the contractions mounted, and Danielle writhed and rolled on the bed. The epidural wasn't starting. "What is happening? Why isn't it working?" she pleaded. With her first baby she'd had an epidural, and it had started working immediately.

An hour passed. Danielle and her husband repeatedly told the nurses that the epidural wasn't working. Eventually, the anesthesiologist returned, and though he tried to fix the epidural, it still didn't take effect. Around this time, Danielle's midwife checked her cervix and saw that Danielle's son was crowning—that it was time to push. "I knew it!" Danielle said. She was furious; she'd been treated as if she were crazy, she felt—as if the pain were only in her head—when in fact she'd been dilating rapidly. And now she had to go through pushing without any pain relief. That wasn't what she wanted, and she didn't think she could do it.

Despite her fear, and her anger, Danielle got her son out with one push. Her providers seemed proud: *You did it!* They told her. But she was so angry she didn't want to hold her baby. The nurses, midwife, even her husband seemed a little shocked. What no one seemed to recognize is that her baby didn't—he couldn't possibly—make up for how she'd been overlooked, and made to feel as if there were something wrong with her for expressing the pain she'd been in. Rather than feel more "womanly" for birthing unmedicated, she told me, she felt victimized. Then, making matters still worse, the epidural *did* kick in—about half an hour after her son's birth, trapping her in bed and on the labor floor; she couldn't leave until she could stand up, and she couldn't stand until she could feel her legs.

A 2022 study by anesthesiology and obstetrics professor Joanna Kountanis and colleagues found that what's important about women who feel pain during childbirth is how mothers feel *about* their pain, and how their providers communicate with them overall. Feeling positively about pain, and "heard" by her providers, protects a mother from developing PTSD.[2] By contrast, if she feels negatively about her pain, and if she feels coerced by her providers and not heard, she is more likely to develop PTSD. It's a good explanation for why the pain of not being listened to can resonate so long after the physical sensations have stilled. The pain is over—except it isn't.

Danielle's son is three now, and she's mostly over it, she told me. She was in the driver's seat of her car while we talked, her son kicking in his car seat, moaning that it was time to go. Though she didn't develop PTSD, she had trouble connecting to her son for the first week at home—to being in love with him. And she was angry for a long time.

As her experience shows, and as Kountanis's study demonstrates, pain that's dismissed isn't eradicated by a happy ending, a healthy baby, or even when the pain fades from the body. That's because physical pain isn't ever entirely physical: it's mental and emotional, in part because of the feelings that can accompany it: negative ones, like fear, terror, sadness, grief; positive ones, like ecstasy, pride, or empowerment, as an athlete feels at pushing through mile twenty-two of a marathon, or a mother screaming through a contraction. These emotional and psychological dimensions of pain are why addressing pain isn't only about numbing the body. Nor is it even always possible to do so; up to 30 percent of epidurals do not work, which is what happened to Danielle and to me during labor (another example of *nobody tells you*). But a birth with little labor pain isn't necessarily a good birth. In studies of mothers, like Dr. Anne Drapkin Lyerly's work, women point not to pain relief but to having agency; feeling connected to others; and feeling that the experience of birth is respected as the stuff of a good birth.[3] By contrast, what makes for a traumatic birth, according to a 2017 study of some 748 women whose births were traumatizing, is being lied to or threatened, violated, having knowledge of one's own body dismissed, and providers "prioritizing their own agendas over the needs of the woman."[4]

Yet when it comes to pain in America, including the pain of childbirth, we tend to address it the same way: aggressively, and with a pill. The financialized, medical model of birth promotes this approach: epidurals are widely available, don't require much personal understanding of the patient, and are relatively quick to administer. The mother needn't have any relationship whatsoever with the anesthetist for the analgesia to work. By contrast, as Rothman observed in chapter 5, the value of other relationships, the encouragement and feeling of safety that nonmedical experts can provide, isn't so widely recognized or rewarded—though that's the whole logic of a doula, whose support, evidence shows, can ease pain and promote vaginal birth.

But childbirth demands more than a medical approach to pain relief, one that means tending to a mother physically, emotionally, and mentally. "Birth is smelly bloody dirty messy bestial, whether it is vaginal or surgical there is no easy way out," writes Mai'a Williams. "The epidural can ease the pain but not the existential fear."

This means that providers have a steep task before them: they must both recognize and credit the pain a laboring person experiences in her body, while also respecting what's going on in her mind. They have to be mindful that a person's prior experiences, their cultural and personal definitions of pain, and whether they feel safe or anxious in the hospital, all contribute to the pain a person feels during birth.[5] And in doing so, they have to be careful not to fall into the woman-pain trap: attributing the pain a woman expresses to her emotions—not to her body—above all.

JENN BRAY-LUONG IS ONE OF the many women I interviewed for this book whose pain was dismissed when she had a baby. What she went through caused her so much pain, and so much trauma, that she never wants to be pregnant again. For that reason alone, her story is important to tell.

But Jenn's experience isn't only about the physical pain that her doctor dismissed. It's also a story of what she was expected to bear, an example of how women are believed to have a higher pain tolerance than men. It's a story of the tacit expectations providers have of women of color; Jenn's mother, who came with her to many of her appointments, is Latina. And it demonstrates that emotional support and human company can lessen the pain and fear brought on by a painful and frightening situation.

Jenn, thirty-seven, is the kind of mom who always seems to have it together. She's prepared for birthdays and Christmas with mom-and-me matching outfits, or customized T-shirts for the whole family. She usually has her nails done: sexy red, Robin's-egg blue, sparkly purple. She's short—five one on a good day—with dark hair that reaches her shoulders. Outspoken. She has a ready smile. And while she projects an almost exuberant friendliness, Jenn is tough. She met her now-husband, Greg, in the middle of his messy divorce. Despite the many reasons his ex gave her to keep moving—the rigors of family court, bankruptcy, Child Protective Services—Jenn was unwavering. And what's more, despite the challenges of integrating their families, despite not having much in the way of cash flow—she works in financial aid at a college; he as a professor at another—soon after they got engaged, she and Greg decided to have a baby together.

At the time, Jenn was already a mother to M, her daughter with her first husband. She'd had a C-section for that birth because of high blood pressure. At the time, Jenn didn't understand why people said that C-sections were traumatizing. Her physicians had been kind: during the surgery, she said, her anesthesiologist had held her hand. And her recovery was swift; within her first few days at home she was walking up and down the stairs of her town house, though her physicians had told her not to.

While she'd planned to have a repeat cesarean with her next baby, the surgery happened earlier than she'd expected: she went from a prenatal checkup to the hospital because her blood pressure was so high. Her son, at only thirty-four weeks, was born small but healthy. And her cesarean appeared to go well.

But the pain she felt after this surgery was nothing like her first operation. While she was still in the hospital, she told this to the nurses, doctor, and midwives she saw. It hurt most on her right side, which a provider told her made sense; that's where the surgeon stood and did most of the work. This seemed plausible, but Jenn wasn't entirely convinced. The pain was so bad that even oxycodone—which Jenn initially hadn't wanted to take, because it had been so constipating after her first C-section—did not help.

At home over the next few days, Jenn's pain got worse. By the time she dragged herself to her post-op appointment, about a week after the surgery, she could barely walk.

By now, she was certain something was wrong. She couldn't even walk into the exam room on her own. She couldn't get comfortable on the exam table. She half sat, half reclined. She told her doctor that she was in tremendous pain.

Her physician, someone she'd seen during the pregnancy and disliked, told her that her incision looked fine. Great, even. "You're doing fine," she told Jenn. "If you're still in pain, I'll prescribe you a few more oxycodone."

Jenn said, "Okay—well, but it really is, like, burning pain."

"It looks good," her doctor repeated. "But if you have any signs of infection, call the hospital."

Jenn wasn't persuaded. "I know my own body," she said. She resolved that, if it still hurt that much in a couple of days, she'd go straight to the hospital. She wouldn't even bother calling her doctor. There was no reason to; her doctor didn't listen.

WOMEN, WHETHER THEY KNOW IT or not, have a "credibility deficit," writes British philosopher Miranda Fricker. Because society largely sees women as overly bound up with their bodies, and overly emotional, they're not consistently treated as capable of identifying or relaying trustworthy, reliable information. Partly as a result, providers conceive of women's pain as psychological rather than physiological. Women are more often prescribed antianxiety medication than men; even postoperatively, they're more likely to be prescribed sedatives, rather than pain relief.[6]

This set of assumptions about women's minds, and their bodies, has a long history. It came to especial prominence in the late nineteenth century, when hysteria emerged as a disease that physicians believed emanated from women's "very nature." Hysteria, linked to women's reproductive organs, could manifest as sexual frustration, sexual licentiousness, headaches, depression, feebleness, dyspepsia, palpitations—a broad array of sometimes contradictory symptoms.[7]

Hysteria gradually disappeared as an official diagnosis during the twentieth century (along the way, it shifted and became a diagnosis applied to men after World War I, like Septimus Smith in *Mrs. Dalloway*). But women's credibility deficit persisted. This "impairment" has often been cited as a reason to bar women from public life. "Many women may possess the knowledge and authority but they seldom can convey this through their voices," said the president of ABC News in the 1960s, explaining why women weren't fit to be news anchors. "Her voice is naturally thinner, with less timbre and range. It's not as appropriate for reporting crucial events. For hard-core news, the depth and resonance of the male voice are indispensable."[8]

Yet even when it comes to reporting on the "crucial events" of labor and childbirth—events so very uniquely embodied—women's voices don't carry. As a consequence, too often when women express pain, their providers don't listen.

LIKE SO MUCH OF WHAT can go wrong between patients and providers, this dismissal of women's pain isn't only an interpersonal phenomenon. It's systemic, effectively built into the US's dismal system of prenatal and postpartum care. Before the baby, the average birth parent has no time off from work. Then she gives birth and returns to work an average of two weeks after.

No matter how you give birth, no body heals in such a short time frame. "At the minimum—the *minimum*—it's thirteen weeks," Helena

A. Grant, the nurse-midwife formerly of Brooklyn's Woodhull Hospital, told me. But really, "it's eighteen months" for full and holistic healing, she says. Yet the impact of paid leave on new mothers' physical well-being has not been widely investigated. The majority of studies focus on the mother's emotional benefits of paid leave—as if the need to restore after birth were only psychic. Or as if it were possible to restore the mind without caring for the body, or to restore the body without caring for the mind.

Grant connects the US's physically punishing lack of paid leave to the legacy of slavery. "As a Black woman, I feel like it comes from seeing the tenacity of women who were brought here, enslaved, and forced to do plantation work and breed," she says. "Have a baby and get right back to work." In time, that legacy became harmful for all American women, she says, promoting capitalism at the expense of human life.

That expectation is even reflected in the built environment of hospitals. Caroline, a mother in New York, had an episiotomy during her son's birth in 2018. A few days after she was discharged, she had to bring him to another hospital for light therapy to treat his jaundice, where the only thing to sit on was a hard bench. "Do you have a sitz bath?" she asked. "My doctor told me to soak my wound in warm water every six hours. I'm going to be here for the next twenty-four hours. I have to stay here because I'm breastfeeding." The staff, she remembers, looked at her with amazement. They'd never fielded that request before. Though the facility is "set up to give care to newborns, it had zero considerations" for birth parents, says Caroline.

Growing up, I was impressed with stories of women in my community who'd graded final exams, or completed their master's theses, during labor. In these tales, the women finished their work and dashed to the hospital just in time for the baby to be born. I thought that these stories were a testament to women's fortitude, how tough and organized and hardworking they were—all values my community prized. I didn't see these stories as the inevitable result of the pressures of living in a society that doesn't give people time off to have babies, a society that fails to recognize procreation as life's most magnificent form of production. My interpretation of these stories—that women are made from tougher stuff—is an example of the ways that women adopt and embody "a cultural self that we become but which we seem to have been all along," as gender theorist Judith Butler writes.[9]

What's sad, and also inevitable, is that my friends bounce this attitude off one another all the time. For instance, my friend who's an engineer and had hyperemesis gravidarum during both her pregnancies went to work throughout. She'd vomit in the trash—multiple times a day—and then calculate the particulars of installing portable toilets at construction sites. Other times she was hospitalized for dehydration; in her second pregnancy, she went to the hospital almost weekly for IV infusions, for hydration. She reminds me of these details when her husband, sick with a "man cold," moans and refuses to drag himself out of bed. I respond with awe at her fortitude, semi-outrage at the lack of his, but also, a sense of realized expectations: *Of course he doesn't carry on as you did.* Women are strong. Men are weak. (Also, we are Holocaust descendants, she reminds me, made to endure.)

My friend's take on her husband's coping with pain, her coping with hyperemesis, my response to both, are emblematic of what Judith Butler calls the "sculpting of the original body into a cultural form": we're tougher because society says we're tougher.[10] The belief comes from the culture at large, from the history of slavery, from the medical system, but at the same time, dangerously, it feels so very natural that it's as if it's coming from within us.

But this isn't because women have a higher pain tolerance than men, another myth that may shape how women's pain is treated—or ignored (though estrogen does play a role in pain perception). It's because of our disproportionate domestic responsibilities. We can't stay home to tend to our bodies because we have to use our sick days to take care of sick children, or kids who are home from school or day care for some other reason. The US doesn't have any other system for providing this essential care. A commercial that ran incessantly during my childhood: "Moms don't take sick days. Moms take DayQuil."

Jessica Grose's book *Screaming on the Inside* makes a similar argument. A story my librarian friend Madeline told me about that book is emblematic of its main ideas: she ordered it for the library but was too overburdened with the demands of her job, single-parenting her daughter, and recuperating from a physically incapacitating birth to read it. Instead, she used the book to prop up a monitor on her desk, and stared at it while she did her physical therapy, before returning it to the library a few months later, without even having an opportunity to read it.

TWO DAYS AFTER JENN HAD told her doctor about her extreme pain—when her son was less than two weeks old—her incision started to look infected. It was raised, red, swollen, and inflamed. She showed her mother, who Jenn says has a "big mouth" and doesn't "sugarcoat" anything.

"What the hell is that?" her mother asked. This was a Saturday, and Jenn thought she'd wait until Monday to call the doctor. But the next day, she knew she shouldn't wait any longer and went to the ER. The physician there did a sonogram and found multiple nodules filled with pus. He drained the largest one. But they couldn't take care of all of them, the physician told her—she'd need to follow up with her OB.

The following day, the incision looked worse. Jenn went back to her doctor's office, and saw yet another doctor—the one who was supposed to do her cesarean in the first place. He told her that he needed to cut it open and drain it. First, he squeezed her wound, which Jenn says was awful—it oozed fluid, the pain burrowing into and waving through her abdomen. Then he numbed her—this was now the second time she'd had a needle in her belly in as many days—and reopened the incision.

"You're going to have to pack it," he told her.

"What?" she said.

"You're going to have to pack it yourself."

"You want me to stick stuff inside of me?"

Yes. The physician apologized and seemed to feel bad. He suggested that she go to the wound care center in the hospital where she'd given birth—though he warned that they might not be able to see her for a few days.

Jenn's mother was incredulous. "You want her to do what?" she asked. She was skeptical of doctors, with good reason; on two separate occasions over the past few years, she'd gone to the ER with chest pain and was sent home. Both times, she was, in fact, having a heart attack. "You really want her to pack this herself?" she demanded of the doctor. "I can try to help her, but neither of us have a medical background. Are we going to make the incision worse? What if we make the infection worse?" The doctor looked at her. "You better show me how to do this because I'm going to have to help her. She just had major surgery."

Jenn was glad her mother was with her. Her mother could be tough. "It's really not that bad," the doctor told her. "Just do the best you can."

"'Do the best you can'?" her mother said. "I'm not a nurse."

The practice sent Jenn home with instructions to change the dressings twice a day. She did her best, but the first night, fluid oozed through the bandage, soaking through her underwear, her clothes—so much fluid that she put down a towel to protect the mattress. But packing the wound was worse. She was to use a large Q-tip to shove iodine-soaked bandages, which stank, into her open wound. Then she had to bandage it again.

Her mother tried to help but couldn't. "I don't want to mess up anything for you," she told Jenn. She wasn't squeamish—Jenn says that if she'd needed it, her mother would change her diapers for her—but that didn't equip her to inflict so much pain on her daughter.

Reluctantly, Jenn turned to Greg to help. Their relationship was still kind of new, and there's that feeling you have with a newish partner: Can I really ask him to help me with this? Will he reject me? And even if you know he won't, there's the desire to protect the relationship from that kind of medical need—medical bodily modesty. So in the end, because she found the wound cleaning was so traumatic, and so shameful, she decided she'd do it alone.

She made a plan: First, she made sure someone—her mother, her brother, Greg—could watch the children. Then she took an oxycodone, waited half an hour for it to take effect, and closed herself in the bathroom. She told her family not to come in, no matter what kinds of sounds they heard. She turned on the bathroom fan to give her more privacy. Then she unwrapped the gauze, stared into her incision, and rooted around in it with the sterile pads and the Q-tip. It was so painful, she cried and retched. After she was finished, all she could do was lie flat.

"The burning pain. I will never forget that pain," she tells me now. "That was the worst pain I ever felt in my life."

UNLIKE BLOOD PRESSURE, TEMPERATURE, OR heart rate, there is no objective measure of pain. While pain may be visible from a person's expression or posture, or from her vitals, it isn't always. And in fact there is evidence that nurses mistakenly expect people reporting moderate to severe pain to show it in visible, quantifiable ways, through increased heart rate, for example, or grimacing—in other words, they believe that patients' bodies will relay evidence that backs them up. That's what happened when I was in labor. The pain was excruciating, but my body didn't seem to tell the story as the providers might have expected. And because pain is subjective, the only way to know with certainty if a person is in pain is to ask, a point that the anesthesiologists I talked with emphasized.

But as we learned in the previous chapter, in Western medicine, history-taking—listening to a patient's experience of her symptoms—was demoted by the early twentieth century in favor of what physicians could divine through their gaze, training, and technologies designed to visualize pathology, from stethoscopes to blood cultures. As a consequence, for "many modern physicians," writes Stanley Joel Reiser in *Medicine and the Reign of Technology*, "facts" technologically derived about a patient hold greater authority than "facts" elicited from a patient's narrative of her illness.[11] By design, a person's account of her symptoms—including pain—is less true, and less authoritative, than what Reiser calls "technologically generated facts."[12] If a physician can't see it, according to the structure and ideology of Western medicine, it can't be that useful. Seen by this light, it's not only women who aren't reliable narrators; no one is a "credible reporter" of their own body.

The problem of pain's invisibility to physicians is effectively what NIH researcher Dr. Mitchell S. Max pointed out in a famous editorial he published in 1990 in the *Annals of Internal Medicine*. Rather than call for reforming how Western medicine recognizes and investigates a person's symptoms, or suggest expanding space for the subjective, Max sought to fit pain into allopathic medicine's objective, visualized practice. He argued that hospitals and physicians needed to implement structures to quantify and visualize pain, much as the stethoscope and laboratory had developed more than a century earlier to identify and visualize pathology. Shortly after Max's editorial, and as he recommended, patients' pain levels began appearing on their hospital charts. But simply visualizing pain in this way wasn't sufficient, Max argued. And so in 1995, the American

Pain Society—which Max led at the time—reconceived pain as "the fifth vital sign."[13]

Awarding pain this status, which professional organizations including the American Medical Association adopted, shifted clinical guidelines and practice. By 1999, the VA mandated that clinicians ask every patient about their pain; California adopted a similar regulation.[14] As a consequence, some providers asked patients about pain at virtually every encounter. And in 2001, the Joint Commission, which rates and accredits hospitals, began including how well hospitals managed pain in its assessments of hospitals.[15]

By design these changes swept in the era of widely available, and aggressively prescribed, opiate pain relief. Rather than focus on selling oxycodone only to people with cancer pain—previously the target audience for opiates—Purdue Pharma believed it could reach the fifty million Americans living with "nonmalignant" and "chronic pain."[16] These people would become repeat, possibly lifelong customers, rather than people dying from cancer who used morphine only at the end of life. As Patrick Radden Keefe concludes in his book *Empire of Pain*, "OxyContin would be a drug for everyone."[17]

In this climate, by the mid-1990s, prescribing opiates after C-sections became "standing orders," says Dr. William Camann, an obstetric anesthesiologist at Brigham and Women's Hospital in Boston. "Everybody got narcotics. Absolutely everybody," whether mothers asked for them or not. That was the case not only at Brigham and Women's, but at most hospitals throughout the United States. By this point, the Joint Commission effectively tied hospital assessment to such use of opioids, even though evidence shows that most women don't need opiate pain relief after C-section (though women who birth addicted to opioids will need far more). Instead, what they do need postpartum, they rarely get, like paid time off or physical and occupational therapy. But prescribing opiates is far simpler and cheaper than these more expensive, one-on-one, personal therapies.

Opioids after C-sections also "introduced" untold millions of mothers to a highly addictive medication that they may not have used previously. For years, many new moms—more white women than women of color—left the hospital with such large prescriptions that, according to one study from the *Journal of Anesthesiology* in 2021, they had an average of seventeen leftover pills banging around their medicine cabinets.[18] Such standing orders produced inadvertent, tragic outcomes: according to a 2016 study, approximately one in three hundred mothers who weren't opioid-dependent when they had their C-section continued to take opiates a year after the operation.[19] (Lisa Marie Presley got hooked that way, as she recalled in her foreword for Harry Nelson's book *The United States of Opioids*.) In the paper, the researchers speculate that there may be something special about that first year postpartum. It "may be a period of vulnerability," they write.[20]

May be a period of vulnerability. It's emblematic of our spectacular failure to see new motherhood for what it is that such a significant, widely cited NIH study would teeter, lexically, about the vulnerability of the first year of motherhood. As if there were insufficient evidence to prove it.

I HAVE OFTEN DESCRIBED MY birth as getting hit by lightning. Reporting this book, I've come to find that my experience is rare, but not as impossibly rare as I'd thought. Without going looking for people who'd had a C-section with inadequate pain relief, or even a traumatic birth, I met an academic, an obstetrician, an aesthetician, a teacher, and two midwives who'd had the same experience. Each time I heard this, my heart pounded with somatic recognition: you have suffered, too.

But it wasn't until I had nearly completed this book that I could locate much information about the frequency of pain during C-section. Not many researchers had collected data about it; like so much of birth, from the names of many great midwives, to the impacts of cesareans, this phenomenon wasn't recognized as sufficiently important for academic recognition or inquiry. Partly that's due to the kinds of materials available to healthcare scholars, who often rely on data drawn from insurance billing codes, or malpractice suits, to figure out how often a complication or event occurs at the population level. But insurance billing codes do not recognize pain during C-section. And because it's very difficult to win a case on the grounds of pain and suffering—or to win enough to make such a case worth litigating—such cases only rarely show up in malpractice databases. As we learned in chapter 1, "something is [only] visible when somebody recognizes it as relevant," as scholars Turrini and Bourgain write. By this measure, women's untreated and underrecognized pain is not relevant. And yet, every year, some number of people get hit by lightning.

To find out how many, Dr. Ruth Landau, an obstetric anesthesiologist and professor at Columbia, has begun to ask women directly. In our Zoom conversation, the afternoon after she'd been on call all night, Landau wore bright red lipstick and told me that the issue quite literally keeps her up at night.

For this study, Landau and colleagues surveyed 399 women who'd had C-sections about whether they'd experienced pain. She crafted questions with input from Susanna Stanford, a British woman who had pain during her cesarean and now works with anesthesiologists to research it—and raise awareness so that no other woman ever endures the same traumatic birth experience she did.

The researchers surveyed the women within hours of their cesareans. Slightly more than 10 percent of the mothers Landau and her colleagues polled (46 of 399 people) reported having pain during their C-sections. While this number was lower than expected, it remains concerning, Landau says, adding that she believes the real figure of pain during C-section to be higher, at her institution and elsewhere. One explanation for this "low" rate was that the anesthesia team knew about the study being conducted and knew that women were being surveyed about the anesthesia care they received during the operation. Everyone was focused on improving the women's experience and reducing pain during C-section—which is the researchers' overarching goal beyond the study period.

The study also looked at the medications that the women were given during the operation. A third received extra intravenous medication, including pain medication (opioids), midazolam (an antianxiety medication), dexmedetomidine (for post-op shivering), and other medications (for itching, nausea, or vomiting).

While 11 percent of women had reported intraoperative pain, an examination of the anesthesia records revealed that 15 percent had received pain medication. Some of them had not reported pain, and some women with pain did not receive pain medication. This shows a mismatch between women's experience and recall of pain and receiving pain medication, a finding that could be due to pain medication actually preventing pain (a good thing). Another possible explanation is that, though some women expressed discomfort during the surgery, which prompted the anesthesia team to give medication, the women did not actually remember the pain. A few women had received midazolam, which can wipe out a person's memory of events occurring during surgery, as the twilight sleep medications did a century ago. (About 5 percent of women received anxiety medication only, and a handful of these responded, "Not sure," when asked if they felt pain during their C-section.) Midazolam is also useful in the OR for another reason: in addition to calming anxiety, Landau explained, it shuts a person up. A quiet patient is an easy patient. But a quiet patient can still be feeling pain.

Landau is adamant about not using antianxiety medication during cesareans. In fact, she tells me, she was shocked to see how widespread its use is in the US—she was born and raised in Switzerland and attended medical school there—and instructs her residents not to use it. Birth is something that a person wants to remember, she says. And she believes other kinds of nonpharmacologic care—tone of voice, holding a mother's hand, asking her if she is okay—are essential tools physicians should use to attend to patients' anxiety. For instance, in the OR she asks mothers if they are cold and if they'd like a blanket. And while a nurse will offer to do it for her, Landau typically fetches the blanket herself. Doing this is very important, she stresses. It is part of how she cares for the patient, a way to address fear and discomfort without a pill.

When she said this, I thought about what nurse-midwife Holly Smith told me about epidurals. That perhaps the reason the epidural level in the US is so high—around 70 percent nationally, upward of 90 percent in some hospitals—is because it's indicative of a lack of other kinds of support.[21] If we were to bring the epidural level down, that would indicate not simply that mothers were refusing epidurals for the sake of feeling birth, she suggested, but that they were getting other kinds of help through labor. This support definitively matters: if they feel lonely or "unsupported," according to a recent review of studies on labor pain, mothers "report more suffering associated with their pain." By contrast, if women are supported and encouraged, they see their pain as productive.[22]

Epidurals are neither inherently good nor bad. Having had back labor, twice, I could praise God for them. And yet I would have, in some way, preferred to avoid them. I'm not alone in that; studies suggest that even though mothers may go into birth not planning to have epidurals, many end up having them nevertheless.[23] They are widely believed to slow labor down, though there isn't sufficient evidence that they do when compared with unmedicated labor. And anecdotally, according to some midwives I spoke with, they appear to reduce a baby's movements—the twisting, the shifting a baby does as it makes its way out of its mother's body—that can help make labor and birth happen (though this could also be because an epidural keeps a mother from moving very much).

In a way, we rely on epidurals as we have relied on opiates to treat chronic pain: a blanket, pharmacological approach. It's notable, in fact, that one of the researchers who developed opiates also developed epidurals. And to be sure, there are times when opiates and epidurals are essential and necessary. But it's likely that for some cases of chronic pain—as surely for some births—a person could reduce her pain, and would be better off doing so, by making use of other tools. Doula support during labor is one non-pharmacological example, and there's ample research that such care lowers C-section rates and use of epidurals, while also increasing mothers' satisfaction with labor.[24] The very idea of doulas is to implement the kind of support women had from their communities before birth transitioned to the hospital. In that sense, doulas are a modern take on what we would have if we still birthed with other women, in multigenerational communities.

But attending to women's pain could also be rectified by the simple but radical decision to ask women how they feel and to listen to the answer, as Landau's study suggests. While "more work remains to be done to see how to prevent pain and further improve women's experience," Landau wrote in an email, "at this point, setting expectations and asking women if they want to receive medication by applying 'shared decision-making' rather than having the anesthesia team make assumptions seem to be the best strategies."

During my C-section, when I told the OB, "I felt that," he responded: "You'll feel pressure." But rather than phrase that as a question—Do you feel pressure?—he assumed he knew what I felt.

My OB wasn't trying to hurt me. What he did was much more ordinary than that: he didn't ask, and when I spoke, he didn't listen. Until that point, I hadn't understood how dangerous it was to be seen as a female subject; I'd always thought of myself as a reliable narrator.

PAIN DURING C-SECTION, LANDAU TELLS me, has long been an open secret among anesthesiologists. In part that's because no one wants to be seen as being at fault or as performing poorly at their job. But there's also a reticence to share the possibility of pain because no one wants to scare women.

"You aren't supposed to mention any ghastly things to pregnant women," writes playwright Sarah Ruhl in her memoir *Smile*. "By some tacit agreement, the elders don't tell young women about all the crappy possible outcomes of pregnancy, and they certainly don't mention them to pregnant women." When I first tried to publish an essay about the pain of my C-section, I encountered that agreement explicitly; an editor at a national publication wrote me, "in this department, we aim to tell stories that help people live better lives and what happened to you seems like an outlier experience that hopefully will happen to very few other people." Kindly, but please: Shhh! You're scaring the ladies!

Another editor, another national publication, who killed a reported piece on the topic: "I just want to make sure that we have the reporting we need to make the case that this is a pervasive issue unique to women having [C-sections] that isn't getting the attention it should and, if that's the case, that we're giving women a really clear understanding of what's going on here and not just spreading fear about what could happen."

One thing about pain is that people—even good people who believe you—don't want to look directly at it. It's frightening. This kind of witnessing suggests that such pain is possible. It's similar to how in the 1950s, Israeli psychologists who were treating Holocaust survivors didn't believe some of what their patients told them. The stories were too horrific. To countenance such pain in the world means that it could happen to someone else—maybe even to you.

But avoiding public conversation about pain during childbirth can be really damaging. Not only does it expose others to the same potential hurt, but it isolates the patients who endure it. Ironically, it creates more pain.

Providers who avoid discussing the possibility of pain during C-section also—perhaps unwittingly—demonstrate the inadequacy of the informed consent process. In the UK, providers mentioning pain during C-section is standard practice, Dr. David Bogod, a retired consultant in anesthesiology who now serves as a medico-legal expert, told me. In the US, it isn't. Bogod believes, in part, that some practices don't include the possibility of pain during cesarean because of the risks of one way of dealing with it: converting to general anesthesia. General anesthesia is riskier than regional anesthesia. A mother who delivers via C-section under general is more likely to die, to lose greater quantities of blood, and to develop severe postpartum depression, requiring hospitalization.[25] As a result, "the whole discussion [of C-sections] becomes wider," says Bogod. By investigating the possibility of pain during C-section, and the subsequent need for general anesthesia, the fuller scope of the operation's potential risks—specifically ones posed to the mother—come into view.

THE LIMITS OF WHAT PAINKILLERS alone can and can't do are evident when you consider how pain is processed and experienced by the body. Western thought is dominated by a Cartesian perspective, meaning that we believe, and behave, as if the body and mind are distinct and disconnected from each other. The traditional model of pain further reinscribed this division, by assuming that a person feels pain because of "injury, inflammation, or other tissue pathology," writes Ronald Melzack, a pioneering researcher on pain.

Yet we have ample evidence that pain is far more complex, and neither entirely biological or psychological. In 2001, Melzack published a seminal article arguing for a neuromatrix model of pain, which he conceived "as a multidimensional experience produced by multiple influences." Among the sources of pain he maps are a person's "synaptic architecture"—the nervous system—which is unique, and itself "determined by genetic and sensory factors." Melzack also described how the brain, and other emotional inputs throughout the body—feeling stressed, for instance, which activates cortisol—further shape pain, by provoking biological responses. That emotional-physical relationship may work the other way around, too;

researchers have found that untreated pain in the body can lead to post-partum depression.[26]

And when it comes to childbirth, pain has still another dimension: an association with ecstasy, says Brigham and Women's Camann. That's distinct from pain that's associated with suffering: the pain of a broken arm, say. "You don't see anybody who's had a broken arm [that says], 'I'm really happy with this.' That just doesn't happen, but does happen in labor. The whole mental aspect of the suffering part makes it a different kind of pain." For that reason, the pain of childbirth is often thought to be "worth it."

But when that pain is too much—maybe because of a C-section, or another painful pregnancy complication—it consumes your soul. You can't reach the ecstasy part. Which is what the wider world often fails to countenance: It might be painful, but now that it's over, don't you feel ecstatic? This denial of the multidimensional elements and impacts of pain is itself a form of dismissal—what happened to Danielle, and to me, and to many others—that causes lasting harm.

Yet what's tricky about the complexity of the relationship among body, mind, pain, and provider, is that when women express pain, they are more likely than men to be told that the problem is in their heads. And while women in general are more likely than men to be considered unreliable and overly emotional, pregnant women are especially vulnerable to that stereotype. Even hyperemesis is still treated by some corners of the medical establishment as an emotional problem, a subconscious desire to eradicate the pregnancy, to the extent that it's treated at all. Yet part of pain really *is* mental and emotional. Which is why treating it isn't always about an analgesic.

In all, to effectively treat pain—its many dimensions—requires listening closely to the person feeling it. That's emblematic in a story that the obstetrician Nicole Calloway Rankins told me about a woman who'd come into one of her hospitals. The woman, who's Black, was in excruciating pain and near the end of her pregnancy. She'd previously gone to another hospital about her pain. The physicians there had told her she was experiencing pelvic symphysis pain, which is caused by joints separating during pregnancy. But they didn't examine her. And they told this woman—who'd been planning a birth-center birth—that only birth by C-section would help it.

Rankins asked the woman to describe her pain. She listened closely. The woman said it was around her tailbone. Then Rankins examined her and found an abscess around her rectal area. A surgeon drained it. The woman felt "miraculously better."

The story, Rankins says, shows two disturbing problems with the woman's treatment. "One, they weren't listening to what she was saying. And two, they didn't even lay hands on this woman to see where this pain was."

AFTER A FEW DAYS OF closing herself in the bathroom to pack her wound, Jenn could not take it anymore. She called the wound center at the hospital and told them she needed help. The nurse she spoke with sounded shocked that she'd been expected to care for her wound on her own, because of its complexity.

At each visit to the wound center, before anyone touched Jenn's wound, she was given a shot to numb the area. Then she lay back on an exam table, while multiple nurses and a doctor tended to her. Clearly, part of the providers' job was "to distract you," says Jenn. It worked. "I felt like it didn't hurt as much because they were talking to you during it." They also covered her with a blanket, so she wasn't exposed if someone walked in.

For the next four weeks, Jenn drove to the wound center four times a week. Cleaning and packing the wound took an hour; changing the dressing took fifteen minutes. Jenn bonded with some of the nurses, especially one who'd also recently had a baby boy. That nurse had teared up when Jenn had described what she'd had to do and how upsetting it was. Every visit after that, she and the nurse exchanged pictures of their babies. The relationship meant a lot to Jenn, she told me. It speaks to the fact that mothers—everyone, really—needs a multidimensional response to their pain, not only the numbing effects of a shot or a pill. For Jenn, this relationship gave her the opportunity to be seen as a mother rather than only a body with a problem.

After a month, Jenn's incision became infected again. She went for another round of ultrasounds, took antibiotics—every six hours, this time—and saw her OB. The OB suggested reopening half of the incision, again.

Jenn refused.

Her mother, who'd come with her to the appointment, backed her up. "No," she said. "If you're going to do that, it has to be at the hospital. Doing this in a room—it's gross, she's in so much pain. Why would you put her through that? You're going to have to put her through some kind of anesthesia—something. She's been through so much and it's not fair. She's home with two babies and dealing with this."

The OB listened. "It seems that you don't want to do this," he told them. "Why don't you wait, come back in a couple of days, and we'll see how it looks with the antibiotic." He didn't seem convinced that it would work but was willing to try.

After a few days, Jenn's wound improved. The antibiotics worked. Several weeks later, she had her last day at the wound center. She brought cupcakes and cookies, and an Easter basket for the nurse she'd bonded with—the one who'd cried with Jenn when she learned that she'd been told to pack her own wound. Then she hit a small gong, a ritual that shows that you're done with your treatment.

The physicians and nurses at the wound center, she said, "took a really traumatic experience for me and made it better. It was so hard. They were so good to me," she told me, tears running down her face. "And I didn't feel like that in my own doctors' office."

Neither of Jenn's pregnancies had been easy; the high blood pressure took a toll. And now she and Greg have four children in their blended family, which is a lot of kids. But the trauma of this birth is definitive. "After this C-section," she told me, "I never want to be pregnant again." She also has not been to the doctor since her wound healed, because she is too afraid to go back.

A year after the birth, Jenn still has stabbing pains and itching on the incision, sensations that she didn't have after her first C-section. The scar is a lot bigger, and the side where it was infected looks like a bullet wound, she says. Although Jenn has heard that her scar looks good, she disagrees. "I don't think it looks good. It looks like there's a hole in my body," she says. "I wish somebody would have said, 'It doesn't look great.'"

Such acknowledgment would confirm what she knows to be true and make her feel seen—what she's gone through, what she has to live with still. She sees the scar every day. She brings it with her wherever she goes.

In that way, the scar is a physical emblem that stands in for the other aspects of the birth that aren't visible but that have left their mark.

WHEN I FINALLY LEFT THE hospital five days after the birth, on a bright, too-warm February day, I was on such serious painkillers that I didn't feel as if I were in my own life, more as if I were watching a movie. I sat in the back of the car with my daughter and watched sunlight streaming through the leafless trees. Ostensibly, I sat back there to keep her company, but I could hardly stay awake.

At home, my friend Lisa had left a balloon tied to the porch railing. I felt too sad to look at it. Its cheer underscored my loneliness, how bizarre and terrible the birth had been. No one asked, but if they had, I would have said, I don't know if, or how, I'll ever be okay.

Sometime that day my husband picked up my prescription for Percocet. In that way, I was like most white women after childbirth: I was sent home from the hospital with more opioid painkillers than I needed. I was afraid of them, of addiction, so I stopped taking them early on.

The team that prescribed me those opioids was following protocol: uncontrolled pain after birth can cause significant, long-standing, even lifelong problems, like chronic pain. And yet the opioids did not dent the fear, terror, isolation, shame, and grief I was feeling. But I didn't have language for any of that. In fact, after the operation, and for several weeks thereafter, I mostly stopped talking. I didn't know how to speak about what had happened. I didn't even know such a thing was possible. As Sarah Ruhl wrote: "The elders don't tell young women about all the crappy possible outcomes of pregnancy."

Despite the pharmacological attention paid to my physical pain, that response was deeply inadequate. No one made me an appointment with a therapist to talk to about what I'd endured. Instead, some of the people who knew what had happened acted as if it were over, like the doula who came by, played with my daughter, and coached me: "Isn't this fun?" she asked. A few days later, at an early follow-up to investigate a greenish bruise that bloomed on my torso, the size of a softball, the physician established I didn't have an infection and left it at that.

What I needed was for someone to recognize and respond to my psychological distress: how it felt that no one had stopped the surgery to help me. Partly as a consequence, and though my physical pain eventually abated, the shock and terror never really went away. Instead, they worked their way into the tissues of my body, and into my nervous system, where they took up residence and alchemized into other problems: nervousness, touchiness, hypervigilance, jumpiness, anxiety, heart palpitations. A feeling that I was always about to get pulled over and taken away.

It's possible that neither my providers nor even my family knew how to address this aspect of my pain. Modalities like EMDR—a therapy that combines talk with embodied intervention, including rapid eye movement, meant to help the brain to reprocess traumatic memories—were not as well-known then as they are now. Maybe the moral injury I'd experienced was so shocking that my family got trapped by their own stress response: they neither fought, nor fled, but froze. Which to some degree did help, because it kept us in the present: my parents and my husband let me cry, without telling me to stop, or buck up, or feel grateful for my healthy baby, which I needed.

Those first few months our door was always open to people bringing food, washing dishes, holding the baby, keeping me company, helping with breastfeeding, delivering gifts. It could have been a slow-unfolding party. But I was too hurt to experience it this way. I'd stopped crying all the time, but I wasn't better. I'd gone numb. My physical pain was passing—it bothered me, but I could live with it. But no one addressed the fear I'd experienced at being abandoned on that table. And this fear of abandonment in a medical setting—despite all of the therapy, and the conversations with friends and family, and writing this book—is still with me. The PCA pump, the opiates I was prescribed—none of that could touch it. It wasn't meant to.

One day after we'd been home for a few weeks, I felt a moment of insight when I realized that, with people always coming and going, my house was like a shiva house. I told this to my husband. Like, *I get it now!* I couldn't understand why that seemed puzzling to him, when it felt so true to me. I see now that at the time he didn't know what or who had died. Though he'd been there, he didn't understand what damage the pain, and the denial of that pain, had caused. That would come later, once I'd relearned to speak.

10

C-SECTIONS AND POSTPARTUM MOOD DISORDERS

THE EDINBURGH POSTNATAL DEPRESSION SCALE (EPDS) IS A TEN-ITEM questionnaire typically administered to mothers during their third trimester and at their six-week postnatal visit.[1] It has been translated into more than sixty languages and is the most common method of screening mothers for postnatal depression in the world.[2]

The questionnaire includes statements such as "I have been anxious or worried for no good reason," "I have felt scared or panicky for no very good reason," and "I have blamed myself unnecessarily when things went wrong." In response, one must answer "no, never" or "no, not at all"; "hardly ever" or "not very often"; "yes, sometimes"; or "yes, most of the time." Each of these answers earns a point value: 0 for no, never, or no; up to 3 for yes, most of the time. The highest possible score is 30. A score of 12 or 13 is the widely recommended cutoff point to identify people with severe depression.

The idea of using a questionnaire to identify depression is simple, even elegant. In that way it resembles another attempt to quantify and visualize an experience that's subjective and internal: pain. And according to studies of its efficacy, the Edinburgh Postnatal Depression Scale does a decent job of identifying mothers with postpartum depression, catching about three out of four mothers experiencing these difficulties—at least in English-speaking countries.

But the EDPS's tidiness belies the messiness of its application. First, although the United States Preventive Services Task Force recommends that all pregnant and postpartum women be screened for depression, not everyone is.[3] Only 40 percent of mothers attend their six-week appointment, and not all who do are assessed.[4] Nor is there widespread agreement about what cutoff to use to refer someone for treatment. Set the cutoff too high, and you'll miss people, especially if they're high functioning. Too low, and you'll expose people to medications they don't need, or ensnare people who are okay, with potentially disastrous results. For instance, when the state of California began instituting these mandated questionnaires, providers called 911, as one mother recounted. The country's inadequate care for people with mental illness, coupled with deeply entrenched white supremacy, means that in some settings, mothers who confess to these feelings—particularly if they are Black—risk having their babies removed from their care.[5]

But depression isn't the only way that mothers' mental health can be affected postpartum. Other postpartum mood disorders include anxiety, psychosis, and post-traumatic stress disorder. And while the scale can identify people with anxiety, it doesn't differentiate between anxiety and depression.[6] (Anxiety can also be hard to spot because it can be hard to distinguish from, say, doing lots of research and asking a lot of questions, which can feel "normal," one obstetrician pointed out to me.) The scale also does a poor job at identifying people suffering from PTSD because of their birth, in part because such symptoms don't necessarily crop up by six weeks.

Despite the scale's having been substantiated by research, many communities, particularly communities of color, say that the language of the questions does not resonate with how mothers would describe their feelings. Black mothers, for instance, may say "they be snapping out," licensed social worker and lactation consultant Jabina Coleman pointed out at her talk on perinatal mood disorders at the Perinatal Health Equity Initiative's New Jersey Birth Equity Conference. It's essential to consider who validated the language in EDPS, she said, and among what groups. Likewise, it's important to note that different communities may find it more or less acceptable to even express such feelings.

There also isn't an established, standardized protocol of what to do with or about these scores, or even with a response other than "never" to question ten: "The thought of harming myself has occurred to me." In that way, what happens after a person scores positively for a postpartum mood disorder largely depends on her provider's judgment and knowledge of mental health resources; what resources exist; and whether the mother can access medication, psychotherapy, inpatient or outpatient care, or other interventions—a big "if" in a country with virtually no universal postpartum support. And while access to therapy and psychiatry has improved since the pandemic, with insurance companies now covering video therapy, for example, access is still difficult for many mothers, particularly women who are low-income or on Medicaid. A critical lack of Black providers also complicates Black women's access to mental health providers—even among women who have insurance.

As a metaphor for how inadequate perinatal mental healthcare can be, I thought of the purported communication protocol for Bernie Madoff's Ponzi scheme. His company phone number, my friend Rebecca G told me, would ring to a phone in an empty room in Riverdale. I kept picturing this phone, its ring echoing off empty walls, not even a voicemail picking up. To some degree, this is what can happen after screening positive for a perinatal mental health problem. A provider might try to call to get resources for a mother who needs help, but there is no apparatus, no single organization or agency, designated to pick up the phone—which means that in some places, because of our country's paucity of mental health resources, there is no one on the other end of the line.

ALTHOUGH THERE HAS BEEN MENTION of psychological distress during and after pregnancy since antiquity, the first study about postpartum depression (PPD) did not appear until 1968. Brice Pitt, a British psychiatrist who'd personally struggled with depression,[7] was inspired to research it by a health visitor—a woman, unnamed, tasked by the National Health Service to check in at home on mothers who'd recently birthed. She approached Pitt with the observation that she often "found newly-delivered mothers to be depressed." She wanted to know "why this happened and how to give help," Pitt later wrote.[8] So he launched a study assessing mothers' depression at the start of the third trimester and then again, six to eight weeks after birth. He developed a questionnaire because his team did not have enough time to interview the mothers. The questions evolved. The format stuck.

Pitt found that most mothers showed more signs of depression after birth than before—even women whose scores didn't climb to depressive levels. In that sense, his findings demonstrated the impact of a new baby, the hard-won wisdom of all new parents: that there's joy alongside hardship in this most profound and irrevocable transition. And he found that about 10 percent of the new mothers surveyed developed postpartum mood disorders, though he believed that to be an underestimate. The data are similar now, in the US, though some estimates put the figure at one in seven new mothers.[9]

The detached language in Pitt's study is striking: how straight it is, how plainspoken, how clean his outsider's take on the up-and-down feelings: "Mood was often labile." Labile, from the Latin *labi*,[10] which means "to slip or fall." That hell most often strikes at night: "Any diurnal variation took the form of greater distress in the evenings." The punishing self-talk: "Guilt was mainly confined to self-reproach over not loving or caring enough for the baby." Reading this seminal paper, I thought, this is why we need what writer Jazmina Barrera calls the literature of motherhood, to animate the clinical description of the terror, the chaos, the absolute invertedness of the postpartum period. Here, for instance, is Pitt on the estrangement from who you once were, that former self racked on the shoals: "Many felt quite changed from their usual selves, and most had never been depressed like this before."[11] Put another way, from Rachel Cusk's *The Bradshaw Variations*—a husband's take on his wife after she gave birth: "He remembers the way her old life died, went over the cliff and smashed itself on the rocks, unfinished."[12] Because even if one doesn't develop a perinatal mood disorder, being postpartum contorts the mind.

I remember becoming convinced after my son's birth that Bruce Springsteen's song "Dancing in the Dark" was actually about postpartum motherhood. I listened to it on repeat and did a close analysis of its lyrics ("I ain't nothin' but tired / Man, I'm just tired and bored with myself / Hey there, baby, I could use just a little help").[13] Yeah, it was funny, but I was also really sure of what I'd recognized, this deep truth about Bruce Springsteen's hit song hiding in plain sight—but also the real truth about being postpartum. I remember believing that I needed to share my newfound insight with the world. I called several friends and shared my analysis with them with great excitement. They humored me ("That's great!" "That's funny!") and still I felt misunderstood. I needed to be seen, and I couldn't understand why no one else seemed as convinced as I was by my vision about the song, which really was an indirect way for me to talk about how I was feeling.

At the time of Pitt's study, postpartum depression was as common as it was overlooked. "It is well known that women are often depressed after child-birth, but only those ill enough to be admitted to hospital have received much study," Pitt wrote.[14] It is a similar situation today; maternal deaths grab the headlines, for these are the absolute worst-case outcomes. But there is a wide spectrum of life, of experience, of mothers sort of hitching along, dragging themselves and their babies onward, between the extremes of thriving and death. Some of these mothers have full-blown postpartum depression; others are having a difficult time. Taken together, these stories receive little attention. They are complex problems without tidy answers, though some of the potential solutions would cost money or attention that the US has largely been unwilling to spend on mothers and children.

So while there are many stories devoted to maternal mortality that showcase the fatal impacts of mistreated physical problems like hemorrhage and preeclampsia, they belie the fact that mental health is actually a leading cause of pregnancy-related deaths. Suicide accounts for one out of five postpartum deaths, a surprisingly high number given how little public attention these deaths command.[15] Despite the Cartesian certainty that the mind and the body are distinct, as this data demonstrates so devastatingly, when it comes to new mothers' lives, they could not be more interdependent.

THE CONVENTIONAL WISDOM ABOUT POSTPARTUM mood disorders is that they are caused by hormones: that estrogen and progesterone plummet after birth, causing psychiatric symptoms. Or, as psychiatrist and associate professor at Mt. Sinai School of Medicine Thalia Robakis puts it, "'The hormones be making the ladies crazy.'" Robakis, who holds an MD and PhD in neurobiology from Columbia University's Vagelos College of

Physicians and Surgeons, explains that researchers were so convinced of this relationship between hormones and psychiatric symptoms that they spent two decades trying to prove it was so. But the results from these efforts have been "zero across the board." Consequently, we have "twenty years of negative data. People couldn't believe the answers, so they kept asking the question over and over again," she says. "And the answer is no."

I ask if researchers kept pursuing the relationship between hormones and psychiatric symptoms because of long-standing beliefs that women are hysterical. We were talking over Zoom on a bright spring morning. Dr. Robakis put up her hands in a frustrated *Yup maybe* shrug. (After our talk, I'd realize that I had my blouse on inside out. "You're researching motherhood," a friend joked, "and so you're living motherhood as praxis.")

The reality is that hormone shifts *do* play a role in postpartum mood disorders, Robakis says, but likely only in a small subset of women, perhaps around 12 percent of mothers (though she clarifies that, to her knowledge, there's no good way to establish this other than through careful interviewing and with hormonal treatment, and that the actual number may be higher). But even among this group, it isn't the "absolute level of the hormone" but the mothers' "cellular response" to the rapid changes in progesterone and estrogen, she says. These mothers may develop severe mental illness, such as bipolar spectrum disorders, because their cells do not tolerate the precipitous hormonal drop. But that's a very different mechanism, she explains, than hormone levels specifically causing psychiatric symptoms.

For the bulk of mothers with postpartum mood disorders—as with psychiatric illness in general—the causes are "multifactorial. It's not all one thing," says Robakis. Postpartum depression and anxiety are caused by stressors including "lifestyle changes, sleep deprivation, role transition," and the availability—or lack thereof—of social support. As further evidence of this, Robakis points out that the incidence of postpartum mood disorders varies "quite a lot interculturally." It is highest in low- and middle-income countries where women have very little economic or social power, she says, and lower where there is more social support. That "suggests we could make more progress [preventing and reducing postpartum mood disorders] by having more types of psychosocial supports" during pregnancy and postpartum, she says.

Yet in the US, Robakis points out, we exhibit a "total refusal to acknowledge the life-changing nature [of birth] and enormous demand required to sustain new and entirely helpless life. We treat it like some kind of short-term medical condition, as if you were to break your wrist. You have to be out to recover for four weeks, then you come back four weeks later with a sling." Similarly, new mothers are told to come back in four weeks, to simply "'Get a nanny, get a day care.' It's so at odds with the reality of the life transformation of having a baby."

"Our cultural expectation is that you'll be sad and depressed," says Dalecia Young, a doula in Anchorage. As an exercise, Dalecia says, Google the word 'postpartum.'" In the pages of search results, she asks, how far do you have to go to get to something that's not postpartum depression? In such a climate, why would a person go looking for help, she says, "if it's normal to be sad?" Perhaps this expectation is another reason I didn't get more help postpartum. What happened to me was extreme, but lots of women come out of birth feeling sad.

While this type of depression or anxiety can be debilitating and impair a mother's relationship with her baby, it's important to point out that it differs from severe mental illness after birth. The latter, Robakis says, may be a biological response that we cannot prevent. "I'm not sure that better supports might change that." But better support for the vast majority of people who are somewhere in the middle, between thriving and severely ill, would indeed make a difference.

PITT'S 1968 STUDY OF PPD found no statistically significant difference in the rates of depression between vaginal and cesarean birth.[16] Some recent studies haven't found a difference, either, asserting that it's the meaning-making of the birth that matters, whether a mother found the birth to be a "negative" experience. "Trauma really is in the eye of the beholder," affirms Renee Racik, a Washington-based perinatal mental health counselor and doula with more than twenty years of experience. Sometimes, at a birth, she thinks, "'Oh my God, this person is going to be so traumatized, they had [every intervention] under the sun.'" But in talking with her clients she tries to be "neutral and see how they felt about it. Sometimes they would not be traumatized the way I was."

At the same time, there is some research that has found that C-sections do increase the likelihood of postpartum depression, particularly if the cesareans weren't planned.[17] Still others slice the data even further, finding that it's specifically mothers who had a cesarean for nonreassuring fetal heart tones who were more likely to develop postpartum depression.[18]

In some of this research, the increased risk of PPD is anywhere from twice to more than three times as likely for C-section moms than for mothers who had a vaginal birth. At a personal level, this makes sense. No matter why a mother has an unexpected cesarean, it simply wasn't the plan. It was probably stressful and may have been frightening. And that unexpected operation creates other unexpected difficulties: a longer stay in the hospital, more follow-up medical appointments, and potentially more pain, some of which are also factors that increase the likelihood of postpartum depression. There's also the stress, uncertainty, and frustration of being debilitated, even temporarily, by an unplanned cesarean. And there's virtually no standard post-op physical or occupational therapy about how to complete daily tasks like diapering, dishwashing, or laundry.

Still, it's worth pointing out that one of the best predictors of postpartum mood disorders is preexisting mental illness. Like any chronic health condition, leaving it untreated during pregnancy only spells more potential problems after birth.

Reading studies about postpartum mood disorders and C-sections, with their well-intentioned conclusions—heartfelt pabulum along the lines of "further research is needed to see how clinicians can do a better job of helping mothers"—I kept thinking of the cascade of consequences, the changes set in motion after a C-section, that receive little attention compared to the cascade of interventions. "Would it help if mothers who'd had unplanned C-sections had the chance to see a provider right away, to help them process the birth? Like a psychiatric first responder?" I ask Robakis. In theory, she says, sure. But preventive care in psychiatry is tough. "You run into funding and access issues. And we can't even fund interventive care for people who are already suffering." In such a climate, "trying to figure out who's at risk, and prepare them, is challenging."

I offer that I've found it useful, personally, when therapists have suggested a reframing of past events, or alternative ways to understand them—highlighting that I did try to advocate for myself, for instance, when I had my baby. Robakis notes that that is most effective when the reframing comes from the person, not the therapist.

"Okay, but are there resources like that?" I ask. "Soon after birth? Someone with whom a person could share their birth stories, who could help them see aspects that might not otherwise be visible?"

There isn't, she acknowledges, but maybe there should be. "People have an enormous need to work through their birth story, even if it was a good one. Everyone comes in and needs to go over it, and get it out, and make sense of it," she says. And while she's typically seeing people who are struggling, Robakis notes that even mothers who are "feeling well usually have a need to process their birth stories." Nevertheless, in a traditional postpartum appointment, there isn't much space to do so.

"Emplotment" is what historian Hayden White called this process: putting nonfiction events into a storyline, so that they form a complete narrative.[19] He was writing about history, and how in affixing a narrative structure to real events from the past, historians effectively fictionalize what's happened. The narrative structure itself demands this; real life isn't a story, but we sort and structure its telling as if it were, to give it shape and meaning. And the generic storytelling structures we've built, like the tragedy, comedy, or the epic, further shape our understanding of these pasts, by providing a container for them—that is, by turning them into one or another type of story from which to extract a moral: Here is a lesson of caution, or here is a lesson of heroism. Here is a lesson of buffoonery. Here is what a challenge or a villain or a hero looks like.

The archetype of American birth is well-known: your water breaks, you rush into a taxi, huff and puff at the hospital, out comes the baby. It's the result of emplotment that leaves out so much, an epic without an implied hero: the mother. Perhaps what we need is less emplotment. A story that doesn't begin in labor, but during pregnancy, when you are a cyborg-like, not-one-but-not-two person. And a different kind of narrative structure to hold our births. Certainly nothing like the American archetype. Messier, more like a dream, maybe, with elements from all the classic genres—comedy, epic, tragedy. Not an airtight narrative. And, therefore, a much truer tale than the current American master narrative holds it out to be.

ONE OF THE BIGGEST PROBLEMS standing in the way of better postpartum care is how poorly insurance reimburses for it. Under Medicaid and most private insurance, prenatal visits, birth, and postpartum care are typically bundled into a global payment that a doctor receives after the baby's birth. In these bundles, postpartum care consists of a single, six-week visit. That means unless a person has a specific diagnosis, like an infection, a physician or midwife isn't reimbursed for an additional postpartum visit. "If we want to make a living then we have to do volume. And if we have to do volume, that means I don't have enough time in my day to focus on postpartum women. They come for their six-week checkup, they get their birth control, and they're out the door," says Dr. Clara Surowitz, the obstetrician in Lakewood, New Jersey, whose 3 percent C-section rate is the lowest in the state. "So all of the things that come up, like pelvic pain and postpartum depression and anxiety and nursing problems and all these things, they just do not get addressed."

Increasing the amount Medicaid reimbursed would help; in New Jersey, a doctor's typical reimbursement rate for nine months of prenatal care, birth, and a postpartum visit is only $2,500. So would reconceiving the postpartum period as the fourth trimester, and holding insurance companies accountable for reimbursing multiple visits besides the six-week checkup along the way, as initiatives such as UNC's 4th Trimester Project are doing.

Postpartum visits from other providers, like doulas, are another potential solution. Yet stingy compensation for doulas appears to be a feature of the majority of new state bills aimed at using Medicaid to cover them. "In states such as New York, prenatal and postpartum visits (which average about 2 hours per visit) are reimbursed at $30 per visit," writes Dr. S. Michelle Ogunwole and her colleagues in a 2022 paper on these proposed laws.[20] Doulas are limited to eight visits total; for working at a birth, they're paid $360. Taken together, according to this framework, "the maximum a doula can earn for services spanning multiple months is $600." Such fees do not constitute a living wage, which makes it difficult to recruit and sustain a diverse doula workforce.

There are other, even simpler ways to reduce stress during pregnancy and the postpartum period, which can help to prevent or reduce postpartum mood disorders. Most basically: giving pregnant and postpartum people money. The Healthy Baby Prenatal Benefit in Manitoba, launched in 2001, gives low-income pregnant mothers up to $81.41 CAD in their second and third trimesters.[21] This modest sum prevented very low birth weights by 19 percent; prematurity by 17 percent; and shortened mothers' hospital stays following vaginal birth, all factors that can increase the likelihood of postpartum depression.[22] The way that money works isn't magic: "I was getting the $80 a month [check], which was totally the difference of me eating or not, so that helped tremendously," one mother who received the income told reporters.[23] Like pain, financial strain narrows the sky of the possible. All you can focus on is how you're going to pay for that next box of diapers.

Similar initiatives are underway in San Francisco and Philadelphia; in 2024, the latter will be enrolling 250 mothers in a guaranteed income pilot program based in three neighborhoods with very low birth weights.[24] The women will receive $1,000 a month, either through a reloadable debit card or direct deposit, during the second and third trimesters of pregnancy and for the first year of parenthood. They'll also be able to choose from a "menu of voluntary supports, if they would like them or not: doulas, lactation support, a safe sleep program that gives out pack and plays, financial counseling," says Dr. Stacey Kallem, director of the Philadelphia Department of Public Health's Division of Maternal, Child, and Family Health. But mothers aren't required to take part in those supports. "The whole point is guaranteed income is unconditional—it's not asking you to do anything." Critically, and because the program was designed with community members, it isn't just for people under the federal poverty line. Even people above that threshold, Kallem says, "still aren't making enough to get by and thrive and raise a family in Philadelphia."

The standard critique is that free money will entice people to have babies. Kallem said that she heard such feedback during a recent press conference. She responded by emphasizing the program's evidence-based conceptual model: extra money during pregnancy will help reduce stress and prematurity; it addresses social determinants of health, like housing and nutrition, though it cannot solve them. These are all sound reasons for the program and the only way for a government agency to respond to such criticism. But as I kept thinking of this critique, playing it in my head, I also thought: *But so what? So what if this kind of support will inspire people to have more babies? And equip them to better be able to care for them?*

Drill down far enough, and any negative response to that shows what we might call a eugenic mind-set: what types of people deserve to have more children; whose children benefit society; what kind of person we want more of. If you then take the perspective that the parents are irresponsible, that the reason they need this support is they can't handle their money, you'll confront another damaging myth: that the people in poverty are poor because it's their fault; that if they don't want to be poor, all they have to do is work, or work harder. But as the evidence on pregnancy and postpartum mood disorders demonstrates, adding stress—say, by requiring mothers to go back to work—doesn't really help anyone. Certainly not mothers or their babies, who are shown to benefit physically and emotionally from paid parental leave.

IN *BEING MORTAL: MEDICINE AND What Matters in the End*, Atul Gawande writes movingly and persuasively about the utility and comforts of hospice and palliative care that enable people to die at home. It's a tempting model for birth, too, that other gateway. But it seems unlikely that American mothers will embrace home birth en masse, because of the financial imperative—one might say necessity—to birth in the hospital. Then there's our broad embrace of epidurals, with about 70 percent of mothers opting for one during labor, which isn't achievable at home or in a birth center.[25]

But birth's setting in the hospital, and the fact that the vast majority of providers don't see mothers in their homes, exacerbates the gulf between what physicians see and the messy, leaky, and exhausting reality of recovering from an unexpected operation while also caring for a new baby. As an example, back at home after my daughter's birth, I couldn't find underwear that I could comfortably wear with my incision. I'd been reusing the three mesh pairs I'd come home with from the hospital. They were bloodstained. They smelled. I felt embarrassed to ask my husband to wash them. But I couldn't—I couldn't even get out of bed alone.

To be unable to clothe yourself in such a basic and intimate way makes the rest of the world come to a stop. Yet when I went to the doctor to check my stitches, I never mentioned this drama, which colored the arc of my days. Nor did he ask how I was getting on with such quotidian tasks as getting dressed. I mean, I was wearing clothes, right? I don't know that he would have even had advice if I'd told him about the underwear problem. And I probably would have felt embarrassed if he had asked. But he certainly would have been more likely to have found out about it if he'd come to my home—if he'd sat with me on the sofa or visited me in my bed, where I spent most of my time.

My mother is the one who solved this. She ordered a pack of the hospital-mesh variety underwear, which in my whacked-out state never crossed my mind as a possibility—that these underwear exist and can be purchased by people who aren't in the hospital. She knew to do this because I told her about it. Besides her, I don't know who I would have told.

Likewise for breastfeeding. Isolated at home, mothers don't have support about how to learn to breastfeed—which can be daunting for any new mother, but can be especially difficult for C-section mothers, who are less likely to initiate breastfeeding than mothers who birth vaginally. Compounding matters, C-section mothers' milk may also come in later than mothers who birth vaginally, a lag that researchers speculate may be due to maternal stress, or less oxytocin, which is thought to "impair" the "hormone pathway" needed to develop the capacity to secrete milk.[26] Breastfeeding plays a role in postpartum depression: mothers who have postpartum depression wean earlier than mothers who don't. But depression can compound isolation, making it even harder to leave the house to get help.

Postpartum home visits are typical after a birth-center birth, or from a home-birth midwife. But even keeping birth in the hospital, home visits are initiatives we can feasibly adopt, akin to the National Health Service's health visitor program that launched contemporary academic inquiry into postpartum depression. New Jersey, which has one of the nation's highest rates of maternal mortality, is initiating one such program: totally voluntary, up to three visits in three months, for everyone—regardless of insurance.[27]

However, the design of this program is potentially problematic. It is set to be housed in the department of Children and Family Services, which administers the state's foster care system. And nurses are mandated reporters. Evidence shows that Black mothers are far more likely to be referred to social services than white mothers. "Not everyone knows what it means to be a guest," professor and interim associate dean at the University of Washington Monica McLemore pointed out in a talk she gave at the New Jersey Birth Equity Conference. She suggests, instead, a space in the community where people can come to have those visits, rather than in their homes.

THERE ARE MANY MODELS OF how to offer culturally appropriate postpartum care that makes mothers feel safe, while providing the kind of care that can help some mothers to stave off, or recover from, postpartum mood disorders. In China and India, women may stay at home while their mothers, families, or hired caregivers cook and care for them. Australia, Israel, South Korea, China, and other countries also have new-baby hotels that include nurseries for babies, lactation support, meals, and cleaning services. These range from basic to luxurious properties, with varying degrees of governmental recognition and support. In Israel, which has socialized medicine, the government will in some cases pay for three nights at a basic mother-baby hotel, for example. And in Australia, some private health insurance programs will pay for new mothers—with the blessing of their obstetricians—to transfer from the hospital to a nearby luxury hotel, where midwives are available twenty-four hours a day.[28]

Boram Postnatal Retreat, a new, high-end mother-baby hotel in Manhattan, offers similar care: food, lactation support, housekeeping, massages, a nursery for the babies so mothers can sleep. The cheapest prepackaged visit is $2700 for three nights, or $900 a night, a price tag that makes it easy to dismiss as a luxury for the privileged. But the care and respite are protective; they can help prevent a woman from developing postpartum depression in part because they guard a new mother's sleep. Thalia Robakis says that, depending on severity, her first-line recommendation for clients with postpartum mood disorders is to develop a sleep-protection plan—to outsource one feeding to someone else so that the mother can have at least a five-hour stretch of sleep at night. (In retrospect, one reason I didn't develop PPD is probably because after several weeks of not sleeping and trying to nurse, my husband and mother took turns feeding the baby at night with pumped milk or formula, while I slept.)

And although Boram has been described as the first hotel of its kind in the US, Kimpatorin (from the Yiddish term referring to a woman who has recently given birth) homes in the States, Austria, the UK, Australia, and other countries with Haredi Jewish communities have been providing this support for many years, if less luxuriously. Like Boram, these mother-baby hotels have nurseries, food, lactation support, and community. Some only allow women; others permit men to visit. They eschew traditional advertising—or virtually any advertising—subsisting mostly on word of mouth. Representatives from one hotel didn't want to be interviewed because of the ways that Haredi communities are often stereotyped in the mainstream media (to wit: the word *Haredi* comes from the verb "to tremble"—as in, to tremble before God—but these communities are often called ultra-Orthodox, which connotes fundamentalism). And while the woman I talked with wouldn't share how much the hotel charges, she said, "It's not like the Boram [costs]—I can tell you that."

Dina Shalom, who works as an NHS dentist in Manchester, in the UK, stayed at a Kimpatorin hotel in Llandudno, Wales, following the birth of her third child. The hotel is a big country house overlooking the sea in North Wales. Food is provided, as is the washing up. Staff care for babies in a nursery, bringing them to mothers if they want to nurse, or feeding them formula or pumped milk. It's also free; if it hadn't been, Shalom says, she wouldn't have gone. Yet the rest is transformative, particularly if people have other children at home: "I went purely to sleep," she told me. "There is no other demand of you. That's the whole point." And because the only other people there are also new mothers, there's a social aspect to it as well—if you want.

The problem with a high-end option like Boram is that it's an uber-capitalist response to a problem that maybe isn't best addressed by capitalism, but instead by the interdependence fostered by community, as Angela Garbes points out in her 2022 book *Essential Labor*. During the pandemic, mutual aid programs emerged and came to prominence—such as community fridges stocked with free food or raising funds for people behind on their rent. Mutual aid is one of the best parts of living in a religious community; in Lakewood, the Haredi Jewish community where

Surowitz lives, people donate money to a community pot, and then when it's their turn to need it, they get the help they need for free: housecleaning, people dropping off meals, a high school student who comes to help with the older children. It is easy to dismiss this kind of support by saying, well, in traditional religious societies, women's reproductive value is so highly prized that of course they're going to make birth nicer. It's similar to how easy it is to brush off a service like Boram as a privilege for the wealthy. The truth is, secular society can learn from the interdependence that religious communities foster. Particularly when it comes to childbirth—a matrix of complex, human needs that capitalism, and technology, can't solve alone. Meeting these basic needs reduces a mother's stress, which in turn may help to soften or reduce postpartum mood disorders.

When I talked to Dina Shalom about what the postpartum period looks like in the US, she audibly gasped. No health visitors; no midwifery visits; no paid leave. "It's barbaric," she said. "It shouldn't be expected. How are women putting up with it?" For that matter, she wondered, "How do people even have children?"

11

VBAC

STARTING AT THE VERY BEGINNING OF MY SECOND PREGNANCY, I
worried that I would die. *Possibly I'm afraid of death because part of me died
when I had C,* I wrote to a friend. Even though I'd revived, or recovered,
or reawoken in the same body, that most material evidence of my survival,
I didn't fully believe it to be true. I see now that I felt as if I'd irretrievably
lost my "self." This can happen to people who are traumatized, but I didn't
know that. Nor did I know that I could—and would—recover it.

From the beginning, I also worried far more about my own life than
about my baby's. This uneven worry manifested most intensely when I
thought about whether to try for a VBAC or to schedule a repeat cesarean. I understood the choice between the two as choosing whose life to
prioritize. That's because, statistically speaking, a VBAC was safer for me.
Its chief risk is uterine rupture, an unlikely but potentially catastrophic
outcome that occurs in less than 1 percent of births (and slightly higher
among mothers who've had two cesareans).[1] About 5 percent of uterine
ruptures result in the baby's death, so small a group that it is difficult to
study.[2] By contrast, a repeat cesarean carried all of the risks of a second
operation to me—needing a blood transfusion, dealing with an infection,
to say nothing of unbridled pain or death—but was safer for the baby.

Though I had absolute clarity that my life was most important, I was
ambivalent about saying so out loud. An essay by the writer Ayelet Waldman had made the rounds a few years earlier, about how she loved her
husband more than her children. "An awkward fallout lingered," Nathan
Heller wrote in the *New Yorker,* including a "gauntlet of domestic criti-

cism, hate mail, and [*The Oprah Winfrey Show.*]"³ My feelings about my upcoming birth were even more scandalous, I thought: I loved myself more than my child.

My mother, not a synagogue-going person (one rabbi from the synagogue we attended jokingly told her she had "unlimited cuts" for skipping services), told me that the Talmud would agree with me when it came to prioritizing my life over my baby's. Indeed, in Jewish law, "the woman's life always takes the precedent until the child is born," Shana Schick, the Bar-Ilan University lecturer, said—as the Talmud demonstrates in its description of embryotomy. In fact, there's no question about whether it's permissible to kill a baby to save its mother's life. "Before it's born, it's not a nefesh," or soul, she said. It only becomes a soul when it takes its first breath. At the same time, she explained, the fetus isn't a nothing; there are midrashim that teach that it learns all of the Torah while the mother is pregnant, only to forget it at birth. What I wish I could have seen, at the time, about this interpretation of pregnancy, is that the US's prevailing medico-legal understanding of the fetus—one that awards it rights equal to or even surpassing its mother's—is neither universal nor inevitable, nor is it the product of my own culture.

TO BE SURE, I DID feel better having God on my side. That gave me ethical and religious cover. But I would have prioritized my own life nevertheless, so much so that it was almost embarrassing how set I was on exercising my bodily autonomy. I was already a mother and thus schooled in the maternal expectations of acting as the lifeguard, the vessel, the guardrail. I understood why maternity clothes so often resemble silly-printed baby clothes: you are not supposed to have an identity separate from the baby; you are to subsume your identity to the baby. Knowing all of this, to voluntarily take on a risk for my next baby seemed outlandish, improper.

The research I did about VBAC only amplified those feelings. I learned that it wasn't always easy to find a provider who'd support VBAC, or even access a hospital that would tolerate such a birth. Many resources emphasized the potential for VBAC to go wrong and cause a disastrous outcome for the baby, without getting into the bad things that a repeat C-section might cause. In online support groups, women in my same position questioned how a person could possibly take a risk like uterine rupture. How selfish, some said, when you could just schedule a cesarean. Earning a "vag badge" couldn't possibly matter that much. Against such declarations, my desire to prioritize my own life seemed shameful and wrong, a violation of the basic tenet of maternity, and one into which I had already been inculcated: *I exist to protect you.*

These concerns bled into my marriage. I asked my husband if he would blame me, or think me selfish, if I had a uterine rupture and the baby died or was brain damaged. He told me that this was a decision we were making together. That he wouldn't blame me. That he loved me. I knew he meant this. But I also knew that you can't predict a response to tragedy. It was like motherhood. You couldn't possibly know how you'd respond, what it would feel like, until you got there yourself.

Toward the end of my first trimester, news of a novel coronavirus started making headlines. By the middle of my second trimester, it had reached New York. My brother and my mother both contracted the virus early on and became severely ill. Already afraid of dying, I believed that if I caught COVID it would finish me. I started my lockdown early, canceling classes before my university did, avoiding supermarkets, and postponing a prenatal appointment. When I was twenty-six weeks pregnant, then-governor Cuomo announced that mothers in New York State must birth alone.

Throughout the pregnancy I'd had recurrent dreams that I was lost in a hospital's subterranean parking lot. It was dark, I was alone, and I would never get out. Cuomo's ruling seemed to confirm the spirit of these nightmares; when I pictured my husband dropping me off at the hospital to have the baby, I didn't think I would be able to get out of the car. Birth alone was something I could not survive. I sat at the kitchen table and wept. And I told my husband that I wanted an abortion.

"As a society we have a tendency to measure motherhood, not in extended narratives, but by a set of signal moments that we interpret as emblematic summations of women's mothering abilities," writes philosopher Quill Rebecca Kukla. "These 'defining moments' tend to come very early in the mothering narrative—indeed many of them come during pregnancy or even before conception."[4] By this measure my thoughts and needs, my mother-character, had failed the ultimate test. But it was one of the most true moments of my motherhood. I wanted my baby, and I valued my own life more than my baby's—so absolutely that I would end his life to protect my own.

At the time, I experienced these intense feelings as my own set of problems to work through. I had to get my head together, I told myself. Friends made similar comments: It's a mental game, they counseled. Don't lose your nerve. This was true, but also, only partially so. I'd fallen into a similar trap during my first pregnancy: doing birth correctly seemed to be my responsibility; I just had to make the right choices. Though I'd already started thinking about writing this book, I didn't see the resemblance between this pregnancy and my first one. I was too overcome by my anger: the C-section felt like a never-ending problem with ceaseless complications. I couldn't just be pregnant, then go into labor and have the baby; I had to have a plan for how the end of pregnancy would go.

What I didn't see was that the feelings I was having—guilt about exercising bodily autonomy—reflected the US's ongoing and intensifying cultural and legal battle for fetal rights. I didn't see that questions about whose life, and whose body, commands greatest value, about who is entitled to make decisions about these bodies, are at stake in all conversations related to reproduction, from abortion to access to midwifery to VBAC.

In that way, though VBAC may seem like a niche issue, one that affects only a small subset of women—the nearly four hundred thousand mothers in the US each year who've already had a C-section and go on to have another baby—it lays bare the restrictions and obstacles that encircle all pregnant women, no matter where, or whether, they plan to see their babies to the other side.[5] In other words, what I had experienced as an entirely private matter had very much been shaped by the ways that we talk about, legislate, and control reproduction. But I was at once too angry, and too deeply inculcated within this ideology, to see this at the time. Instead, in the moment, I longed for an escape. I wished to God I could just skip the birth part.

AT THE NATIONAL AND STATE levels, VBAC is legal. But a patchwork of official and tacit restrictions in virtually every state makes it difficult and, in some places, effectively impossible to try for one. According to a study by the International Cesarean Awareness Network from 2011, the most recent year for which information is available, about 1 in 5 hospitals refuse to permit VBAC, an estimated 800 of 4,500 hospitals.[6] These hospitals cluster in the southern and rural parts of the country—places where, even before Roe's overturn, it was also difficult to have an abortion. Thus, as with abortion, the potential to VBAC is only a "symbolic" possibility given that, on a practical level, not all people can access it.[7]

Hospitals defend so-called VBAC bans out of a stated concern that they don't have the personnel available—obstetricians, anesthesiologists—to do an immediate cesarean, should a person attempting a VBAC need one because of uterine rupture. Others only permit VBAC in mothers with a "proven pelvis": a mother who's already had a prior vaginal birth, which makes a subsequent vaginal birth more likely. Then there are physicians who refuse to attend VBACs, because they prefer to do repeat cesareans out of convenience or perceived safety; because they haven't seen VBAC that often or have learned that it is dangerous; or because they are frightened of the legal implications of VBAC that goes poorly. As we've learned, medical malpractice lawsuits highly favor harms committed against babies. In this way, too, the comparative economic value of mothers' and babies' lives is so evident as to shape how and with whom women can birth.

Still other providers will do what Victoria Williams, and many others I spoke with, called "bait and switch": tell patients that they can have a VBAC, but then, once the pregnancy progresses, pressure the patient to schedule a cesarean.[8] Sometimes it's by just saying, "So when can we get the cesarean scheduled?" Other times, one labor and delivery nurse told me, doctors will make "any excuse" to do a cesarean. Among the reasons they needed a C-section, mothers who'd hoped to VBAC told me: The baby's too big. Your scar is too thin (there is no evidence about scar thickness and uterine rupture, because it hasn't been studied). Your pelvis is too narrow. You don't want your baby to die, do you? In still other cases, an OB might have been okay with a trial of labor—but then the mother develops a condition, or pregnancy complication, and the provider changes her mind.

But at thirty-eight or thirty-nine weeks, it's too late to transfer to another practice. You're stuck. (In fact, mothers attempting to VBAC are more likely than those going for a repeat cesarean to change providers after thirty weeks.⁹)

Other providers might tell patients from the get-go that they can't VBAC, and end the conversation there, rather than share information with them about where they could have one. "True informed consent means that you offer the patient—the client—risks, benefits, and alternatives," Helena A. Grant says. "People love to leave the alternatives out. When you're not saying that, you're not offering true informed consent. You're bullshitting. And you're doing it because you want the money." The failure to share alternatives with C-section mothers is evident in a study led by Bridget Basile Ibrahim that appeared in *Birth* in 2021: about 14 percent of people who'd planned a repeat cesarean did not even know VBAC was an option.¹⁰

That's what happened to Timbrel Geter with her second baby. Geter, who lives in Louisville, Kentucky, had a physician tell her she needed a C-section simply because that's how she'd birthed her first baby. "I knew that wasn't right," Geter says. "But I just didn't have the courage and support to back myself up." Geter, who's Black, was on her own at the time, parenting and holding down a full-time job that entailed waking up at 4:00 a.m. to catch the bus to get to work. "Maybe if I was working a part-time job, or maybe if I had someone to talk to about it," it would have been different, says Geter. "I was tired, I was scared, I was alone. I didn't have anybody in my corner." Her experience speaks to the ways that the constraints of work, money, and support coalesce to winnow a mother's options—how "choice" accrues to mothers who can afford it—particularly when providers don't explicitly discuss alternatives. And while she ended up having cesareans with her first three babies, it was only for her fourth birth that she was able to VBAC—which she accomplished by showing up to the hospital in labor and refusing a cesarean once there.

What's more, says Geter, providers might present a repeat cesarean as the reasonable option, framing it as something that a mother would want: schedule the birth and meet the baby, rather than wait for labor to start. At the end of pregnancy, when you're so big you can barely see your feet, put on your own shoes, when there is hardly any space left in your body for your own organs, that proposition is hard to resist. "Of course you want to get that fuckin' baby out of you—duh," she says.

And when it comes to deciding whether to VBAC or schedule a repeat cesarean, a physician's impact matters substantially. "We know from the research that people will follow the lead of the physician," says Jen Kamel, who runs the research and advocacy site VBAC Facts. So it matters quite a bit how physicians present the options, she says. If they say things like, "'Do you want a healthy baby?'" or "'Your baby's going to die,'" she says, it's difficult for mothers to pursue VBAC—because doing so would make them seem as if they are "stupid, selfish, dangerous."

As difficult as it can be for a mother to VBAC after one C-section, the options are even fewer for mothers seeking a VBAC after two. ACOG supports VBAC after two cesareans: studies show that the risk of uterine rupture is similar to, or perhaps slightly more than, the risk of rupture after one C-section.[11] Other data suggests that for a VBAC after one or two cesareans, the outcomes for mothers and babies are virtually the same.[12] But even hospitals and birth centers that support VBAC often refuse to offer it to women who've had two cesareans, which is what happened to Victoria Williams, the mother and healthcare administration PhD in New Orleans who'd tried to switch to a midwife-run birth center; she couldn't because she'd had two previous operations.

In that way, the quest for VBAC can very much resemble access to abortion: wanting one; struggling to find someone who will attend one; being railroaded into what other people believe to be best for you and your family. What happens next depends on where you live, your resources, your race, and some degree of luck, like which provider is on call when you go into labor.

I used to think it was luck that had brought me to Lena, my midwife. She lived a few blocks away from me. Before I was pregnant, I'd see her walking her dog on a steep hill in our neighborhood. She wore funky clogs and gorgeous, dangly earrings, the kind of accessories I'd admired but didn't think I had the style to pull off. She was friends with a friend of mine, and so I got to meet her long before I considered getting pregnant again. At these meetings she projected big energy without being overbearing, reflective of a constitution that equipped her, when necessary, to stay up all night.

But once I started to see her for my pregnancy, Lena, who works for a large health system, did something that I didn't even know could be done, which was vital to earn my trust: she told the schedulers only to schedule me with her, to the extent that they could. Over the course of my pregnancy, I saw her for every visit except three—and one of those was with the maternal fetal medicine specialist who did my eighteen-week anatomy scan. I now know that she doesn't just do this with me; she does this with many of her pregnant patients—the ones who want to stick with a single provider.

At these visits, Lena and I got to know each other. We talked about my first birth and my fears of death. When we talked, she sat on a stool and listened, staring into my eyes—not at her laptop. She also cared about the other things going on with my body, the pregnancy miseries that wouldn't kill me but still caused suffering, like varicose veins (try horse chestnut, she counseled) and symphysis pubis pain (try a symphysis pubis belt, which provides pelvic support). No OB, or midwife, had ever listened to me like this during my first pregnancy; the point of those prenatal visits had been to ensure that I didn't gain too much weight and that, while I contained her, my baby stayed alive. This kind of care, I was learning, was different. It was true midwifery care. I was so, so lucky, I told myself, to have found Lena.

But as Keisha Goode, the sociologist and historian of birth at SUNY Old Westbury, pointed out to me, what often looks like luck really isn't luck. Because it wasn't luck that had brought me to a predominantly white town, or luck that had enabled multiple white midwives to live in it. Not luck that gave us access to the town pool, where my daughter befriended Lena's niece, which is how I found her. Not luck that shaped how we perceived each other—two white women, out for a walk—when we ran into each other in the neighborhood. Not luck that influenced how Lena understood my fear, aggression, indecisiveness, the ways that I wasn't an agreeable or obedient patient.

Much of what we take as luck, especially at the beginning of prenatal care, Goode says, is actually the result of "social determinants of health: your education, your employment." When it came down to my prenatal care, my midwife, and my birth, she said, sure—I was in the right place at the right time. And, "there's so many other things that happened before that."

IN 1989, ANGELA CARDER, A twenty-seven-year-old who'd had cancer and periods of remission since she was a teenager, became pregnant. Tragically, just into her third trimester, her cancer returned, this time in her lung; the tumor was inoperable. Her cancer specialist advised the hospital to treat her with chemotherapy, but the hospital administration balked. They were concerned about chemotherapy's effect on the fetus.[13] Then Angela deteriorated rapidly, faster than anyone had anticipated. She was expected to live for only a few more weeks. Because she was only twenty-six weeks pregnant, and given her "weakened condition," her physician believed that her baby likely wouldn't survive a cesarean. Carder elected for palliative care—pain medicine—to make her more comfortable, knowing she and her baby would not survive.

Her husband and parents agreed with her choice. But George Washington University Hospital, concerned about the rights of the fetus, convened a hearing. "Even before the hearing was over," her mother later told reporters, "they started prepping her for surgery—she was already in so much pain."[14] Judge Emmet Sullivan, who'd not met Angela, said, "I have an obligation to give that fetus an opportunity to live." Angela, who was intubated, mouthed soundlessly to her doctor, "I don't want it done. I don't want it done." He scrubbed in but refused to operate. Another physician performed the surgery.

Two hours after birth, her baby, Lindsay Marie Carder, died. This was one of the last things that Angela learned before her own death, days later.

"They wrote her off," her father later said. "It's like they said, 'You're as good as dead and we're taking the baby.'"[15]

Cases of forced C-section—when a doctor or hospital obtains a court order—are rare. But as legal scholar Michele Goodwin writes in *Policing the Womb*, "the collateral consequences that flow from even this small sample of cases cause serious alarm."[16] Moreover, such cases are "'capable of repetition,'" and have occurred in nearly every state in the country. And they fly against nearly a century of settled law about medical ethics and bodily autonomy, demonstrating that the courts will make exceptions in established law when it comes to pregnant people's bodies.

To understand how much these cases go against settled law, lawyer and MD Julie Cantor gives me a hypothetical. Imagine, she says, a five-year-old is dying of liver disease. The child's parents are both perfect matches to donate a portion of their livers, and let's pretend that we know the operation will be successful. But the parents refuse. Now, imagine if a hospital tried to get a court order to operate on the mother—or the father—without their consent, to save the five-year-old child. "Do you know what would happen if you went to court to get that order?" she asks.

I hazard a guess. "They'd say no?"

"The court would say no. And they would turn to all kinds of cases about the right to refuse care and the right to control your body," she says, beginning with the 1914 case *Schloendorff v. Society of New York Hospital*. The opinion, written by Justice Benjamin Cardozo during his tenure on New York's highest court (he was subsequently appointed to the Supreme Court of the United States, a helpful historical marker of the high esteem in which he was held), holds that in a medical setting, operating on someone—even so much as touching them—without their consent is assault. Such law established that people of "adult years and sound mind," she says, have the right to refuse care. Medical providers cannot so much as touch patients without their consent.[17] This precept, she explains, is one of the four core tenets of medical ethics.

The point, Cantor says, is that pregnancy is not an exception to consent. And it cannot be an exception unless we carve out those who are pregnant as a lesser class of citizen with fewer civil rights than those who are not pregnant, an issue that Cantor says raises serious concerns about equal protection of the law under the Fourteenth Amendment to the Constitution of the United States.

Goodwin argues that it's essential to see cases of forced cesarean as emerging from the same logic and legal precedents that seek to control women's reproductive capacities: prosecutors who craft deals with courts in exchange for women being sterilized; physicians who obtain court orders to keep a pregnant woman on bed rest; judges who punish women for using drugs during pregnancy.[18] Critically, though "legislators seek to justify their attacks on reproductive rights as a means of safeguarding women," Goodwin writes, such surveillance and control isn't making birth any safer.[19]

"Part of why we're in the mess we're in," says Lynn Paltrow, founder and former executive director of Pregnancy Justice, is that the fight for reproductive rights "isn't just for abortion or, you know, access to VBAC. We have not evolved to a place in which we regard pregnancy, the capacity for pregnancy, as human health."

UNTIL THE 1970S, US LAW held that charges of murder or manslaughter could only apply to a child born alive.[20] Since then, some thirty-eight states have adopted feticide laws, meaning that if a pregnant woman is killed, and her fetus dies, too, those deaths can be tried as two separate crimes.[21] At the federal level, the United States passed the Unborn Victims of Violence Act in 2004, which "amends the United States code to protect unborn children from assault and murder," making it punishable to harm or kill a fetus as an entity distinct from its mother.[22]

It seems heartless, perhaps even venal, to argue against such laws. And as far as we know, Paltrow told me, the nation's first feticide law, in California, wasn't devised by an antiabortion figure. But the Catholic Conference and other antiabortion groups have seen subsequent laws, which enshrine fetal rights and fetal personhood, as "part of a very long-term strategy to overturn *Roe*," Paltrow says. By devising new laws to recognize fetal rights in an array of legal contexts—including tort law and murder statutes—these groups recognized that they could eventually change culture, and law, and overturn *Roe*. And as these laws emerged, their architects sought yet more terrain, Paltrow told me. Where feticide laws once focused on fetuses after viability, new laws seek to enshrine fetal rights as early as fertilization. Or these groups changed the language of existing law, to redefine categories like "'child' or 'person'" to include fetuses. Still others are no longer billed as feticide laws; they're simply laws against murder, which rhetorically puts feticide in the same category as murder against a person who has already been born.

These laws explicitly state that they can only be used to apply to someone who *isn't* pregnant who kills a fetus—meaning that they aren't intended to be used against women who have abortions or miscarriages. Nevertheless, says Paltrow, even before the *Dobbs* decision, prosecutors charged women under those laws when women had miscarriages or stillbirths and admitted to using methamphetamines or fentanyl.[23] A prosecutor in Indiana even charged a woman with feticide for attempting suicide while pregnant.[24] These laws aren't exclusively applied in states against abortion rights: in California in 2019, Chelsea Becker, who birthed a stillborn baby at 8.5 months pregnant, was charged with murder because she'd used methamphetamines during pregnancy.[25] A court ultimately exonerated her, but only after she spent sixteen months in jail.[26]

These same philosophies are at play when a physician or hospital seeks a court order for a cesarean against a mother's will. If institutions or physicians "are seeking to justify an action against a person, they will cite anything," says Paltrow. "As claims of separate, interested human rights for fetuses were developed, doctors could fall back on [those claims] to justify whatever coercive or forced intervention they did."

This logic is evident in what happened in 2013 to Renate Dray, an observant Jewish woman in Staten Island who sought a VBAC after two cesareans. (One reason she pursued the VBAC is because she wanted a large family; multiple C-sections limit family size.) Although her obstetrician agreed, he wasn't on call when her labor started. The obstetrician at the hospital, Dr. James Ducey, decided to operate anyway, and against her objections. Subsequently, in court, Ducey argued that the State of New York's courts had found that a viable fetus's well-being was a sufficient reason to ignore a mother's vocal objection to medical treatment—so long as the treatment does not present a "serious risk to the mother's well being." Such logic demonstrates a belief that repeat C-section does not pose a "serious risk," he argued—even though, in Dray's operation, Ducey lacerated her bladder. As of fall 2023, the case has not been resolved.

"It's quite shocking," says Paltrow, that lower trial courts "agree with this framework": that it's acceptable to overrule a mother's objections to maintain her fetus's well-being. "If not at the beginning of pregnancy, at least at a certain point in pregnancy, you lose your civil rights."

IN THE HISTORY OF C-SECTIONS, access to VBAC is a relatively recent issue. It only became possible in the early twentieth century, once physicians began doing cesareans on people who could also, theoretically, birth a baby vaginally.

"Once a cesarean, always a cesarean," the famous dictum, comes from a lecture by Dr. Edwin B. Cragin later reprinted in the 1916 *New York*

Medical Journal. Then chair of the Department of Obstetrics and Gynecology at Columbia University's College of Physicians and Surgeons, Cragin issued his pronuncation in a talk he gave about how obstetrics can best safeguard mothers' and babies' lives. The measures he discussed included handwashing; using forceps only after sufficient dilation; and taking mothers' blood pressure to assess for eclampsia. He also argued that cesarean use "should be exceptional and infrequent,"[27] and avoided when possible—even for conditions like eclampsia and placenta previa.[28] His reasoning was that once a woman had a cesarean, her uterus—weakened by the surgery—would be more likely to rupture in a future pregnancy and labor.

VBAC has likely existed as long as there have been C-sections on women who could have vaginal births. Articles in medical journals from the 1930s describe mothers who spontaneously birthed their babies in the operating room awaiting their repeat cesareans. Still, until the 1970s, only about 2 percent of American women who'd had cesareans went on to VBAC.[29] The pressure to change came partly from a feminist movement determined to make birth more mother-centered, from demanding partners be allowed in the birth room, to resisting routine and often punitive interventions like restraints and enemas. Then, in 1983, Nancy Wainer Cohen and Lois J. Estner's book *Silent Knife: Cesarean Prevention & Vaginal Birth After Cesarean* centralized mothers' objections to repeat cesareans as the default "choice." Some of the book engages the over-adulation of a vaginal birth "completely free of medical intervention," which can make it easy to dismiss. Yet their arguments about VBAC still ring true: "We are told we are too young, too old, too short, too small, too nervous, too weak, too high strung, too overconfident to have a VBAC," they write. "What we really are is *just right.*"[30]

Around the time that Cohen and Estner published their book, the National Institutes of Health, alarmed at the nation's 18.5 percent C-section rate, convened a committee that advocated for VBAC as one way to reduce the nation's C-section rate.[31] Repeat cesareans were the second-most-likely reason for a C-section at the time. Importantly, the committee pointed out, surgical technique had changed since Cragin's recommendation. A low-transverse incision, the "bikini" incision that is now common, which was first adopted in the 1930s, makes uterine rupture less likely.

For the next two decades, as rates of cesarean birth increased, VBAC became more common, too. By the mid-'90s, nearly a third (28.3 percent) of mothers in the US who'd had prior C-sections went on to have VBACs. The next year, that number started to decline; by 2006, the number of VBACs in the US plummeted to 8.5 percent.[32]

The VBAC decline is typically traced to a growing awareness of the potential of uterine rupture, thanks to two publications that appeared in the *New England Journal of Medicine* in 1995 and 2001, respectively. The latter study found that mothers who'd attempted a VBAC were more likely to have a uterine rupture than those who'd elected a repeat cesarean; it was even higher among women who'd had their labor induced, especially with prostaglandin, like cytotec.[33]

A persuasive editorial accompanied the 2001 *New England Journal of Medicine* (*NEJM*) study. "After a thorough discussion of the risks and benefits of attempting a vaginal delivery after cesarean section, a patient might ask, 'But doctor, what is the safest thing for my baby?'" The writer concluded, "My unequivocal answer is: elective repeated cesarean section."

During this same period, ACOG also issued bulletins about VBAC, recommending that institutions that offer it have "resources for emergency delivery immediately available."[34] The widely interpreted meaning of "immediately available" was that physicians—the obstetrician and anesthetist—could reach the unit within ten minutes. Some hospitals did not have such immediate access to anesthesiologists or obstetricians, and thus stopped offering VBACs. At least one hospital stopped offering VBAC because it did not have an anesthesia provider dedicated specifically to labor and delivery. Other hospitals defined that recommendation to mean that an obstetrician has to be in the hospital continuously while a person attempting to VBAC labors—an effectively impossible requirement, given that labor could last days.[35]

The swiftness of the decline in VBAC recalls the way that the profession responded to the pivotal 1998 study about breech birth: it effectively abandoned the practice in favor of cesarean section. It also says a lot about obstetrics: the expectation that pregnancy and birth are pathological; that the "risks of pregnancy" are best dealt with through "invasive techniques," says Dr. Nicholas Rubashkin, the associate professor at University of California San Francisco. It demonstrates a deeply entrenched fear of liability. And, too, there's the real fear about uterine rupture, which after one cesarean is about one in two hundred, or slightly less than 1 percent. Still, it's worth noting that the "immediately available" standard doesn't apply to births in general—though the risk of an obstetric emergency, like cord prolapse, is about as likely as uterine rupture.

But the precipitous drop in VBAC also says something unique about the atmosphere regarding mothers and birth in the United States. Because though European obstetricians had access to the same data regarding uterine rupture, the plunge in VBAC rates that occurred here did not happen in Europe, where rates of VBAC have always been higher. In fact, though VBAC seems to have declined in some European countries since the late 1990s, including Ireland, elsewhere in Europe and over the same time period it became more common than repeat cesarean.[36]

Thus it is critical to understand the precipitous drop in VBACs in the US in light of other pressures: specifically, the successes of the antiabortion movement's efforts to criminalize all pregnant people as potential murderers. By the mid-'90s, when the VBAC rate started to fall, the US had seen about twenty years of "antiabortion rhetoric that claimed that abortion is murder," Lynn Paltrow told me. As part of this approach, antiabortion activists characterized people who get pregnant as criminals, she says. "If you say, 'abortion is murder,' you can't avoid it. . . . Those same people who have abortions, you're calling criminals, murderers, are the people that give birth." At the same time, she says, such rhetoric advanced the argument that "we should adopt the fiction that fetuses are already separate when they're still inside." Taken together, it's not surprising that our culture would become hostile to VBAC, or to mothers who hope to have them.

The breadth and depth of this cultural logic is evident in that closing line of the influential 2001 *NEJM* editorial that advocated for repeat cesarean sections. "'What is the safest thing for my baby?'" the author, an obstetrician, imagined a mother asking him. But there was no counter question, the other mirror, the one that drove me through my second pregnancy and birth: What is safest for me?

WHEN BRITTANY MERIWETHER WILLIAMSON BEGAN looking for a provider who would attend her VBAC in 2018, she knew that no hospital would take her. She had had too many previous sections—three—and her

BMI was too high. So even as she pursued prenatal care from an obstetrician in South Carolina, where she was living at the time, she found an underground midwife who would come to her home to attend the birth.

Brittany wasn't against a cesarean if she needed one, but only if it was medically necessary. She'd had a C-section for her second birth, following a VBAC attempt at home, because of a partial placental abruption. But she says her first and third C-sections weren't medically necessary—for either her or her baby—and her experiences in the hospital had been so poor, so coercive, she didn't want to go near one for this birth.

Brittany was careful to conceal her plans for her birth. She told her obstetrician that she was okay with a fourth cesarean. But she didn't want to schedule it. She'd come in for the operation when she went into labor. She did so because she did not want to get kicked out of the OB's practice and wanted to have regular prenatal care.

Brittany is a nuclear engineer, charged with figuring out how to safely store nuclear ordnance left over from the Cold War. She has spent most of her seventeen-year career at the Savannah River Site in Aiken, South Carolina, where, from the 1950s until 1988, the US manufactured plutonium and tritium to make nuclear weapons.[37] The leftover materials are unstable, and require a team of engineers, including Brittany, to calculate what to do with them. For one recent, yearslong project, she did the math to figure out how to ensure that several hundred barrels of nuclear waste, which the military had packed up for a one-way trip to the Waste Isolation Pilot Plant in New Mexico, did not explode en route.[38] Talking with Brittany, I thought about how her line of work is a strikingly good metaphor for how some physicians and even some mothers feel about people who attempt VBAC after multiple C-sections. Both the mothers, and their uteruses, are unstable, potentially explosive, and need to be contained.

Brittany is white. She wears glasses, her wavy brown hair framing her face. And she's straightforward, a bearing that reflects her training as an engineer. When I asked if she had been frightened about pursuing a vaginal birth at home after multiple cesareans, because of the risk of uterine rupture, she told me that she wasn't. "Not really. As an engineer, I'm matter of fact. I understand the risks and statistics. I plan, and have a contingency plan." For this baby, her contingency plan—if the home VBAC didn't work out—was to go to the hospital.

To find an underground midwife, says Brittany, "you have to know somebody who knows somebody." Brittany had an acquaintance who'd had a baby with this midwife under similar circumstances. She gave her her number, and the acquaintance passed it on to the midwife. Then the midwife called Brittany. They met about four times during her pregnancy and talked about potential complications and emergencies. Yet Brittany didn't even know her full name until a few weeks before the birth. "That's the only way they stay under the radar." If the midwife advertised or disclosed her identity to the wrong person, she could be prosecuted for practicing medicine without a license.

This midwife, Brittany told me, chooses to remain unlicensed. She's a certified professional midwife, which means that she learned the profession through apprenticeship, not through a master's degree, like a certified nurse-midwife (CNM). As we learned in chapter 5, these midwives are more widely regulated, and prosecuted, than certified nurse-midwives—a legacy of nineteenth- and twentieth-century efforts to bring midwifery under physician and hospital control, and to wrest birth from "amateur" and into "professional"—and male—hands. As a result of this regulation, some CPMs choose to go unlicensed, so that they can attend births that a license would prohibit them from attending: VBAC after multiple cesareans, twins, or breeches. (Some state laws restrict VBAC at home altogether, or limit it only to VBAC after one cesarean, which means that a CNM could not legally attend such a birth, either. And if a CNM attended a VBAC after multiple cesareans that had a bad outcome, she'd get called in front of a midwifery board—and would likely lose her license.)

Even licensed CPMs face pressure from insurance carriers, which often charge high premiums for midwives who attend VBAC.[39] "I've personally been quoted between $1,800 and $4,500 per VBAC," Elke Barnes, a midwife based in Tacoma, Washington, told me. At the end of the year, the insurance carrier would ask, "'How many VBACs?' And they raise your rates accordingly. Every year you'd pay an extra $20,000 or something." As a consequence, some midwives won't offer VBAC, even if they legally could. Others "go bare"—they don't carry malpractice insurance, says Barnes, because "it's completely cost-prohibitive" to do so and attend VBACs. And while physicians can theoretically attend VBACs at home, doing so can also endanger their admitting privileges, so in practice, few do.

Malpractice insurance can be cost-prohibitive for nurse-midwives as well; Lena, my midwife, used to attend home births in another state; due to high costs, she carried medical malpractice insurance, a requirement under state law, for everything except birth. "Were you scared?" I asked her. "I should have been," she told me, but she wasn't. She had confidence that she knew when to transfer a person to the hospital; by the time she was doing home birth, she'd already attended 3,500 births as either a labor and delivery nurse or a midwife and knew what could go wrong.

Other mothers in Brittany's situation will have an unattended or unassisted birth at home, because they can't find or afford a midwife who will attend to them. "Women of color do this to protect themselves," Dalecia Young, the doula in Anchorage, told me. "A lot of them are VBAC and they're not getting a better choice." Such mothers are often excoriated in the mass media. One news story from 2020 that went viral described a mother who said she "brainwashed [herself] with the internet" into seeking an unattended birth; she had a stillbirth at nearly forty-five weeks.[40]

"I don't want to see anyone winging it," says Barbara Stratton, a former ICAN of Baltimore chapter leader who reversed a VBAC ban at Frederick Memorial Hospital in Maryland in 2006. Yet, she says, "I completely understand why some people choose it. I would think that they probably are ones who don't have a good birth option . . . It's the mess in the medical community forcing that behavior and the women are doing it for that reason."

Other mothers who seek unattended birth "feel safer giving birth at home with no skilled professional, than giving birth with any of the licensed skilled professionals available," says Hermine Hayes-Klein, an attorney who filed an amicus brief on the Renate Dray case. That's why Jonea, a "wild birth" influencer on Instagram, had her third baby at home with only her husband in attendance. A *USA Today*/ProPublica investigation, "Lost Mothers: Maternal Mortality in the US," had come out while she was pregnant, about the dangers that Black women in particular encountered giving birth in the hospital. Jonea, a nurse who is studying to be a nurse-midwife, is Black; she sent the article to her husband. "I was like, 'This is why I don't want to go back to the hospital, or the birth center that runs under the same exact regulations,'" she told me. "It just clicked for him in that moment, that where he was putting his faith of safety in the system was not where it should have been." Birthing with professionals, she said, "wasn't the safest option. We were choosing something safer. Even if it felt scary at first."

"There's too many" people who choose unattended birth "to say they're all crazy. It's the culture," says Hayes-Klein. "It says a lot. We're desperate."

BRITTANY, WHO HAD A HISTORY of going past her due dates, went into labor at forty-two weeks and three days. Labor took twelve hours. She relished staying home rather than going to the hospital. She sent her children to her mother's house. The midwife, midwife's assistant, Brittany's husband, and a doula tended to her. She labored on a birthing stool and pushed for two hours. Her daughter, says Brittany, was "born perfect."

Then Brittany started to hemorrhage. The midwife gave her a shot of Pitocin, which Brittany does not know how she obtained. She also advised her to go into the hospital for a blood transfusion. Brittany asked her if she would die if she didn't. No, the midwife told her. But you'll probably be pretty weak for a while. Still, Brittany refused. She worried that she would have been admitted, and possibly separated from her baby; that the circumstances of her birth might have brought her to the attention of Child Protective Services. "If I really thought that there would be no negative consequences from the hospital, or the administration of the hospital, or my OB, or the government, then yeah, I totally would have gone in for a transfusion," she said. "I'm not against the transfusion. I was against the hospital."

The next day, Brittany called her OB's answering service to tell them that she'd had her baby. Her OB called her back. She expressed deep concern about Brittany, because of how weak she sounded. Later, she'd tell Brittany that she almost called the police to do a well check. But she didn't, she said, because she knew Brittany would never forgive her.

Brittany saw her OB for her six-week postpartum checkup. At the appointment, she told her that she'd planned the home birth all along.

Her OB said that she hadn't needed to lie to her. That she would have supported Brittany in having a VBAC at the hospital.

"I think I believe her," Brittany told me. But she wasn't sure. At the hospital, there was a complex of systems beyond her control that could spin out. And who knows, says Brittany; her OB said that she'd have supported her VBAC, but perhaps at the last minute she would have changed her mind.

I DIDN'T SIGN OFF ON the paperwork for a VBAC until about three weeks before my due date. I was alone, because of COVID, and meeting the OB, Dr. M, for the first time. I lay back on the exam table so that he could listen to the baby's heartbeat and measure my fundal height. He didn't even suggest checking how dilated I was—a welcome surprise. And he gave me his hand to help pull me back up—the way that my midwife, Lena, did, too.

To talk, we moved to his office. It struck me that where Lena had a "room," as the nurses called it, Dr. M had a corner office, with windows, a bookshelf, and a desk. I sat on the other side of it.

Dr. M was tall and broad-shouldered, and laconic, with gray stubble growing in around the edges of his mask. I had the feeling he'd spent the night on call at the hospital. It was early June 2020, and more likely he was exhausted from the stresses of doctoring in a pandemic. He reminded me of a New York City cop, someone who'd see you smoking pot at the park and tell you to move along rather than give you a ticket—someone who knew what was worth panicking over, and weed wasn't it. It's an association that demonstrates my privilege, but that's also revealing of how I felt in his office—as if I were in trouble. I was a little afraid of him.

"Have you read any of this yet?" he asked, handing me a packet about the risks of a VBAC.

"No," I said. I glanced at the statements that I had to initial: "I understand that VBAC is associated with a higher risk of harm to my baby than to me." "If my uterus ruptures during my VBAC, I understand there may not be enough time to operate and prevent death or permanent brain injury to my baby."

"I'm sorry to have to go over this with you," he said. "What happened the last time?"

How a person responds to a story like mine reveals a lot about them. Maybe they're a voyeur for pain and want to dwell on the trauma. Others are unable to hear beyond the medical outcome, that both my baby and I survived. Sometimes—like the last time I'd met an anesthesiologist, before a colonoscopy—providers didn't believe me, and tried to correct what I was saying, because the shock of what I'd endured—surgery without anesthesia—was too incomprehensible. Dr. M listened, heard my pain. Saw it, but didn't stare.

We talked about what would happen if I went over forty weeks, and he said that he wouldn't automatically schedule a cesarean—something that other practices counsel. "We'll do whatever's safe," he said—words that would take on another shade and a deeper meaning the more I learned about him. He rose to signal the end of the conversation. "Next time I'll see you, you will probably be in labor."

"I'll be a lot more hysterical then," I said, throwing myself under the bus. And for what? I wondered. I didn't feel hysterical at all. Nervous, yes. But calm. I knew exactly what I wanted, had expressed my wishes, but somehow I still felt I should apologize for them: my decision to pursue a birth that elevated my own life at the possible—though remote—expense of my baby's.

"Nah," he said. "You won't." He'd read my type. I'm a fighter, but not a freaker-outer. Not externally. As I'd pegged him, he'd pegged me: I knew what to panic over, and this wasn't it. I wondered if there was something to that effect in my chart.

I didn't know that Dr. M's closing words—next time I'll see you, you will probably be in labor—would turn out to be right.

12

SOLUTIONS

WRITING A BOOK TAKES A LONG TIME, AND WHEN IT'S A BOOK ABOUT real people, many of the book's characters don't stand still. People included in these pages have changed jobs and completed dissertations. Others—and among the happiest changes that occurred as I was reporting this book—got pregnant again and had more babies.

Kate, the Anchorage mom we met in chapter 1, struggled with multiple miscarriages over several years following her son's birth. At dinner, her husband asked—while Kate was out of the room—whether C-sections can cause miscarriages. The answer is probably, though it's impossible to know what caused Kate's. Kate and her husband were devastated over these losses and, she told me, contemplated not trying again. But then, in fall 2023, Kate let me know that she was twenty-six weeks pregnant.

While VBAC had once been important to Kate, she no longer felt that it was so essential, she told me; she'd gone through so much already for this baby—she didn't want to take any chances with the birth. And she felt better about her first birth overall, thanks partly to a conversation about birth, and cesareans, she was part of in Anchorage during summer 2022. Her experience shows how important it can be to examine, discuss, and better understand C-sections. And that doing so isn't tied to any "right" outcome (like VBAC or repeat cesarean), other than greater knowledge, peace, and self-acceptance. She gave birth to her son by repeat cesarean section the week I finished writing this book.

Timbrel Geter, the mother in chapter 11 who had been coerced into three cesareans, also became pregnant again. Timbrel had had her fourth baby, a VBAC, after showing up to the hospital in labor. Because she perceived that she'd get little support in the hospital, she planned to have this baby—which she intended to be another VBAC—at home. While this book was in production, she did.

Justine Richardson, who had an unplanned epidural and cesarean, and whom we met in chapter 7, also had another baby. She wanted to VBAC, and her physician—a different provider than from her first birth—supported her decision. But the pregnancy wasn't easy. She developed tachycardia, or a fast heart rate, in the first trimester, and hyperemesis gravidrum as well. One day after her due date, she decided to be induced, with what she described as "low and slow" Pitocin. Her nurse was "an absolute cheerleader," she says, and helped Justine, who opted not to have an epidural, get into different positions. She really seemed to Justine to believe that she could do it.

After about twelve hours of labor, Justine was dilated to a six, or an eight; she doesn't quite remember. Her doctor told her that there was a C-section coming up in the OR in a few hours. "If we don't do your C-section now, you will be laboring until midnight. I am really started to get worried about that," he told her. He may have been nervous because of the baby's projected size—nine pounds, eight ounces—and the possibility that the baby's shoulders could get stuck. (In the end, the baby weighed about eight pounds, ten ounces—the same as her first; the ultrasound's projection was off by nearly a pound, showing how unreliable such technology can be.)

Justine decided to go for the C-section. She'll never know if she needed to or not, she told me. But the operation itself was much more humane than her first one. She told the resident assisting her physician about her previous birth trauma, and asked her to help make the surgery a positive experience. The resident listened and held Justine's hand. Both the labor and the operation felt healing, she said.

Justine's story is emblematic of the simple changes that can make C-sections better: more support and encouragement during labor and in the operating room.

While the medical resident played that role for her, and though doulas are most often used as a means to promote vaginal birth, they can also be important to mothers who have C-sections. Emily Likins-Ehlers, who uses they/them pronouns, became a C-section doula after their cesareans, and now accompanies birthing people to the operating room. Similarly, Denise Bolds, of Black Women Do VBAC, trains doulas to assist mothers to prepare themselves specifically for surgical birth. There will be many people in the operating room, but none is that focused on a mother's comfort or humanity, she says. A doula can coach a mother to prepare for the surgery; to breastfeed afterward; to cope with the operation's psychological impact; even to navigate getting onto the narrow gurney the mother lies upon for the operation, Bolds pointed out.

So-called gentle or family cesareans are also meant to further improve mothers' experiences during surgical birth. Although they differ depending on the hospital and surgeon, typically they make the surgery feel more like the birth that it is, and honor the birthing person's desires to participate more fully in the experience. This might include lowering the opaque drape to a clear curtain when the baby is born, so the mother can see the birth; allowing the mother to help lift the baby up and out; and giving the mother the opportunity to hold the baby skin-to-skin immediately.

To accomplish this, some hospitals will put the newborn on the mother's chest, with a heavy blanket on top of them both; others, particularly if they're planned, will instruct the mother to wear a kind of tube top to the surgery, so that the baby can be fitted inside it after its birth. Still others will leave one of the mother's arms free—putting both the IV and blood pressure cuff on a single arm, and placing EKG leads on her back—so that she can hold her baby. A gentle C-section might also include options for the mother to control the lighting and music in the operating room. It's important to note that even facilities that don't advertise "gentle" C-sections can, and may, offer these accommodations, and that a birthing person who is interested in these options ask for them.

But a gentle C-section can't make up for or negate the circumstances leading to the operation. Brittany Meriwether Williamson, the mother from chapter 11 who had her fourth child, after three cesareans, at home, had a gentle C-section for her third surgical birth. The actual operation was lovely, she told me; but she'd been so strong-armed into having the cesarean that she counts it as her most traumatic birth.

Nor can a gentle C-section take away from the severity of the operation. To be sure, ensuring mothers can have more autonomy during surgical birth is important. But cesareans aren't "gentle." They're a serious operation: "It's organ surgery," Jenn Stone, a physical therapist, pointed out. And even an operation that goes perfectly, or gently, can be uncomfortable—a person might have a lot of nausea, for example.

No matter what kind of cesarean a person has, we can also do a better job of taking care of mothers during their recovery. Justine Richardson's story is emblematic of that need. Her recovery wasn't simple: she developed postpartum preeclampsia, as well as PUPPP, a skin condition that causes itchiness. She had to be on blood pressure medication for several weeks following the birth. She was also in more pain this time, too, perhaps because the surgeon removed two ovarian cysts during the surgery. And though Justine received the medical help she needed to deal with these conditions, she still would have benefited from care that recognized the operation's effects on her emotions. Tellingly, one of the last times we spoke, Justine was feeling sad when she contemplated having another baby. A VBAC after two cesareans "is an option in the future. But I don't know if I'll pursue it or not. My C-sections permanently changed my family planning and my body." While she'd always believed she'd have a large family, with visions of many grown children around the Thanksgiving table, "based on how incredibly painful those two C-sections were, and the difficulty of the second pregnancy," she let go of that dream.

TO BETTER CARE FOR MOTHERS' complex needs after C-sections, some of the experts I talked with recommended interdisciplinary teams in the hospital—because an obstetrician, or midwife, cannot possibly adequately address all of the different kinds of emotional and physical healing that a new mother faces. Importantly, interdisciplinary teams that include physical or occupational therapists can help mothers heal from a cesarean and prevent further injury as they're recovering. But absent these hospital-based teams, and because medicine is so siloed, obstetricians and midwives may not even think to make the referral to physical or occupational therapy, says Carlin Reaume, an occupational therapist and assistant clinical professor at the University of the Pacific. Which is common, says Karen Brandon, a physical therapist in California. Maternal health seems only to "matter to the metrics if it's at a level of harm that would kill you," she says.

But even interdisciplinarity has its problems. P. Mimi Niles, the assistant professor at NYU and midwife, noted that it can become hierarchical. And that the "many specialists" model is still fractured, and not holistic.

Improving care for all moms, before and after a C-section, also requires changing how providers treat patients. Rei Shimizu, assistant professor of social work at the University of Alaska Anchorage, suggests making racial-awareness training "a continuing education requirement: if you want to keep your MD, you must go through racial bias training." Such education isn't only "for the white people. It's across the board," she says. "I'm Asian. When I see an Asian doctor, I almost have an affinity with them. Sometimes that affinity gets betrayed. They've had to survive in a system that requires them to be a certain way and lean in to whiteness. They've internalized some of that. Sometimes I feel even more betrayed," she says, because Asian providers violate her expectation of being seen as a whole person—not according to the stereotypical outlines of her race. And yet, as much as racial awareness or implicit-bias training is important—it increases people's knowledge of their own biases—there are no evidence-based examples of such programs' efficacy for lasting behavioral changes (at least not yet).

Identifying new paths for redressing obstetric racism, and obstetric violence, is also part of improving care—because it can lead to systemic change. Deborah Fisch, the Michigan attorney and vice president of the Birth Justice Bar (formerly the Birth Rights Bar Association), points out that absent sustained damage to a baby, or substantial physical injury to the birthing person, medical malpractice litigation will rarely produce any real remedy. To that end, she noted, activists are encouraging people who've experienced obstetric racism, or obstetric violence, to file a complaint with the Office of Civil Rights (OCR) in the US Department of Health and Human Services. A person doesn't need a lawyer to file such a complaint; the process does not involve any court system. But OCR has the power to investigate acts of discrimination and hold providers accountable, though it won't award financial compensation for any damages

a person experienced. For that, says Fisch, you have to resort to malpractice, "and that is very difficult. But if you're after systems change—which
we know is actually a reason that many people file suits," a civil-rights
complaint may be more effective. (To her point, only about one in four
people who bring malpractice lawsuits say they do so because they need
money.)

Group prenatal care is another solution to improve the experience
of pregnancy and birth, and that may also bring down the number of
medically unnecessary cesareans. In this model, expectant mothers meet
as a group of about eight to twelve people. These appointments can last
about an hour and a half to two hours. The appointment includes a health
assessment—checking each person's blood pressure and the baby's heart
rate—as well as education and support. What's significant about the
group prenatal care model is that mothers benefit from support from their
provider and from the community of other mothers—a kind of harkening
back to the social support that got left behind when birth became medicalized and moved into the hospital. According to a 2017 meta-review
of such programs in *BMC Pregnancy and Childbirth*, the model reduced
preterm birth among low-income and Black women.[1] Black women and
teenagers also reported "increased satisfaction with care" according to
the study, among other improvements. Another study from 2017 that
compared mothers in group prenatal care with mothers receiving traditional prenatal care found that those in group prenatal care had a lower
C-section rate (14 percent birthed by C-section compared with 25 percent
of mothers in the other group).[2]

Unfortunately, one of the greatest difficulties in implementing this
type of care is financial: it is difficult to bill for. This obstacle demonstrates
how the financialized nature of medicine creates obstacles to improving
care—even implementing evidence-based models that improve people's
physical and psychological experiences of pregnancy and birth. According
to Tammea Tyler, the CEO of the Centering Healthcare Institute, a nonprofit that promotes CenteringPregnancy, a type of group prenatal care,
as of 2021, some fifteen states participate in the payment strategies necessary to offer group care. Because these payment strategies are as essential
as they are difficult to navigate, Tyler wrote in an email, "understanding
the reimbursement policies, medical codes, and how they work together is

just as valuable as clinical care itself." (To her point, evaluations of mothers participating in the CenteringPregnancy model have shown lower rates of C-section and epidurals, and higher rates of non-pharmacological pain relief, than women who'd received individual care and birthed in the same clinic.[3]) Last, a novel program initiated by the administrators of 32BJ, a labor union in New York of some two hundred thousand members, shows how benefits managers can encourage mothers-to-be to seek maternity care that's not overly, and unnecessarily, medicalized. Cora Opsahl, head of benefits for 32BJ, found that members, the majority of whom are "Black and Brown," had worse birth outcomes than white mothers. They were also are more likely to have cesareans. She observed that even though the union membership skews older—there were only 1,500 births in 2020—childbirth played an outsized role in healthcare costs.

Opsahl asked hospitals in New York for their data about maternal mortality and morbidity, NTSV C-section rates, whether they permit doulas or offer lactation support. In looking at this data, Opsahl recognized that hospitals with the best maternity care weren't necessarily the ones that charge the most for birth. With her colleagues, she designed a program to encourage union members to go to hospitals with the highest-value maternity care: those with the best outcomes. If they go to one of the "five-star" hospitals in the 32BJ program, mothers do not pay anything for prenatal care or delivery. These hospitals don't necessarily have a reputation as elite; they include Elmhurst Hospital Center in Queens, Jacobi Hospital in the Bronx, and Metropolitan Hospital in Manhattan. But, says Opsahl, "We know that when we send our moms there, they're not going to have unnecessary C-sections. They have a lower risk of maternal mortality, and of a bad outcome." She adds, "We do this because then we know that the members have a high-quality doc, and are going to a high-quality hospital." When we spoke, in spring 2023, about two hundred mothers had participated in the program, which started in 2020. So far, the initiative has a 100 percent satisfaction rating, says Opsahl, as measured by the mothers' assessments of where they gave birth, and whether they received the care that they wanted and needed. By encouraging expecting mothers to go to these hospitals, Opsahl also saves healthcare costs. That benefits everyone in the union: in doing so, she says, "there's more money left over wages."

These initiatives demonstrate that there is no single way to improve birth or reduce C-section rates. That a surprising number of thoughtful, evidence-based measures to do so are already in motion. And that the people who can effect these changes aren't only in medicine.

STILL, FOR MOST MOMS, THE struggle to have a good birth is felt at the bedside: whether she is permitted to eat during labor; whether she's permitted to move around, or must be constrained by the tethers of EFM. If she'll have her water broken or be pressured into accepting Pitocin or an epidural. Partly for this reason, some moms bring a birth plan with them, which—depending on the circumstances—providers might honor to the best of their abilities, or utterly ridicule. These "micro battles," notes P. Mimi Niles, "have become front and center" in the story of birth.

But the real battle of how and whether mothers are empowered in birth takes place far from the person in the bed, says Niles. It occurs in the executive suite and the statehouse. And these decisions often have to do with what's known as midwifery integration: if, how, and to what degree midwives can practice in a given place or healthcare system.[4] This matters, because a wealth of research shows that midwifery care is associated with lower primary C-section rates in low-risk pregnancies and higher VBAC rates.[5] Across the world, "maternal and perinatal outcomes are better in jurisdictions where midwives are regulated and have the legislative authority to practice to their full scope across birth settings," conclude Saraswathi Vedam and colleagues in a paper on midwifery integration in the US.

Investing in midwives, according to the *Lancet* series on midwifery, "is crucial to the achievement of national and international goals and targets in reproductive, maternal, newborn, and child health." But in the US, midwives often face obstacles that bar their entry to practice—like CPMs, who can't even be licensed in very US state—and that constrain their autonomy. To achieve midwifery integration requires amending these barriers, which in turn shape how and with whom people birth. That's not just an abstract idea, it's evident in the data: In another study, Vedam and colleagues assessed states' midwifery integration—which includes regulations on midwives, the availability of Medicaid reimbursement, and midwives' authority to write prescriptions, among other metrics—and found associations between those states with a higher degree of midwifery integration and lower rates of C-sections, as well as lower rates of preterm- and lower-birth weight babies. States with greater degrees of midwifery integration also "correlated strongly with lower rates of neonatal mortality and race-specific neonatal mortality," the researchers wrote—meaning, the greater the midwifery integration, the less likely infants born in that state are to die in their first four weeks of life.[6]

Some of the barriers to midwifery are enacted at the state level, like CPM licensing or whether Medicaid reimburses midwifery care. But Niles also points to hospital and health system executives, who determine who has admitting privileges—and whether to extend those to midwives. Such leaders also decide who to name faculty or sit on the bylaws committee. Who has full voting rights, which is important symbolically and practically: lacking voting rights in a hospital, as CNMs often do, puts them at the bottom of the hierarchy; it also makes it impossible for them to have a say in how the hospital operates, says Kathryn Ault, a certified nurse-midwife in Homer, Alaska. With full voting privileges, midwives can make recommendations to the operating board of the hospital about who stays credentialed, for instance, and can draw attention to physicians who might intervene too frequently or cavalierly. That's why, to see real change for midwives—and, by extension, the ways that birthing people experience birth, "it has to happen at the C-suite level," says Niles. "Those are the decision-makers."

Such changes are essential to changing hospitals' cultures of birth. Without that kind of cultural shift, midwives can't work according to the midwifery model of care—that is, treat pregnancy as a physiologically normal experience and promote a low-intervention approach to birth that values personal support and human touch, rather than relying exclusively on EFM, epidurals, and other technology. But, cautions certified nurse-midwife Holly Smith of the California Quality Maternal Care Collaborative, "A vision for low intervention care, midwifery care, can't exist in a place that doesn't support it. You can't live in something that doesn't support the work you do. Instead, you switch and become a physician extender." Midwives integrated into a hospital or health system's administration can help to bend institutional culture to the midwifery model of care—modulating the ways that physicians and nurses take care of patients, too.

The need for this cultural shift emerged in work led by the California Quality Maternal Care Collaborative to bring down C-sections throughout the state. When the CQMCC first came together, in 2015, data showed that the number of C-sections in California hospitals varied widely—from about 12 to nearly 70 percent of all births. At first, midwife Holly Smith told me, the group approached this problem "from a very medical point of view, which is to say, 'We've overdone interventions, so now what are the reverse interventions we can do to reverse cesareans?'" But once midwives, nurses, and—in particular—doulas got involved, the conversation shifted, to focus on the "culture of care that . . . leads down the road to quickly and easily choose C-sections over vaginal birth." In part, that culture pivoted on avoiding "any risks" to the baby, and—as a result—considering the mother merely as a "vessel for this baby coming out." To that end, the CQMCC advocated creating a "culture of normalcy, where we actually treat most pregnancies and births as low-risk unless otherwise indicated." And, she said, even in the presence of indicators that a birth is higher-risk, to create a supportive system that is "not going to intervene unless we absolutely need to." So CQMCC put together a tool kit for hospitals to promote vaginal births from which hospitals could implement. The two most effective tools, and the ones that participating hospitals used most, were working to change the culture within the hospital, and transparency about physicians' cesarean rates.

By 2019, California's NTSV C-section rate fell from 26 percent in 2014 to 22.8 percent. Mothers who gave birth in hospitals that participated in the collaborative were less likely to have a cesarean than mothers who birthed elsewhere. What's more, although cesareans are touted as being safer for babies, the initiative appeared to have made birth safer for babies, too: the rate of "severe unexpected newborn complications," a study in *Obstetrics and Gynecology* found, fell from 2.1 to 1.4 percent among hospitals that took part in the initiative.[7]

But there's one thing that didn't change: the inequitable rate of cesareans between Black mothers and mothers from all other ethnic groups—even though the number of C-sections fell in each demographic. That gap, Smith says, "did not close at all. . . . We need a different system of care to address this."

MIDWIFERY INTEGRATION WOULD SURELY POINT out the need for health systems to hire more midwives. But that alone would not increase or diversify the midwifery workforce. Such workforce development will take time. "You cannot mass-produce midwives," Niles says. "It takes time to train us—as it should. We get better as we age—as we should." Yet in recent years, philanthropies have focused on training doulas, which is much faster—you can train a doula in a weekend—and cost-effective. Because where you can train ten midwives for $1 million, says Niles, you could train a thousand doulas for the same amount. And while doulas are important, they cannot—do not—provide midwifery care. We need to understand and respect the time and money it takes to train a midwife if we wish to transform birth and bring down the number of unnecessary cesareans.

Niles also points to the role that the federal government can play in such training. Presently, it does not subsidize hospitals to train midwives—though it does subsidize medical residencies, by giving money to hospitals to train doctors. As a consequence, hospitals do not have a financial incentive to train midwives. "The catalyst for midwifery training is all internal" to each midwifery service, says Niles. "There's no system lever to say we are committed to training ten midwives a year. Our director says, 'Who's going to take a student?'" she says. That's "very different than the contracts the hospitals have, the structural mechanism to build a physician workforce."

Growing and diversifying the midwifery workforce would also address the paucity of maternity providers that's a legacy, in part, of state legislatures' decimation of traditional networks of midwifery throughout the South and in rural areas throughout the rest of the country. After the states legislated midwives out of practice, obstetricians and nurse-midwives did not move in to serve these communities. With the closure of obstetric units since the 1980s, hastened in part by hospital systems' consolidation, so-called maternity deserts have only gotten worse. Today in the United States, about 6.9 million women have no or low access to maternity care, which represents about half a million births each year;

among them, 1.2 million women live in a county that lacks a hospital or birth center that provides obstetric care, and without a single certified nurse-midwife or obstetrician.[8]

Needing to travel long distances for obstetric care has been shown to increase the likelihood of bad outcomes for mothers and babies. The paucity of available care can also make it virtually impossible to access VBAC, which is one reason the rates of VBAC are so low. The care that's available is also too often out of step with what mothers need. Thus, the rates of near-misses and maternal deaths, of stillbirths and infant mortality, are still stubbornly high. And by most accounts, obstetric racism, which is only beginning to be measured, is quite high, too. "By tossing out these [community] midwives, we've tossed out entire communities that desperately need that care," says Jamarah Amani. "It's lifesaving care. It's life-affirming care. And the rest of the world recognizes this."

But building up the number of nurse-midwives who practice in hospitals is not the only solution or totality to midwifery integration, Amani points out. Midwifery integration also requires easing restrictions that CPMs face—the midwives who learn primarily through apprenticeship—and building up respectful relationships between CPMs and hospital-based providers, should a CPM need to transfer a laboring person. Doing so would expand the number of places where a person could have a baby with a midwife: at home, at a birth center, or in the hospital. If we can recognize these different kinds of midwifery care and expertise, then we can transform the way we birth. Because part of bringing down the C-section rate is making it easier, and more affordable, for mothers who want to birth out of the hospital.

This itself is radical, because it requires fundamentally reimagining what kinds of knowledge can make for a good, safe birth. What bodies produce the knowledge, what bodies possess it, and the meaningful ways to transmit it. It requires recognizing that there are people who are experts in nonhospital birth—that such expertise is legitimate and possible, and isn't only found or obtained in the formal classroom. It means going back to the kinds of knowing about birth that we fenced off when obstetrics took over from midwifery—when, as Barbara Katz Rothman said, obstetrics colonized birth—and listening to the communities from whom birth was taken away.

But midwifery integration alone can't solve birth. Alicia D. Bonaparte, the Pitzer sociology professor, points to all that happens before an expecting mother enters the consulting room, from environmental pollutants that contribute to infant and maternal mortality to policies that have systematically underfunded schools and hospitals in Black communities, to name but two. These injustices comprise the architecture of American society, by design. Consequently, you "can't say, 'Hey, midwife. Hey, doula. Fix this thing,'" says Bonaparte. "You can't make them be the scapegoat for why things aren't getting better."

"It is a societal shift that needs to happen," says midwife Jamarah Amani. People say, "'Oh, wow, Black maternal mortality is terrible,'" she says. "We can change it. Here's how: give people paid time off. We can make sure everyone is insured, not just during their pregnancy, but from birth to death, because that protects the entire life cycle. We can make sure that there's adequate access to training and education programs, specifically to repair the damage that has been done to communities of color, who forever knew how to take care of themselves, and were systematically disconnected from that knowledge," she says. "All of these things are fixable and for sure will lead to dramatic reductions in C-section rates, as we relearn how to support physiologic birth."

IN THE LATE 1970S, HARVARD cardiologist Dr. Bernard Lown noticed that the patients he treated with heart disease who'd had balloon angioplasty and bypass surgery didn't seem to be faring any better than the ones who'd not had an operation, and who'd managed their disease with diet and exercise. So he decided to design a study to formally measure the outcomes of his more conservative approach to coronary disease. It may sound pedestrian, or even abstract, but Lown was wrecked with anxiety over the study, his former Fellow, Dr. Vikas Saini, told me. Invasive procedures like balloon angioplasty and bypass surgery were widely popular at the time. Lown was going against established practice. And while Lown believed he'd hypothesized correctly, he wouldn't be sure until the study was over. Even more than risking professional opprobrium, for embarking on this almost anti-American, noninterventionist manner of treatment, he worried about his patients. If he was wrong, he might have been humiliated. But his patients—they were the ones who'd truly suffer; they could die.

In the end, and as we now know, Lown was right. A less invasive approach sometimes really is better when it comes to treating heart disease.

The same medical model that encourages and rewards invasive treatments for heart disease shapes how and why physicians recommend C-sections to "treat" slow or stalled labor. The ideology undergirding the model, that the risk of invasive procedures is worth the outcome, describes how physicians will advise mothers with low scores on the VBAC calculator to schedule a cesarean—rather than counsel them how to improve their chances at vaginal delivery. Even the widespread use of electronic fetal monitoring, which is responsible for identifying questionable fetal heart tracings, is a natural outcome of this model.

That's why to bring down the number of C-sections requires reimagining the American health system to one that isn't financially driven to promote costly surgeries, tests, and invasive interventions. This new system also has to eradicate volume-driven incentives for physicians—see forty patients a day, earn a bonus—and move to "global budgets." A global budget, Saini explains, means that a region, or an entire state, is given a set amount of money to use to provide healthcare to people who live there.

In practice, this would work so that an institution in a defined region—say, the Hudson Valley—cares for one hundred thousand people. "Insurance premiums on those one hundred thousand people are, let's say, $10,000 each. One hundred thousand people multiplied by $10,000 is $1 billion. Say to that provider system, here's a billion dollars," says Saini. It's then up to the local system to care for those people within that budget.

Of course, a system would be incentivized to do more with less—to spend only $900 million, not $1 billion. This is why Saini argues for "global budgets under public control," so that budgets are "a matter of public record and public review." In other words, if the system saves $100 million, the savings don't all belong to that system. "If it's publicly run, the public could say, 'We're going to take some back, and invest in childcare and nutrition programs,'" the very kinds of preventative care, and systemic support, that are critical to maintaining people's health—emotionally, physically, spiritually.

Saini also advocates for a universal single-payer system that funds global budgets nationally but is administered regionally for as much local control as possible. In theory, this system could help with cost control for procedures. As it stands, cost variability is a major aspect of cesareans, whose costs can vary from $8,312 to $70,098 according to a study of hospitals in California—and can even differ wildly in the same city.[9] "Create public accountability and oversight and give the doctors, hospitals, and provider networks enough flexibility on how they're going to do that without answering to insurance companies, or anybody else, but to their own communities."

Naturally, he cautions, the process of making this work is complicated. And he says that while Medicare is pushing for such arrangements, for-profit institutions are "milking it for all it's worth." But if we could successfully design such a system, "it would be the envy of the world."

It may sound impossible, like something that would never happen in our lifetimes, and certainly not in the US. But it already has, Saini says. "The Southcentral Foundation," says Saini, in Alaska. "They show it can be done."

I TRAVELED TO ALASKA TO try to understand why the state has a relatively low C-section rate: 22 percent. There are many reasons: it has the highest rate of out-of-hospital births in the country, which represent people who have babies in birth centers or at home. Evidence shows that low-risk mothers who birth in those settings are less likely to have an intervention, including a cesarean.[10] There are also demographic explanations for the state's C-section rate: about one in five people in Alaska are Alaska Native, and these communities are young: the average age of Alaska Native and American Indians in Alaska is twenty-seven, and younger mothers have lower C-section rates.[11] But the state's C-section rate may also be a result of the structure and mission of the Alaska Native Tribal Health Consortium (ANTHC), a socialized system that provides free healthcare for Alaska Native people—an example of the kind of system Saini imagines that's already been implemented in the US.

What's important to understand about the ANTHC is that it is owned and run by Alaska Native people through a federal policy known as tribal compacting. Members of the board come from fifteen regional

Tribal health organizations from across the state. By contrast, I have no idea where the members of the board of UnitedHealth Group, which owns Optum, a multinational company that recently cannibalized most of the physician practices I see, come from. Three have worked for, or led, financial services companies. This qualification demonstrates a key aspect to Optum's strategy: to make money.

Thea Agnew Bemben, a consultant in Anchorage, says that it differs from the rest of the US's medical system. Alaska's Tribal Health System is much more holistic and has greatly expanded access to behavioral health care. By contrast, the traditional American medical system quite literally has its roots in what she described as "a patriarchal white supremacist system," with a Cartesian approach that separates the body and the mind. "To instead say, 'Your culture and your mental health is part of your physical health,'" is profound. These health organizations, she says, are "creating a care model based on that."

As to be expected, birth also looks quite different in Alaska's Tribal health system. The Alaska Native Medical Center (ANMC), a hospital in Anchorage run by the ANHTC and the Southcentral Foundation, sees the second-most births in Alaska. Many of these births have already been designated higher-risk. Because of the remoteness of much of Alaska, and the lack of perinatal emergency care, a mother whose doctor or midwife believes she may have a problematic labor, or may need a cesarean, is sent to Anchorage at around thirty-six weeks.* She stays with family or in a hospital-provided room (not in the hospital, but in a homelike setting) and awaits labor to start.

Yet ANMC has a C-section rate of only 11 percent. The two other hospitals in Anchorage have C-section rates comparable to other hospitals in the US: 33 percent (Providence Alaska Medical Center); 40 percent (Alaska Regional Hospital).

There are many reasons that the ANMC's C-section rate is so low. First, doula Dalecia Young points out, promoting vaginal birth is a method of harm reduction, because Alaska Native mothers are disproportionately more likely than other mothers in the US to hemorrhage postpartum.[12] (In a typical cesarean, mothers are already more likely to lose more blood

---

* Or the closest hospital providing emergent birth care, like a cesarean section.

than in a typical vaginal birth.) Midwifery is also integrated into the practice so that, even before pregnancy, people see midwives for basic well-woman care—rather than gynecologists. That continues throughout pregnancy. Young, who is Iñupiaq, noted that "even if you risked out you can see a nurse-midwife in the hospital. If you're high-risk, you can still be attended by midwives [along with physicians]. It's much more collaboration of care as you move through the system." This kind of care is what Helena A. Grant made a similar argument for in one of our early conversations: every woman deserves the touch of a midwife.

"Every place has things to complain about, but it's different than other hospitals," Young told me. For instance, she says, "care at ANMC is more humane. So much about hospital births is identical. But they are primarily midwives at ANMC. You can have both." ANMC also has a "more graceful" approach, says Young—the people who aren't needed right away, like the baby nurse, stand behind a curtain. [A provider] will say, the baby's decelerating, but that's okay, you are doing great right now.

Labor rooms are large, designed to accommodate many people, which is an important part of Alaska Native birth culture. The hospital cafeteria serves food that's culturally appropriate. And Alaska Native doulas advocate for mothers to have culturally appropriate care during birth.

What's more, Young says, is that after birth, "skin-to-skin of one hour is a standard of care—at all births." As a doula, Young has been at births in a variety of environments. She says, "elsewhere, I'm shocked to educate the providers about the golden hour."

Young says that because the people who seek care at the Alaska Native Medical Center are also its owners, "We have a say." At other hospitals, in the mainstream medical system, she says, "the providers' POV" can be, "I'm here to do my objective. I have power. You don't." But at ANMC, you're not "just a patient on a conveyor belt."

She also sees "much more consent sought before touching people" at ANMC. "Like how lactation is initiated. Not roughly of, 'Get the baby on the breast,'" where the emphasis "is on the latch and not honoring this incredible moment." At ANMC, providers "honor the golden hour and baby-led latching."

To some extent, this is care that one might associate with a birth center, as it follows a midwifery model. But it is also an outgrowth of how the care is structured: its priorities, its mission, the people—the stake-holders—to whom the entire system must answer. And one of the AN-THC's missions is self-determination. Autonomy. The right to decide, for yourself, how to live.

REVISIONING BIRTH CAN SEEM OVERWHELMING. And, for people work-ing to improve birth, it can lead to burnout. Brittany Meriwether Wil-liamson, the nuclear engineer who had a VBAC at home, and who has done advocacy work for the International Cesarean Awareness Network, likened it to the ocean: waves of mothers, harmed, just keep washing up. There is seemingly no end to them.

To some degree, I told her, I relate; in reporting the book, I was some-times amazed at how many people around me had stories of C-sections that they didn't really need, or who experienced infections, or who were left feeling anxious about their bodies or at the thought of being separated from their babies. So often, these topics came up just in the course of talk-ing with friends, acquaintances, and coworkers: a secret club with an ever-expanding membership. At the same time, reporting showed me that, too, there are so many people throughout the country—and the world—working to make birth better. Safer. Who honor its beauty. I thought of the phrase from Pirkei Avot, Ethics of the Fathers, in which Rabbi Tarfon says: "It is not your duty to finish the work, but neither are you at liberty to neglect it."

On a warm early spring day in the Hudson Valley, I was running late to meet Jenn Sullivan, the lactation consultant who'd helped me after my daughter's birth and, more recently, after my son's. Jenn has worked as an LC for seventeen years, running groups and visiting peo-ple at home. She's used to seeing people who are in the atmosphere of birth: dazed, traumatized, crying, brilliantly happy, half-demented, like me, when I insisted that Bruce Springsteen was really singing about a postpartum mom.

We hiked around a path in town that cuts through farmland. The red-winged blackbirds had just returned and were trilling in the fields. The wind whipped our hair, blowing off the Shawangunk Ridge, which rose in the distance.

"So," I asked her, "C-sections. What are the solutions?"

"Emphasizing C-section education," she said, immediately. "Because let's face it. There's at least a 30 percent chance you're having one. And no one fucking talks to you about it until you're in there. So," she says. "Let's talk about it."

EPILOGUE

WHEN I'D FIRST GOTTEN PREGNANT WITH MY SON, I'D THOUGHT I'D spend the last months bobbing in a pool. But it was June 2020 and everything was closed. There was nowhere to take the weight off my body. Those last few weeks of the pregnancy, it was so hot I became crepuscular, leaving the house only in the mornings and evenings. During the day, I closed myself in my dark bedroom, AC blasting, and sprawled on the bed, listening to a HypnoBirthing meditation about picturing myself in a safe space. I imagined standing in my garden, limned by peonies and white alliums. I imagined holding my baby's hand, and then letting it go.

It remained an open question who would watch our daughter when I went to the hospital. My mother had broken her ankle a few weeks after COVID clamped down on New York City, then developed pneumonia that nearly killed her. In an entirely uncharacteristic way, she wasn't sure that she could commit—didn't know if she could even get up the few steps into our house. My brother offered to take C, but I worried about getting her there, an hour and change away, while I was in labor. My friend Aidan offered, too. As we closed in on thirty-seven weeks, I wasn't sure what to do. Really I wanted my own mother: her assurance, her faith in me, her touch.

Ultimately, we asked my in-laws, who live in Ohio. They agreed unhesitatingly. They would drive ten hours straight, stopping only for gas, so as not to contract COVID on the way. This was one of the most beautiful and loving gifts I have ever received. They were not my parents, but they would parent me.

Labor started a few days shy of my due date. Early in the morning, my husband and I walked the block, pausing with each contraction. A woman walking her dog smiled at me in a kind of secret way; she knew what was happening. A car drove down the deserted street and another woman leaned out and called out to us, J____, is that you? My husband and I were both startled; we'd been planning to give our baby that name.

We left for the hospital on a Saturday evening—a different one from where I'd had my daughter. The hospital that, ironically, I'd believed to be too "medicalized" when I'd gotten pregnant the first time.

Even as we drove, I wondered if it were too early. My midwife, Lena, was there and checked me in at triage: I was four centimeters dilated, she said. Once admitted, she hooked me up to the electronic fetal monitor and ran a test strip to see how baby was doing, then came back to talk to us. He wasn't looking so good, she said. She showed me the strip: his heart rate wasn't that changeable, more like little ups and downs, like a small pebble bumping down the road. She showed me an example of someone else's baby, whose heart rate was making big leaps, like mountains—these are called accelerations, she said. That baby was very healthy. This is what you want to see. Frankly, this baby was practically showing off.

My contractions had stopped, and she said something about Pitocin, maybe, or breaking my water. Then she stepped out. I started crying. I'm caught in the net, I told my husband. We'd arrived too early, I believed. The baby wasn't ready. These contractions—known as prodromal labor—were a false alarm, a prelude to the big show. I'd had the same thing with my first labor. Later, my husband would tell me that when we'd left for the hospital, his father had told him, privately, "I think she's getting ahead of her skis."

I could see how this was going to go. I wanted to go home. I told Lena that when she came back in.

"Yeah," she said, sounding sympathetic. "Why don't you rest and let's check back in in a bit."

I sat on the bed and tried to calm myself. But all I could see was another cesarean, bearing down on me. I wasn't even going to get a chance to try for a different story.

Lena came back about a half hour later. Baby was looking great on the monitors, she told me. He may have been sleeping before. She felt okay about us going home if that's what I wanted. I felt a little mad at her—why didn't she tell me that he could've been sleeping from the get-go?—as I unhooked myself and we packed up and left the hospital.

Walking through an empty corridor at 1:00 in the morning, still pregnant, I felt as if I were getting away with something, as if someone were going to come after me. But I was also sure we were doing the right thing.

The next few days were portentous, novelistic with their foreshadowing. It was hotter than it had yet been that summer, and it rained every afternoon, as in a tropical place. Nights, the moon was full. Our cat, dying of kidney failure, lolled in the corner of our bedroom, or beneath the bushes outside. On top of everything else, I worried the cat would die while I was having the baby. I wondered when, or if, I'd ever go into labor again. But my body stayed quiet. The baby stayed put.

Three days after we left the hospital, in the middle of the night, labor started again. I knew this time that I was ready, because it was a lot like my first labor, when that had started up for real. My back ached. I rolled around on a yoga ball, folded into child's pose, did cat and cow. I also tried to rest. I knew better than to exhaust myself as I had the first time; then, eager to get things rolling, I'd run up and down the stairs before leaving for the hospital, believing it would speed labor along.

In the morning, I texted my midwife; I was slated to see her anyway for a regular checkup. She told me to bring my hospital bag to the office. By the time I arrived, I'd developed a bad headache, elevated blood pressure, and protein in my urine. I'd also dilated to a six. From the checkup, Lena told me to go straight to the hospital. But this time, she said, "With that blood pressure, and dilated to a six, they're going to want to hang on to you. There isn't going to be the going home and coming back." I knew she told me this because she wanted me to be realistic about what was to come. But she didn't need to tell me; I could feel with my body that this was it.

In the hospital, my husband hung up a drawing of my daughter's. It showed the three of us. I focused on it; it was my talisman. As long as I could see it, I was going to stay alive. I would get home to her.

Though I'd thought I'd go without it, I was grateful for the epidural that took away the pain of my back labor. But it plunged my blood pressure, and I could feel myself passing out. "DOCTOR!" the nurse yelled into the hall. Someone put something into my IV, and I shot back awake, with the speed and momentum of a diver hitting water. After that, I was afraid of closing my eyes. I worried I'd never open them again.

When Lena showed up, sometime in the afternoon, I was completely surprised. I hadn't expected that she would come. She'd worked in the office all day and she wasn't on call. And yet, there she was. Relief washed over me. I'd liked the nurses and other midwives, who'd cared for me as I'd labored all day. They'd set me up with a peanut ball; they'd helped me to turn from side to side. They'd acknowledged what had happened in the first birth but hadn't dwelled on it. They'd believed that I would have that VBAC! But Lena—Lena was different. Lena I could trust.

Lena saw me through labor until I was almost ready to push. We did a few practice pushes. But I could feel that my baby wasn't in the right position. I thought, *This isn't going to work. This is why there are C-sections.* I felt not happy, but at peace; we'd all done our best. I'd been respected and had autonomy. It seemed like the lesson I'd been learning my entire life: it didn't matter how hard I worked at something. If it wasn't set up properly, I could knock my head against it as much as I wanted. But I still wouldn't get what I'd hoped for.

"Is it okay if I try to move his head?" Lena asked. As with my daughter, my baby's head was turned to the side. I hadn't even known that turning his head was a possibility. What I didn't yet appreciate about Lena at that point was that she'd started as a home-birth midwife. For her, a C-section truly was a last resort. She had the hand skills to rumble someone into labor, to get them and their baby well-positioned, and to see them through to the other side.

"Yes," I said.

She tried, but her fingers weren't strong enough.

She left, and a few minutes later, she came back in with Dr. M. "Hello," he said. He'd been right, when he'd told me, in his office: the next time we'd see each other I'd be in labor. How he'd known he'd be on at the hospital at that point, I don't know.

Dr. M, quietly and without crowing about it, put his fingers inside of me and moved my son's head. Later, I'd ask Lena how she persuaded him to do this. It was risky, this move, on a VBAC mom. He'd groaned at her at first, she said. But she'd told him that mom and baby were doing great. And that she had a feeling it would work. They'd worked together seventeen years, starting when Lena was a nurse, before she became a midwife. He trusted her knowledge and her instinct. Her authority. Even though she's a midwife, and he's a doctor.

"How did he even know how to move his head?" I asked her later.

"He trained in the military," she told me. "With midwives."

Later, I found out that he was, for an obstetrician, comfortable right on the edge of risk. He had his own story of birth trauma: his baby had died at birth. And so, the lactation consultant who told me about this cautioned that though he is usually pretty risk-tolerant, he can be very—perhaps overly—cautious in some circumstances. That is: he largely treats birth similarly to the ways a midwife might—as a low-risk event in which to intervene only when necessary—except when his own trauma gets in the way.

Once Dr. M moved the baby's head, everything started to happen very quickly. My water broke, suddenly, in a wave that splashed all over Lena. She needed to change her clothes, and called for towels to mop up the floor of the tiny room. *So this is why she was wearing goggles*, I remember thinking. I was stunned that my body had contained so much fluid.

Then, pushing. The epidural had stopped working, or maybe someone had turned it off, because I thought I was ripping in half. And then my husband told me, "I see the head!" A few more pushes, and then there he was, at 9:17 p.m. on his due date. As a chronically late person who (ironically?) feels stress about trying to be punctual, I felt praised by the universe for this.

My teeth chattered; my whole body shook. We gave him a name that means "God gave."

Hours later, when a nurse came to take me to the postpartum floor, I collapsed into the wheelchair. I was completely depleted by the birth. I worried, then, too, that something had gone wrong; that I had lost too much blood, maybe. Dr. M came in and put his hand against mine. "This is the quick and dirty way to tell if you're anemic," he said. "I'd put you at an eight." (He was right.) "I don't think you're anemic," he said. "I think you're shot." He kept me overnight anyway, because of the staffing, he said: one nurse to one patient. A closer set of eyes on me. Later, after I was released to the postpartum floor, he called to check on me there, too. The nurse who'd coached me through the birth came to see me to congratulate me and ask how I felt. All of this care: from Lena; from Dr. M; from the nurses. I hadn't experienced anything like it the first time. Not until after that birth had gone south.

This was beautiful care, even in a pandemic. If only it had been that way the first time. If only every mother, no matter where or how they birth, could expect such tenderness.

Still, in the weeks to come, I had my own amalgam of postpartum woes: A chronic case of mastitis I couldn't kick. The pinching from stitches of a first-degree tear. Continued experiences with PTSD. All of which is to say, VBAC and the kindest providers didn't fix everything. That first birth still shapes the present. And yet the respectful and personal care I experienced remains a touchstone of what should be possible for every mother.

My mother came to visit a few days after my son's birth. We were taking a walk around the block, our first as a family of four, and my parents drove past us. Mom opened the passenger door even before my father had stopped the car. She jumped out. She had a cane in one hand, and a big black boot on her foot. I hadn't seen her since her seventy-fifth birthday party several months earlier, before COVID. While I'd been getting ready to have a baby, her life had been ebbing: a broken ankle; three days in a hospital at the height of COVID; an operation; COVID; pneumonia. She'd lost twenty, maybe thirty pounds. While I was pregnant, she'd nearly died.

My mother grabbed me, took me into her arms. She held me, her baby. "When I saw you," she told me later, "I forgot that I couldn't walk."

ACKNOWLEDGMENTS

I OFTEN TELL MY STUDENTS THAT SCHOLARSHIP IS A SHARED EN-deavor, and that multiple brains are always better than one. This book is an excellent example of that advice. I am profoundly grateful to the many people who made this book so much better than I could have on my own.

Veronica Goldstein, my agent, pushed me to make the book sharper when it was still a proposal, and led me through the publishing process with wisdom and vision. Julie Will believed in the book from the beginning and saw it better than I could; she guided me to use C-sections to think through American culture in ways I didn't even know I was doing. Helen Atsma welcomed me to Ecco with warmth and confidence. Rachel Sargent gave sage advice about how to start even the most difficult chapters and untangle my deeply muddled renderings of the philosophies of pregnancy. Sarah Murphy encouraged me to make this book smarter, clearer, more cohesive, and deeper, when I didn't even realize there was deeper to go. A dream team—truly—of committed and generous thinkers and editors who guided me with tremendous respect, patience, humanity, and encouragement. I've come out a better writer. It has been an absolute privilege and so very rewarding to work with you. Thank you.

Meghan Holtan provided insight into the Alaska Native health system, sources, a place to stay in Anchorage, and a sharp eye. Lisa Phillips's comments brought the book to the next level and also made me feel that I was capable of finishing it—even when I wasn't sure of that myself. Jessica Slice's perspectives on parenting, disability, and storytelling proved indispensable. Diana Lind (who conceived the term "cascade of consequences"), also a writer and mother, encouraged me through the twin and often simultaneous marathons of writing and parenting; I am so grateful for her friendship and the example she sets. Sarah Yahr Tucker reported with me on inadequate anesthesia during C-sections long before most anyone would speak about the topic. Heather Hewitt was both pacesetter and thoughtful editor. Sylvie Beauvais, Meghan Baudry, and Kate Lewis read early drafts of many of these chapters and provided invaluable advice. Sari Botton and Anica Butler gave me the chance to explore what became some of the book's main ideas in Longreads and the *Boston Globe*, respectively. Brigid Schulte's editorial eye, and a reporting grant from the New America Foundation, did as well.

Jacqueline H. Wolf's books *Cesarean Section* and *Deliver Me from Pain* provided an essential basis for this book. I'm also deeply indebted to work by Rima D. Apple, Janet Bogdan, Deirdre Cooper Owens, Sabine Hildebrandt, Keisha L. Goode, Linda Janet Holmes, Judith Walzer Leavitt, Neil Postman, Stanley Joel Reiser, Loretta J. Ross, Barbara Katz Rothman, Rickie Solinger, Alexandra Minna Stern, Laurel Thatcher Ulrich, and Harriet Washington. Conversations with Alicia D. Bonaparte, Julie Cantor, Nicole Carr, Keisha L. Goode, Helena A. Grant, Linda Janet Holmes, Lynn Paltrow, and Barbara Katz Rothman further sharpened and broadened my thinking. Meghan Blair Turner lucidly and generously explained telomeres to me.

Thank you to the librarians at SUNY New Paltz, particularly in interlibrary loan, and to Arlene Shaner at the New York Academy of Medicine, who located crucial archival texts and guided my research. Nicole Zanchelli and Dana Halladay contributed research assistance. A sabbatical from SUNY New Paltz allowed me the time necessary to write the bulk of this book, and a SUNY New Paltz research and creative projects award provided important funding.

Cordelia Calvert made sure this book reached the wider world. The art and production teams at Ecco worked patiently and thoroughly to create a beautiful design and cover.

Cruz Bueno showed me my blind spots. Sam Manzella fact-checked with such diligence and thoughtfulness, she made me a better reporter. Dr. Amanda Rohn's medical insights and editorial eye made this text more accurate and more profound. Copy editor Janet Rosenberg saved me from truly embarrassing errors. I learned so much from each of you. Any remaining mistakes are my own.

Many parents shared their experiences with me, sometimes opening their homes to me and even allowing me to hold their babies. I'm so grateful to each of you for your candor and vulnerability, and for trusting me with your stories. Even if your name is not in this book, your story helped to shape it.

For their ideas, suggestions, perspectives, cheerleading, and love, thank you to friends and colleagues Kara Belinsky, Sophia Benikram, Greg Bray, Jessica Crowell, Andrea Gatzke, Kiersten Greene, Naomi Kohen, Rachel Margolis, Robin Minkoff, Charlotte Nunes, Danielle Rein, Laura Rowntree, Megan Sperry, Erica Tunick, Madeline Veitch, and Rebecca Wester. Over the past couple of years, Kate Ryan and Aidan Koehler batted around many of the ideas and problems explored in this book. I have done a far better job with this material because of these conversations. In some ways I feel as though we wrote this book together. And when I couldn't see how I would finish (or start) a chapter, our walks in the woods kept me going.

Dave Gerrard—thank you for your belief in me as a writer, and for twenty-five years of friendship; I wish we could celebrate this milestone together.

Bill Weinstein pointed me in the direction of Ashley Montagu and the importance of touch. My writing teachers Leslie Woodard and Michael Koch taught me how to write, and to read; I wish I could show them this book. Jon Jucovy and Mary Roldán showed me what kind of questions I could ask of the past, and Mary Roldán introduced me to the concept of collective memory, which—though I didn't know it at the time—I'd been working on in one way or another for most of my life. Anne Demo taught me to think about photography as both art and rhetoric. Dennis Kinsey and my other professors at Newhouse taught me to be a researcher, and Darin Strauss and other faculty at NYU helped me to hone my craft.

Thank you to all of the people in New Paltz (especially at Moriello Pool) who shared their own experiences with C-sections and birth. These conversations—sometimes even brief ones—helped me to think about the book in new ways and also reaffirmed the importance of talking about birth.

Beth Sirof and Noelle Damon helped to get me to a place where I could write this book without being too frightened of the material. Debbie Healy was first a healer, then a guide, and is now a true friend. Jenn Sullivan and Susie Fenton provided kinship, healing, and perspective.

The staff at the Children's Center at SUNY New Paltz provided a loving and nurturing environment for my children while I worked on this book. Thank you in particular to Marcia Villiers, AnnMarie Callan, Cindy Joao, Erin Rauth, and Belkis Estrella. Thank you to Orna Gorosh, Charlotte Vignoles, and Natalie Nunez, who cared for my children with creativity and love, even in the darkest of COVID times.

My mother, Lynn Somerstein, brought me to writing classes at Columbia when I was a teenager. My father, Mark Somerstein, gifted me his engagement with the past. Both gave me the courage to look at the dark places, a serious work ethic, and the superpower of reading between the lines. Thank you for standing with (and taking care of) me through the joyful and difficult seasons of parenting and writing.

David, Debbie, Ben, Abby, Sam, and Josh Tyler gave me their love, constancy, and delicious cooking. Tom and Karen Lingeman came to our family's aid at the most crucial hour. Ehrin and Ben Lingeman sustained me with their encouragement, curiosity, and sharp insights about the cover. Hazel Correa shared important perspectives about navigating American healthcare as a person of color. Years of conversation with all of you about birth, children, parenting, family, and medicine helped to make this book.

Joe: As I wrote and revised this book, sometimes you articulated ideas I didn't yet know I had. I am in awe at your clarity of vision. Thank you for your great faith in me and for giving (and making) the space I needed to write this book.

To my children: Your smiling faces are the best of any balm. Thank you for your patience; I know it wasn't always easy to have a mother who was writing. But now the book is done. Really, really done!

To my family, I love you.

NOTES

PROLOGUE

1. March of Dimes Peristats, "Total Cesarean Deliveries: United States, 2021," last updated January 2022, accessed September 6, 2023, https://www.marchofdimes.org /peristats/data?reg=99&top=8&stop=645&lev=1&slev=1&obj=1&dv=ms; March of Dimes Peristats, "Low-Risk Cesarean Births: United States, 2017–2020," last updated January 2022, accessed September 6, 2023, https://www.marchofdimes .org/peristats/data?reg=99&top=8&stop=645&lev=1&slev=1&obj=1&dv=ms.
2. Jacqueline H. Wolf, *Cesarean Section: An American History of Risk, Technology, and Consequence* (Baltimore: Johns Hopkins University Press, 2018), 45.
3. Pelin Dikmen Yildiz, Susan Ayers, and Louise Phillips, "The Prevalence of Post-traumatic Stress Disorder in Pregnancy and After Birth: A Systematic Review and Meta-analysis," *Journal of Affective Disorders* 208 (January 15, 2017): 634–45, https://doi.org/10.1016/j.jad.2016.10.009.
4. Susan Ayers and Alan D. Pickering, "Do Women Get Posttraumatic Stress Disorder as a Result of Childbirth? A Prospective Study of Incidence," *Birth: Issues in Perinatal Care* 8, no. 2 (2001): 111–18; Deniz Ertan et al., "Post-traumatic Stress Disorder Following Childbirth," *BMC Psychiatry* 21, no. 155 (2021), https://bmc-psychiatry.biomedcentral.com/articles/10.1186/s12888-021-03158-6#:~:text =One%20study%20showed%20that%20about.
5. Judith Walzer Leavitt, *Brought to Bed: Childbearing in America, 1750–1950* (New York: Oxford University Press, 1986): 268–69.
6. UNICEF and the World Health Organization, "Trends in Maternal Mortality: 1999 to 2008," accessed September 7, 2023, https://apps.who.int/iris/bitstream /handle/10665/44423/9789241500265_eng.pdf.
7. "The Evaluation of the Pregnancy Status Checkbox on the Identification of Maternal Deaths," *National Vital Statistics Reports* 69 no. 1 (January 2020): 1–25, https://www.cdc.gov/nchs/data/nvsr/nvsr69/nvsr69_01-508.pdf.
8. "Detailed Evaluation of Changes in Data Collection Methods," Centers for Disease Control and Prevention, last updated November 21, 2019, https://www.cdc .gov/nchs/maternal-mortality/evaluation.htm.
9. Kathleen Chin, Amelia Wendt, Ian M. Bennett, and Amritha Bhat, "Suicide and Maternal Mortality," *Current Psychiatry Reports* 24, no. 4 (2022): 239–75, https:// doi.org/10.1007/s11920-022-01334-3.

10. Centers for Disease Control and Prevention, "Pregnancy-Related Mortality Surveillance: United States, 1991–1999," *Morbidity and Mortality Weekly Report* 52 (SS-2), February 2003, https://www.cdc.gov/mmwr/pdf/ss/ss5202.pdf.

11. Lindsay K. Admon et al., "Trends in Suicidality 1 Year Before and After Birth Among Commercially Insured Childbearing Individuals in the United States, 2006–2017," *JAMA Psychiatry* 78, no. 2 (2021): 171–76, https://doi.org/10.1001/jamapsychiatry.2020.3550; Hamisu M. Salihu, Deepa Dongarwar, Emmanuella Oduguwa, and Toi B. Harris, "Racial/Ethnic Disparity in Suicidal Ideation, Suicide Attempt and Non-suicidal Intentional Self-harm Among Pregnant Women in the United States, *Journal of Immigrant and Minority Health* 24 (2022): 588–596, https://doi.org/10.1007/s10903-021-01260-1.

12. Anne Case and Angus Deaton, "Rising Morbidity and Mortality in Midlife Among White Non-Hispanic Americans in the 21st Century," *Proceedings of the National Academy of Sciences of the United States of America* 112, no. 49 (2015): 15078–83, https://doi.org/10.1073/pnas.1518393112.

13. Jennifer C. Nash, *Birthing Black Mothers* (Durham and London: Duke University Press, 2021), 12.

14. Patrick Drake, Anne K. Driscoll, and T. J. Mathews, "Cigarette Smoking During Pregnancy: United States, 2016," NCHS Data Brief 305 (February 2018), https://www.cdc.gov/nchs/products/databriefs/db305.htm; Lucinda J. England, Carolyne Bennett, Clark H. Denny, et al., "Alcohol Use and Co-Use of Other Substances Among Pregnant Females Aged 12–44 Years—United States, 2015–2018," *Morbidity and Mortality Weekly Report* 69, no. 31 (August 2020): 1009–14; Elizabeth Armstrong, *Conceiving Risk, Bearing Responsibility: Fetal Alcohol Syndrome and the Diagnosis of Moral Disorder* (Baltimore: Johns Hopkins University Press, 2003).

15. Maeve Wallace et al., "Homicide During Pregnancy and the Postpartum Period in the United States, 2018–2019," *Obstetrics & Gynecology* 138, no. 5 (November 1, 2021): 762–69, https://doi.org/10.1097%2FAOG.0000000000004567.

16. Dorothy Roberts, *Killing the Black Body: Race, Reproduction, and the Meaning of Liberty* (New York: Pantheon, 1997), 23.

17. Iris Jacob, "What I Carry: A Story of Love and Loss," in *Birthing Justice: Black Women, Pregnancy, and Childbirth*, edited by Julia Chinyere Oparah and Alicia D. Bonaparte (Routledge: New York and London, 2016), 90–95.

CHAPTER 1: THE STATE OF THE UTERUS

1. Mauro Turrini and Catherine Bourgain, "Appraising Screening, Making Risk In/visible: The Medical Debate over Non-Rare Thrombophilia (NRT) Testing Before Prescribing the Pill," *Sociology of Health & Illness* 43 (2021): 1627–42, https://doi.org/10.1111/1467-9566.13348.

2. Wolf, *Cesarean Section*, 166.

3. Healthy People 2030, "Reduce Cesarean Births Among Low-Risk Women with No Prior Births—MICH-06," Office of Disease Prevention and Health Promotion, accessed August 14, 2023, https://health.gov/healthypeople/objectives-and-data/browse-objectives/pregnancy-and-childbirth/reduce-cesarean-births-among-low-risk-women-no-prior-births-mich-06.

4. Paul J. Placek and Selma M. Taffel, "Trends in Cesarean Section Rates for the United States, 1970–1978" *Public Health Reports* 95, no. 6 (1980): 540–48.

5. Michelle J. K. Osterman et al., "Births: Final Data for 2021," *National Vital Statistics Reports* 72, no. 1 (January 31, 2023): 36, https://www.cdc.gov/nchs/data/nvsr/nvsr72/nvsr72-01.pdf; Wolf, *Cesarean Section*, 4.

6. Gretchen Livingston, "They're Waiting Longer, but U.S. Women Today More Likely to Have Children Than a Decade Ago," Pew Research Center, January 18, 2018, https://www.pewresearch.org/social-trends/2018/01/18/theyre-waiting-longer-but-u-s-women-today-more-likely-to-have-children-than-a-decade-ago/#:~:text=Overall%2C%20women%20have%202.07%20children,low%20of%202.31%20in%202008.

7. Maria Regina Torloni, Ana Pilar Betran, Joao Paulo Souza, et al., "Classifications for Cesarean Section: A Systematic Review," *PLoS ONE* 6, no. 1 (2011): e14566, https://doi.org/10.1371/journal.pone.0014566.

8. Annelee Boyle et al., "Primary Cesarean Delivery in the United States," *Obstetrics & Gynecology* 122, no. 1 (2013): http://doi.org/10.1097/AOG.0b013e3182952242.

9. Laura B. Attanasio, Katy B. Kozhimannil, Sindhu K. Srinivas, and Kristen H. Kjerulff, "Concordance between Women's Self-Reported Reasons for Cesarean Delivery and Hospital Discharge Records," *Women's Health Issues* 27, no. 3 (2017): 329–35.

10. Bipartisan Policy Center, "Paid Family Leave in the United States," 2020, https://bipartisanpolicy.org/download/?file=/wp-content/uploads/2020/02/Paid-Family-Leave-in-the-United-States.pdf.

11. Shiliang Liu, Robert M. Liston, K.S. Joseph, et al., "Maternal Mortality and Severe Morbidity Associated with Low-Risk Planned Cesarean Delivery Versus Planned Vaginal Delivery at Term," *Canadian Medical Association Journal* 176, no. 4 (February 2007), http://doi.org/10.1503/cmaj.060870.

12. Osterman et al., "Births: Final Data for 2021," 36.

13. Marie Ashe, "Law-Language of Maternity: Discourse Holding Nature in Contempt," *New England Law Review* 22 (1988): 521–59.

14. Isabel Karpin, "Legislating the Female Body: Reproductive Technology and the Reconstructed Woman," *Columbia Journal of Gender & Law* 3 (1992).

15. Ashe, "Law-Language of Maternity."

CHAPTER 2: "NATURAL" CHILDBIRTH AND THE "NORMAL" WOMAN

1. Kathy Lette, "A Natural Birth in the Name of the Environment? Absolutely Not," *Sydney Morning Herald*, July 10, 2022, https://www.smh.com.au/lifestyle/life-and-relationships/a-natural-birth-in-the-name-of-the-environment-absolutely-not-20220704-p5ayvz.html.

2. Saima Kara (@livewildfreebirth), Instagram photo, July 6, 2022, https://www.instagram.com/p/CfrqaoTjmq1/.

3. Renate Blumenfeld-Kosinski, *Not of Woman Born: Representations of Caesarean Birth in Medieval and Renaissance Culture* (Ithaca, NY: Cornell University Press, 2019), 33; Wolf, *Cesarean Section*, 5.

4. Jacqueline H. Wolf, *Deliver Me from Pain: Anesthesia & Birth in America* (Baltimore: Johns Hopkins University Press, 2009), 18.
5. Ibid., 96.
6. Ibid., 98.
7. Leavitt, *Brought to Bed*, 45–48.
8. Wolf, *Deliver Me from Pain*, 48.
9. Ibid., 51.
10. Ibid., 67.
11. Ibid., 71, 140–43.
12. Ibid., 69.
13. Grantly Dick-Read, *Childbirth Without Fear* (London: Pinter & Martin Ltd., 2004), 24.
14. Wolf, *Deliver Me from Pain*, 154.
15. Dick-Read, *Childbirth Without Fear*, 250.
16. Gladys Denny Schultz, "*Journal* Mothers Report on Cruelty in Maternity Wards," *Ladies' Home Journal*, May 1958, 44–45, https://archive.org/details/ladies-home-journal-v-075-n-05-1958-05/page/n45/mode/2up.
17. Wolf, *Deliver Me from Pain*, 179.
18. Schultz, "*Journal* Mothers Report," 44–45, 152–53.
19. Ibid., 152–53.
20. Wolf, *Deliver Me from Pain*, 156.
21. Ina May Gaskin, interview, *Birth Story: Ina May Gaskin and the Farm Midwives*, directed by Sara Lamm and Mary Wigmore (Ghost Robot/Reckon So Productions, 2012), Amazon.
22. Schultz, "*Journal* Mothers Report," 154.
23. Gaskin, *Birth Story*.
24. Ina May Gaskin, *Ina May's Guide to Childbirth* (New York: Bantam Books, 2019), xii.
25. Ibid., 175–76.
26. Ibid., 189.
27. Ibid., 184–85.
28. North American Registry of Midwives, "Legal Recognition of CPMs," updated August 1, 2023, https://www.nacpm.org/legal-recognition-of-cpms-1#:~:text=Alabama%2C%20Alaska%2C%20Arizona%2C%20Arkansas,Carolina%2C%20South%20Dakota%2C%20Tennessee%2C.
29. Osterman et al., "Births: Final Data for 2021."
30. The Farm Midwifery Center, "Preliminary Statistics," https://thefarmmidwives.org/preliminary-statistics/.
31. Gaskin, *Ina May's Guide to Childbirth*, 148.
32. The Farm Midwifery Center, "Preliminary Statistics."
33. Elizabeth C. W. Gregory, Claudia P. Valenzuela, and Donna L. Hoyert, "Fetal Mortality: United States, 2020," *National Vital Statistics Reports* 71, no. 4 (2022), https://dx.doi.org/10.15620/cdc:118420.
34. Donna L. Hoyert, "Maternal Mortality Rates in the United States, 2020," NCHS Health E Stats (2022), https://www.cdc.gov/nchs/data/hestat/maternal-mortality/2020/maternal-mortality-rates-2020.htm#.

35. Michelle J. K. Osterman et al., "Births: Final Data for 2020," *National Vital Statistics Reports* 70, no. 17 (2022), https://dx.doi.org/10.15620/cdc:112078.

36. Gaskin, *Ina May's Guide to Childbirth*, 162.

37. Laura B. Attanasio and Rachel R. Hardeman, "Declined Care and Discrimination During the Childbirth Hospitalization," *Social Science & Medicine* 232 (July 2019): 270–77, https://doi.org/10.1016/j.socscimed.2019.05.008.

38. Rosalind R. Gill and Shani Orgad, "The Amazing Bounce-Backable Woman: Resilience and the Psychological Turn in Neoliberalism," *Sociological Research Online* 23, no. 2 (2018): 477–95, https://doi.org/10.1177/1360780418769673.

39. Gaskin, *Ina May's Guide to Childbirth*, 211.

40. Wolf, *Deliver Me from Pain*, 137.

41. Ibid., 179.

42. George B. Feldman and Jennie E. Freiman, "Prophylactic Cesarean Section At Term?," *New England Journal of Medicine* 312, no. 19 (1985): 1264–67.

43. Stephen A. Myers and Norbert Gleicher, "1988 U.S. Cesarean-Section Rate: Good News or Bad?," *New England Journal of Medicine* 323, no. 3 (1990): 200.

44. Robert D. Vincent Jr. and David H. Chestnut, "Epidural Analgesia During Labor," *American Family Physician* 58, no. 8 (1998): 1785–92, https://pubmed.ncbi.nlm.nih.gov/9835854/.

45. Saraswathi Vedam, Kathrin Stoll, et al., "The Giving Voice to Mothers Study: Inequity and Mistreatment During Pregnancy and Childbirth in the United States," *Reproductive Health* 16, no. 77 (2019), https://doi.org/10.1186/s12978-019-0729-2.

46. Wolf, *Deliver Me from Pain*, 166.

47. Schultz, "*Journal* Mothers Report," 152–53.

48. Marian MacDorman and Eugene Declercq, "Trends and State Variations in Out-of-Hospital Births in the United States, 2004–2017," *Birth* 29, no. 2 (June 2019): 279–88, https://doi.org/10.1111/birt.12411.

49. Elizabeth C. W. Gregory, Michelle J. K. Osterman, and Claudia P. Valenzuela, "Changes in Home Births by Race and Hispanic Origin and State of Residence of Mother: United States, 2019–2020 and 2020–2021," *National Vital Statistics Reports* 71, no. 8 (2022), https://www.cdc.gov/nchs/data/nvsr/nvsr71/nvsr71-08.pdf.

50. Paul Frosh, "Rhetorics of the Overlooked: On the Communicative Modes of Stock Advertising Images," *Journal of Consumer Culture* 2, no. 2 (2002): 147–288, https://doi.org/10.1177/146954050200200202.

51. Samantha Griffin, "The Ina May Gaskin Racial Gaffe Heard 'Round the Midwifery World," *Rewire News Group*, April 26, 2017, https://rewirenewsgroup.com/2017/04/26/ina-may-gaskin-racial-gaffe-heard-round-midwifery-world.

52. American College of Nurse-Midwifery Philosophy of Midwifery, "Our Philosophy of Care," last revised August 2023, https://www.midwife.org/our-philosophy-of-care.

CHAPTER 3: THE ORIGINS OF THE C-SECTION

1. Marianne Hirsch, "Past Lives: Postmemories in Exile," *Poetics Today* 17, no. 4 (1996): 659, https://doi.org/10.2307/1773218.

2. Jeffrey Boss, "The Antiquity of Casearean Section with Maternal Survival: The Jewish Tradition," *Medical History* 5, no. 2 (April 1961): 117–31, https://doi.org/1 0.1017%2Fs0025727300026089.

3. Joseph G. Ryan, "The Chapel and the Operating Room: The Struggle of Roman Catholic Clergy, Physicians, and Believers with the Dilemmas of Obstetric Surgery, 1800–1900," *Bulletin of the History of Medicine* 76 no. 3 (2002): 461–94.

4. Nadia Maria Filippini, *Pregnancy, Delivery, Childbirth: A Gender and Cultural History from Antiquity to the Test Tube in Europe* (London: Routledge, 2021), 96.

5. Katharine Park, *Secrets of Women* (New York: Zone Books, 2006), 154.

6. Alan Frank Guttmacher, *Pregnancy, Birth, and Family Planning: A Guide for Expectant Parents in the 1970s* (New York: Viking Press, 1973).

7. Filippini, *Pregnancy, Delivery, Childbirth*, 140.

8. Park, *Secrets of Women*, 65.

9. Justin Barr et al., "Surgeons in the Time of Plague: Guy de Chauliac in Fourteenth-Century France," *Journal of Vascular Surgery Cases and Innovative Techniques* 6, no. 4 (2020): 657–58, https://doi.org/10.1016/j.jvscit.2020.07.006.

10. Vern L. Katz, "Perimortem Cesarean Delivery: Its Role in Maternal Mortality," *Seminars in Perinatology* 36 (2012): 68–72.

11. Elizabeth O'Brien and Miriam Rich, "The Art of Medicine: Obstetric Violence in Historical Perspective," *Lancet* 399, no. 10342 (2022): 2183–85, https://doi .org/10.1016/S0140-6736(22)01022-4.

12. Vern L. Katz and Robert C. Cefalo, "History and Evolution of Cesarean Delivery," in *Cesarean Delivery* (Amsterdam: Elsevier, 1988), 5

13. Jolien Gijbels, "Medical Compromise and Its Limits: Religious Concerns and the Postmortem Caesarean Section in Nineteenth-Century Belgium," *Bulletin of the History of Medicine* 93, no. 3 (2019): 305–34.

14. Daniel Schäfer, "Medical Practice and the Law in the Conflict between Traditional Belief and Empirical Evidence: Post-Mortem Caesarean Section in the Nineteenth Century," *Medical History* 43 (1999): 485–501.

15. Ibid.

16. Ibid.

17. Ibid.; Gijbels, "Medical Compromise and Its Limits."

18. Adrienne Rich, *Of Woman Born: Motherhood as Experience and Institution* (New York: W. W. Norton & Company, 2012), 134.

19. Saidiya Hartman, *Lose Your Mother: A Journey Along the Atlantic Slave Trade* (New York: Macmillan, 2008), 17.

20. Rudolph Matas, "François Marie Prevost and the Early History of the Cesarean Section in Louisiana," *New Orleans Medical and Surgical Journal* 89 (May 1937): 14; Robert P. Harris, "The Caesarean Operation in the United States," *American Journal of Obstetrics and Diseases of Women and Children* 4 (1872).

21. Schäfer, "Medical Practice and the Law," 488; Katz and Cefalo, "Cesarean Delivery," 4.

22. Katz and Cefalo, "Cesarean Delivery."

23. And he did. He was so well regarded that Napoleon asked him to attend his wife, Empress Marie-Louise, during her first birth.

24. Wolf, *Cesarean Section*, 29.
25. Deirdre Cooper Owens and Sharla M. Fett, "Black Maternal and Infant Health: Historical Legacies of Slavery," *American Journal of Public Health* 109, no. 10 (October 2019), https://doi.org/10.2105/AJPH.2019.305243.
26. Harriet A. Washington, *Medical Apartheid: The Dark History of Medical Experimentation on Black Americans from Colonial Times to the Present* (New York: Penguin Random House, 2008): 101.
27. Thomas Benton Sellers, "Louisiana's Contributions to Obstetrics and Gynecology," *Bulletin of the History of Medicine* 22, no. 2 (March–April 1948): 196–207.
28. Matas, "François Marie Prevost," 619.
29. Ibid., 617.
30. William T. Lusk, "The Prognosis of Cesarean Operations," reprinted from *American Journal of Obstetrics and Diseases of Women and Children* xiii, no. 1 (January 1880): 5.
31. Matas, "François Marie Prevost," 6.
32. Wolf, *Cesarean Section*, 24–26.
33. Joseph G. Nancrede, "Observations on the Caesarean Operation, Accompanied by the Relation of a Case in Which Both Mother and Child Were Preserved." *American Journal of Medical Sciences* (1835), 16: 347.
34. *A Southern Practice: The Diary and Autobiography of Charles A. Hentz* (Charlottesville: University of Virginia Press, 2000), quoted in Stephen C. Kenny, "The Development of Medical Museums in the Antebellum American South," *Bulletin of the History of Medicine* 87, no. 1 (Spring 2013): 53.
35. Kenny, "The Development of Medical Museums in the Antebellum American South," 32–62.
36. Robert P. Harris, "A Study and Analysis of One Hundred Cesarean Operations Performed in the United States, During the Present Century and Prior to the Year 1878," *American Journal of Medical Sciences* nos. 77 (January 1879): 46.
37. Nora Doyle, *Maternal Bodies: Redefining Motherhood in Early America* (Chapel Hill, NC: University of North Carolina Press, 2018), 85; Wolf, *Cesarean Section*.
38. Wolf, *Cesarean Section*.
39. Harris, "A Study and Analysis of One Hundred Cesarean Operations Performed in the United States, During the Present Century and Prior to the Year 1878," 15–16.
40. Harris, quoted in Wolf, *Cesarean Section*, 27.
41. Lusk, "The Prognosis of Cesarean Operations," 7.
42. Franklin Luther Mott, *Golden Multitudes: The Story of Best Sellers in the United States* (New York: Macmillan, 1947), 27.
43. Harris, "The Caesarean Operation in the United States," read in a meeting of the Philadelphia Obstetrical Society on September 7, 1871, and reprinted in the *American Journal of Obstetrics and Diseases of Women* 4 (1871–1872), 421.
44. Edward P. Davis, *Operative Obstetrics Including the Surgery of the Newborn* (Philadelphia: W.B. Saunders Company, 1911), https://babel.hathitrust.org/cgi/pt?id=mdp.39015074002893&view=1up&seq=315&skin=2021.
45. Franklin Newell, *Cesarean Section* (Boston: D. Appleton & Company, 1921), 30.

CHAPTER 4: CASCADE OF CONSEQUENCES

1. Shefaly Shorey, Yen Yen Yang, and Emily Ang, "The Impact of Negative Child-birth Experience on Future Reproductive Decisions: A Quantitative Systematic Review," *Journal of Advanced Nursing* 74, no. 6 (2018): 1–9.
2. I. Gurol-Urganci et al., "Impact of Caesarean Section on Subsequent Fertility: A Systematic Review and Meta-analysis," *Human Reproduction* 28, no. 7 (July 2013): 1945, https://doi.org/10.1093/humrep/det130.
3. Oonagh E. Keag, Jane E. Norman, and Sarah J. Stock, "Long-Term Risks and Benefits Associated with Cesarean Delivery for Mother, Baby, and Subsequent Pregnancies: Systematic Review and Meta-analysis," *PLoS Medicine* 15, no. 1 (2018), https://doi.org/10.1371/journal.pmed.1002494.
4. Ibid.
5. The American College of Obstetricians and Gynecologists, "Placenta Accreta Spectrum," *Obstetrics & Gynecology* 132, no. 6 (December 2018).
6. Jane Sandall, Rachel M. Tribe, Lisa Avery, et al., "Short-Term and Long-Term Effects of Caesarean Section on the Health of Women and Children," *Lancet* 392 (2018): 1349–57, https://www.healthynewbornnetwork.org/hnn-content /uploads/Caesarean2.pdf.
7. Ilan E. Timor-Tritsch and Ana Monteagudo, "Unforeseen Consequences of the Increasing Rate of Cesarean Deliveries: Early Placenta Accreta and Cesarean Scar Pregnancy: A Review," *American Journal of Obstetrics & Gynecology* 207, no. 1 (2012); Wolf, *Cesarean Section*, 6.
8. The American College of Obstetricians and Gynecologists, "Placenta Accreta Spectrum."
9. Kristen H. Kjerulff et al., "Mode of First Delivery and Women's Intentions for Subsequent Childbearing: Findings from the First Baby Study," *Paediatric and Perinatal Epidemiology* 27 (2013): 62–71, https://onlinelibrary.wiley.com /doi/10.1111/ppe.12014.
10. Kristen H. Kjerulff et al., "First Birth Caesarean Section and Subsequent Fertility: a Population-Based Study in the USA, 2000–2008," *Human Reproduction* 28, no. 12 (2013): 3349–57, https://www.ncbi.nlm.nih.gov/pmc/articles /PMC3829579/.
11. Wolf, *Cesarean Section*, 41–43; David L. Barclay, "Cesarean Hysterectomy: Thirty Years' Experience," *Obstetrics & Gynecology* 35, no. 1 (1970).
12. Isaac E. Taylor, "Gastro-Hysterectomy: On the Recent Modification of the Cesarean Section by Dr. Porro," *American Journal of Medical Sciences* (July 1880): 4–17.
13. Edwin Black, "Eugenics and the Nazis—the California Connection," SFGate, November 9, 2003, accessed July 31, 2023, https://www.sfgate.com/opinion/article /Eugenics-and-the-Nazis-the-California-2549771.php.
14. Adam Cohen, *Imbeciles: The Supreme Court, American Eugenics, and the Sterilization of Carrie Buck* (New York: Penguin Books, 2016), 131.
15. Taylor, "Gastro-Hysterectomy," 4–17.
16. Davis, *Operative Obstetrics*, 315.

17. Marita Sturken and Lisa Cartwright, *Practices of Looking: An Introduction to Visual Culture*, 2nd ed. (New York: Oxford University Press, 2009), 106; Brian Wallis, "Black Bodies, White Science: Louis Agassiz's Slave Daguerreotypes," *American Art* 9, no. 2 (1995): 38–61.

18. Donna Haraway, "Situated Knowledges: The Science Question in Feminism and the Privilege of Partial Perspective," *Feminist Studies* 14, no. 3 (1988): 585, https://philpapers.org/archive/harskt.pdf.

19. "The Caesarean Operation," *New York Times*, February 8, 1893, 2.

20. "Successful Caesarean Operation," *New York Times*, May 8, 1895, 5.

21. Wolf, *Cesarean Section*, 4.

22. Davis, *Operative Obstetrics*.

23. "Lady Diana Doing Well," *New York Times*, September 17, 1929, 10.

24. Wolf, *Cesarean Section*, 59.

25. Edwin A. Bowman Jr., *Cesarean Hysterectomy: An Analysis of One Thousand Consecutive Operations from Charity Hospital of Louisiana at New Orleans and the Early History of the Operation* (Dexter, MI: Thomson-Shore, 2009).

26. Alexandra Minna Stern, "Sterilized in the Name of Public Health: Race, Immigration, and Reproductive Control in Modern California," *American Journal of Public Health* 95, no. 7 (July 2005); *No Más Bebés*, directed by Renee Tajima-Peña (Independent Lens, 2015).

27. Dorothy Roberts, *Killing the Black Body* (New York: Pantheon, 1997); Thomas W. Volscho, "Racism and Disparities in Women's Use of the Depo-Provera Injection in the Contemporary USA," *Critical Sociology* 37, no. 5 (2011), https://doi.org/10.1177/0896920510380948.

28. *No Más Bebés*, directed by Renee Tajima-Peña.

29. Newell, *Cesarean Section*, 139.

30. M. Pierce Rucker and Edwin M. Rucker, "A Librarian Looks at Cesarean Section," *Bulletin of the History of Medicine* 25, no. 2 (March–April 1951): 140.

31. Wolf, *Cesarean Section*, 90–92.

32. Robert M. Silver et al., "Maternal Morbidity Associated with Multiple Repeat Cesarean Deliveries," *Obstetrics & Gynecology* 107, no. 6 (June 2006).

33. Ibid.

34. Stern, "Sterilized in the Name of Public Health."

35. Philipp Mitteroecker et al., "Cliff-Edge Model of Obstetric Selection in Humans," *Proceedings of the National Academy of Sciences* 113, no. 51 (December 5, 2016): 14680–85, https://doi.org/10.1073/pnas.1612410113.

CHAPTER 5: THE AMERICAN (MEDICAL) WAY TO BIRTH

1. Leavitt, *Brought to Bed*, 14; Janet Carlisle Bogdan, "Childbirth in America, 1650–1990," in *Women, Health, and Medicine in America: A Historical Handbook*, edited Rima Apple (New York: Garland Publishing, 1990).

2. Bogdan, "Childbirth in America, 1650–1990," 105.

3. Laurel Thatcher Ulrich, *Good Wives: Image and Reality in the Lives of Women in Northern New England, 1650–1750* (New York: Knopf, 1982), 144.

4. Leavitt, *Brought to Bed*, 36.
5. Doyle, *Maternal Bodies*, 81.
6. Ibid., 69–70.
7. Ulrich, *Good Wives*, 126.
8. Ibid., 127.
9. Ibid., 127.
10. Bogdan, *Childbirth in America*, 106.
11. Tamfer Emin Tunc, "The Mistress, the Midwife, and the Medical Doctor: Pregnancy and Childbirth on the Plantations of the Antebellum American South, 1800–1860," *Women's History Review* 19, no. 3 (July 2010): 395–419.
12. Bogdan, *Childbirth in America*, 106.
13. Filippini, *Pregnancy, Delivery, Childbirth*, 88.
14. Ibid., 89–90.
15. Tunc, "The Mistress, the Midwife, and the Medical Doctor," 400–401.
16. Bogdan, *Childbirth in America*, 106–12; Doyle, *Maternal Bodies*.
17. Ulrich, *Good Wives*, 129.
18. Linda Janet Holmes, interview with the author.
19. Linda Janet Holmes, *Safe in a Midwife's Hands: Birthing Traditions from Africa to the American South* (Columbus, OH: Ohio State University Press, 2023), 155.
20. Bogdan, *Childbirth in America*, 107.
21. Leavitt, *Brought to Bed*, 25.
22. Doyle, *Maternal Bodies*, 59.
23. Leavitt, *Brought to Bed*, 39–40 and 117; Wolf, *Cesarean Section*, 45.
24. Paul de Kruif, "Why Should Mothers Die?," *Ladies' Home Journal*, March 1936, 104, https://archive.org/details/sim_ladies-home-journal_1936-03_53_3/page/103/mode/1up?view=theater&q=%22cesspools%22.
25. Rich, *Of Woman Born*, 154.
26. Ibid., 152.
27. Leavitt, *Brought to Bed*, 45–48, 56–57.
28. Irvine Loudon, *Death in Childbirth: An International Study of Maternal Care and Maternal Mortality, 1800–1950* (New York: Oxford University Press, 1992), https://doi.org/10.1093/acprof:oso/9780198229971.003.0022.
29. Quoted in Leavitt, *Brought to Bed*, 61.
30. Leavitt, *Brought to Bed*, 57.
31. Leavitt, *Brought to Bed*, 61.
32. M.H.P., "Obituary: Joseph B. DeLee, M.D.," *British Medical Journal* 1, no. 4248 (June 6, 1942): 711, https://www.jstor.org/stable/20323356.
33. Quoted in Charles R. King, "The New York Maternal Mortality Study: A Conflict of Professionalization," *Bulletin of the History of Medicine* 65, no. 4 (1991): 478.
34. Sherri Broder, "Child Care or Child Neglect? Baby Farming in Late-Nineteenth-Century Philadelphia," *Gender & Society* 2 no. 2 (June 1988): 128–48; Judith Walzer Leavitt, "Joseph B. DeLee and the Practice of Preventative Obstetrics," *American Journal of Public Health* 78, no. 10 (1988): 1352–59, https://doi.org/10.2105%2Fajph.78.10.1353.

35. Morris Fishbein and Sol Theron DeLee, *Joseph Bolivar DeLee: Crusading Obstetrician* (New York: Dutton, 1949).

36. Leavitt, "Joseph B. DeLee," 1353–61; King, "The New York Maternal Mortality Study,"482.

37. Marina Boushra, Omar Rahman, "Postpartum Infection," StatPearls [Internet] (January 2024, last updated July 10, 2023), https://www.ncbi.nlm.nih.gov/books /NBK560804/.

38. S. Josephine Baker, "Maternal Mortality in the United States," *JAMA* 89, no. 24 (December 10, 1947): 2016, https://www.deepdyve.com/lp/american-medical-association/maternal-mortality-in-the-united-states-Xodbt7rDpo?key=JAMA.

39. Leavitt, *Brought to Bed*, 267.

40. King, "The New York Maternal Mortality Study," 481.

41. Ibid., 482–83.

42. Rich, *Of Woman Born*, 137.

43. Thomas Darlington, "The Present Status of the Midwife," *American Journal of Obstetrics and Diseases of Women and Children* 63 (1911). Quoted in Keisha L. Goode, "Birthing, Blackness, and the Body: Black Midwives and Experiential Continuities of Institutional Racism" (PhD diss., City University of New York, 2014), 12.

44. Katy Dawley, "Leaving the Nest: Nurse-Midwifery in the United States 1940–1980" (PhD diss., University of Pennsylvania, 2001), 51–52.

45. F. Elisabeth Crowell, "The Midwives of New York," *Charities and the Commons* 17 (1907): 674.

46. Quoted in Alicia D. Bonaparte, "'The Satisfactory Midwife Bag': Midwifery Regulation in South Carolina, Past and Present Considerations," *Social Science History* 38, nos. 1–2 (2014): 158, doi:10.1017/ssh.2015.14.

47. Yulonda Eadie Sano, "'Protect the Mother and Baby': Mississippi Lay Midwives and Public Health," *Agricultural History* 93, no. 3 (2019): 393–411, https://doi.org/10.3098/ah.2019.093.3.393.

48. Richard W. Wertz and Dorothy Wertz, *Lying In: A History of Childbirth in America* (New Haven, CT: Yale University Press, 1997).

49. Bonaparte, "'The Satisfactory Midwife Bag,'" 158–59.

50. Frances E. Kobrin, "The American Midwife Controversy: A Crisis of Professionalization," *Bulletin of the History of Medicine* 40, no. 4 (July–August 1966): 353.

51. Wangui Muigai, "'Something Wasn't Clean': Black Midwifery and Postwar Medical Education in *All My Babies*," *Bulletin of the History of Medicine* 93, no 1 (2019): 82–113, 10.1353/bhm.2019.0003.

52. Dawley, "Leaving the Nest"; Goode, "Birthing, Blackness, and the Body."

53. Katy Dawley, "Origins of Nurse-Midwifery in the United States and its Expansion in the 1940s," *Journal of Midwifery & Women's Health* 48, no. 2 (2003): 87, https://doi.org/10.1016/S1526-9523(03)00002-3.

54. "Occupational Employment and Wages, May 2022: Nurse Midwives," U.S. Bureau of Labor Statistics, accessed July 5, 2023, https://www.bls.gov/oes/current /oes291161.htm; "2021 Demographic Report," American Midwifery Certification Board, accessed July 5, 2023, https://www.amcbmidwife.org/docs/default -source/reports/demographic-report-2021.pdf?sfvrsn=cac0b1e8_2.

55. Sarah DiGregorio, *Taking Care: The Story of Nursing and Its Power to Change Our World* (New York: Harper, 2023).

56. "Pinkbook: Diphtheria," Centers for Disease Control and Prevention, https://www.cdc.gov/vaccines/pubs/pinkbook/dip.html.

57. Leavitt, *Brought to Bed*, 268; Joseph Gottfried, "History Repeating? Avoiding a Return to the Pre-Antibiotic Age" (class paper, Harvard Law School, 2005), https://dash.harvard.edu/bitstream/handle/1/8889467/Gottfried05.html.

58. David Cutler and Grant Miller, "The Role of Public Health Improvements in Health Advances: The Twentieth-Century United States," *Demography* 42, no. 1 (February 2005): 1–22, https://blogs.ubc.ca/internationalwaters/files/2017/03/The-role-of-public-health-improvements-in-health-advances-the-twentieth-century-United-States.pdf.

59. Leavitt, *Brought to Bed*, 267.

60. Charlotte G. Borst, *Catching Babies: The Professionalization of Childbirth, 1870–1920* (Cambridge, MA: Harvard University Press, 1995), 11.

61. Goode, "Birthing, Blackness, and the Body," 53.

62. Leavitt, *Brought to Bed*, 182.

63. Ibid., 269.

64. Leavitt, *Brought to Bed*, 268.

65. M.H.P., "Obituary: Joseph B. DeLee, M.D."

66. Katz and Cefalo, "History and Evolution of Cesarean Delivery."

67. Jack Gould, "Lucille Ball Adheres to Television Script; Comedienne Gives Birth to 8 ½-Pound Boy," *New York Times*, January 20, 1953.

68. UPI, "Mrs. Kennedy to Have a Caeserean Delivery," *New York Times*, November 18, 1960, accessed via ProQuest Historical Newspapers.

69. Katz and Cefalo, "History and Evolution of Cesarean Delivery."

70. George P. Hunt, "The Day of the Great Baby Chase," *Life*, December 1, 1967, 3.

71. Marek Glezerman, "Five Years to the Term Breech Trial: The Rise and Fall of a Randomized Controlled Trial," *American Journal of Obstetrics & Gynecology* 194, no. 1 (2006), https://doi.org/10.1016/j.ajog.2005.08.039.

72. Helen B. Taussig, "The Thalidomide Syndrome," *Scientific American* 207, no. 2 (August 1962), 29.

73. Ibid., 29–30.

74. Ibid., 35.

75. J. C. Furnas, "That Mothers May Live," *Ladies' Home Journal* 56, no. 11 (November 1, 1939): 58.

76. Yulonda Eadie Sano, "Protect the Mother and Baby," *Agricultural History* 93, no. 3 (2019): 393–411.

77. Sano, "Protect the Mother and Baby."

78. Charlotte Painter, *Who Made the Lamb* (New York: McGraw-Hill, 1965), 166–67.

CHAPTER 6: "HISTORY IS SHOWING THEM HOW TO TREAT US"

1. Kimberlé Crenshaw, "Mapping the Margins: Intersectionality, Identity Politics, and Violence Against Women of Color," *Stanford Law Review* 43, no. 6 (1991): 1244, https://doi.org/10.2307/1229039.

2. William A. Grobman et al., "Prediction of Vaginal Birth After Cesarean Delivery in Term Gestations: A Calculator Without Race and Ethnicity," *American Journal of Obstetrics & Gynecology* 225, no. 6 (December 2021), https://doi.org/10.1016/j .ajog.2021.05.021.

3. "Delivery Method," March of Dimes, January 2022, https://www.marchofdimes .org/peristats/data?top=8&lev=1&stop=355&reg=99&sreg=22&obj=1&slev=4.

4. Michelle J. K. Osterman, "Changes in Primary and Repeat Cesarean Delivery: United States, 2016–2021," *NVSS Vital Statistics Rapid Release*, no. 21 (July 2022).

5. Wissam Arab and David Atallah, "Cesarean Section Rates in the COVID-19 Era: False Alarms and the Safety of the Mother and Child," *European Journal of Midwifery* 5 no. 14 (May 20, 2021), https://doi.org/10.18332/ejm/134998.

6. Osterman, "Changes in Primary and Repeat Cesarean Delivery."

7. Saraswathi Vedam, Kathrin Stoll, and Tanya Khemet Taiwo, "The Giving Voice to Mothers Study: Inequity and Mistreatment During Pregnancy and Childbirth in the United States," *Reproductive Health* 16, no. 5 (June 11, 2019), https:// reproductive-health-journal.biomedcentral.com/articles/10.1186/s12978-019 -0729-2#citeas.

8. Eugene R. Declercq et al., "Listening to Mothers III: Pregnancy and Birth," Childbirth Connection, May 2013.

9. Attanasio and Hardeman, "Declined Care and Discrimination During the Childbirth Hospitalization."

10. "The CATCH Pilot and the PReM OB Scale," Birthing Cultural Rigor, https:// www.birthingculturalrigor.com/thecatchqipilot/.

11. Rebecca F. Hamm, Sindhu K. Srinivas, and Lisa D. Levine, "A Standardized Labor Induction Protocol: Impact on Racial Disparities in Obstetrical Outcomes," *American Journal of Obstetrics & Gynecology* 2, no. 3 (August 2020), http:// doi.org/10.1016/j.ajogmf.2020.100148.

12. Quoted in Linda Villarosa, *Under the Skin: The Hidden Toll of Racism on American Lives and on the Health of Our Nation* (New York: Doubleday, 2022), 75.

13. Villarosa, *Under the Skin*, 75–76.

14. "Black Women's Health Study," Boston University School of Public Health, https://www.bu.edu/sph/research/black-womens-health-study/#:~:text=The%20 Black%20Women's%20Health%20Study,major%20illnesses%20in%20Black%20 women.

15. Arline Geronimus, cited by Villarosa, *Under the Skin*, 80–81.

16. Arline Geronimus, "The Weathering Hypothesis and the Health of African-American Women and Infants: Evidence and Speculations," *Ethnicity & Disease* 2, no. 3 (Summer 1992): 210.

17. Bruce S. McEwen, "Stressed or Stressed Out: What Is the Difference?," *Journal of Psychiatry & Neuroscience* 30, no. 5 (2005): 315–18, http://www.ncbi.nlm.nih.gov /pubmed/?term=16151535.

18. Arline Geronimus et al., "Race-Ethnicity, Poverty, Urban Stressor, and Telomere Length in a Detroit Community-Based Sample," *Journal of Health and Social Behavior* 56, no. 2 (2015): 200, http://doi.org/10.1177/0022146515582100;

M. A. Shammas, "Telomeres, Lifestyle, Cancer, and Aging," *Current Opinion in Clinical Nutrition and Metabolic Care* 14, no. 1 (January 2011): 28–34, https://doi.org/10.1097/MCO.0b013e32834121b1.

19. Fleda Mask Jackson et al., "Examining the Burdens of Gendered Racism: Implications for Pregnancy Outcomes Among College-Educated African American Women," *Maternal and Child Health Journal* 5, no. 2 (2001): 95.

20. "Cesarean Section Deliveries," FL Health Charts, https://www.flhealthcharts.gov/ChartsReports/rdPage.aspx?rdReport=Birth.DataViewer&cid=443.

21. Haim A. Abenhaim and Alice Benjamin, "Higher Caesarean Section Rates in Women With Higher Body Mass Index: Are We Managing Labour Differently?," *Journal of Obstetrics and Gynaecology Canada* 33, no. 5 (2011): 443–48.

22. Anna I. Girsen, Sarah S. Osmundson, Mariam Naqvi, et al., "Body Mass Index and Operative Times at Cesarean Delivery," *Obstetrics & Gynecology* 124 no. 4 (2014): 684–89, https://doi.org/10.1097/AOG.0000000000000462.

23. Sabrina Strings, "Obese Black Women as 'Social Dead Weight': Reinventing the 'Diseased Black Woman,'" *Signs* 41, no. 1 (2015), https://doi.org/10.1086/681773.

24. "AMA Adopts New Policy Clarifying Role of BMI as a Measure in Medicine," American Medical Association, June 14, 2023, accessed August 14, 2023, https://www.ama-assn.org/press-center/press-releases/ama-adopts-new-policy-clarifying-role-bmi-measure-medicine.

25. "Four in 5 Pregnancy-Related Deaths in the U.S. Are Preventable," Centers for Disease Control and Prevention, September 19, 2022, accessed July 24, 2023, https://www.cdc.gov/media/releases/2022/p0919-pregnancy-related-deaths.html.

26. Daniel Dench et al., "United States Preterm Birth Rate and COVID-19," *Pediatrics* 149 no. 5 (2022): e2021055495, https://doi.org/10.1542/peds.2021-055495.

27. Aja Clark et al., "Centering Equity: Addressing Structural and Social Determinants of Health to Improve Maternal and Infant Health Outcomes," *Seminars in Perinatology* 46, no. 8 (2022).

28. Personal communication from Sarah Y. Tucker.

CHAPTER 7: "YOU'D BE NAIVE TO THINK HEALTHCARE ISN'T A BUSINESS"

1. Restore West Virginia Hospitals, https://restorewv.com/hospitals/.

2. Brady E. Hamilton et al., "Births: Provisional Data for 2021," NVSS Vital Statistics Rapid Release, https://www.cdc.gov/nchs/data/vsrr/vsrr020.pdf.

3. William Johnson et al., "Understanding Variation in Spending on Childbirth Among the Commercially Insured," Health Care Cost Institute brief, 2020, 5.

4. Truven Health Analytics, "The Cost of Having a Baby in the United States," 2013, https://nationalpartnership.org/wp-content/uploads/2023/02/cost-of-having-a-baby-executive-summary.pdf.

5. Rie Sakai-Bizmark et al., "Evaluation of Hospital Cesarean Delivery-Related Profits and Rates in the United States," *Obstetrics and Gynecology* 4, no. 3 (March 19, 2021).

6. See, for instance, David Epstein, "When Evidence Says No, But Doctors Say Yes," ProPublica, February 22, 2017, https://www.propublica.org/article/when-evidence-says-no-but-doctors-say-yes.

7. Luna Lopes et al., "Health Care Debt in the U.S.: The Broad Consequences of Medical and Dentail Bills," KFF Health Care Debt Survey, June 16, 2033, accessed August 10, 2023, https://www.kff.org/report-section/kff-health-care-debt-survey-main-findings/#:~:text=Substantial%20shares%20of%20adults%20carry,form%20of%20health%20care%20debt.

8. Colleen Grogan, *Grow and Hide: The History of America's Health Care State* (Oxford: Oxford University Press, 2023).

9. Eileen Appelbaum and Rosemary Batt, "Financialization in Health Care: The Transformation of US Hospital Systems," Center for Economic and Policy Research, September 9, 2021, https://cepr.net/wp-content/uploads/2021/10/AB-Financialization-In-Healthcare-Spitzer-Rept-09-09-21.pdf.

10. Robert Tyler Braun et al., "Association of Private Equity Investment in US Nursing Homes with the Quality and Cost of Care for Long-Stay Residents," *JAMA Health Forum* 2, no. 11 (2021), https://doi.org/10.1001/jamahealthforum.2021.3817.

11. Appelbaum and Batt, "Financialization in Health Care," 79.

12. DiGregorio, *Taking Care*.

13. Appelbaum and Batt, "Financialization in Health Care," 22–23.

14. Ryan K. Masters, Andrea M. Silstra, Daniel H. Simon, and Kate Coleman-Minahan, "Differences in Determinants: Racialized Obstetric Care and Increases in U.S. State Labor Induction Rates," *Journal of Health and Social Behavior* 64, no. 2 (2023): 174–91.

15. Matthew Rae, Cynthia Cox, and Hanna Dingel, "Health Costs Associated with Pregnancy, Childbirth, and Postpartum Care," Peterson-KFF Health System Tracker (July 13, 2002), https://www.healthsystemtracker.org/brief/health-costs-associated-with-pregnancy-childbirth-and-postpartum-care/.

16. P. Preston Reynolds, "Professional and Hospital DISCRIMINATION and the US Court of Appeals Fourth Circuit 1956–1967," *American Journal of Public Health* 94, no. 5 (2004): 710–20, https://doi.org/10.2105%2Fajph.94.5.710.

17. Peiyin Hung et al., "Why Are Obstetric Units in Rural Hospitals Closing Their Doors?," *Health Services Research* 51, no. 4 (2016): 1546–60, https://onlinelibrary.wiley.com/doi/10.1111/1475-6773.12441.

18. Alecia J. McGregor et al., "Obstetrical Unit Closures and Racial and Ethnic Differences in Severe Maternal Morbidity in the State of New Jersey," *American Journal of Obstetrics & Gynecology* 3, no. 6 (2021), http://doi.org/10.1016/j.ajogmf.2021.100480; Severe maternal morbidity defined by CDC: https://www.cdc.gov/reproductivehealth/maternalinfanthealth/severematernalmorbidity.html#anchor_how.

19. "Physician Employment and Acquisitions of Physician Practices 2019–2021 Specialties Edition," Avalere Health, published June 2022, accessed August 10, 2023, https://www.physiciansadvocacyinstitute.org/Portals/0/assets/docs/PAI-Research/Physician%20Practice%20Trends%20Specialty%20Report%202019-2022.pdf?ver=MWjYUAcARbuGP9uxcgQkPw%3d%3d.

20. UnitedHealth Group, "UnitedHealth Group Reports 2022 Results," published January 13, 2023, accessed August 10, 2023, https://www.unitedhealthgroup .com/content/dam/UHG/PDF/investors/2022/UNH-Q4-2022-Release.pdf.

21. Eyal Press, "The Moral Crisis of America's Doctors," *New York Times*, June 15, 2023, accessed August 10, 2023, https://www.nytimes.com/2023/06/15 /magazine/doctors-moral-crises.html.

22. Gerald B. Hickson, Ellen Wright Clayton, Stephen S. Entman, et al., "Obstetricians' Prior Malpractice Experience and Patients' Satisfaction with Care," *JAMA* 272, no. 20 (1994): 1583–87, https:// doi:10.1001/jama.1994.03520200039032.

23. Debra Roter, "The Patient-Physician Relationship and Its Implications for Malpractice Litigation," *Journal of Health Care Law and Policy* 9, no. 2 (1994), https:// digitalcommons.law.umaryland.edu/jhclp/vol9/iss2/7.

24. Margot Sanger-Katz, Julie Creswell, and Reed Abelson, "Mystery Solved: Private-Equity-Backed Firms Are Behind Ad Blitz on 'Surprise Billing,'" *New York Times*, September 13, 2019; Appelbaum and Batt, "Financialization in Health Care," 75.

25. Barbara Katz Rothman, *The Biomedical Empire: Lessons Learned from the COVID-19 Pandemic* (Redwood City, CA: Stanford University Press, 2021), 79.

CHAPTER 8: TECHNOLOGY AND TOUCH

1. Quoted in Michel Foucault, *The Birth of the Clinic: An Archeology of Medical Perception* (New York: Vintage Books, 1994), 164.

2. Ruth Richardson, "From the Medical Museum," *Lancet* (December 23/30, 2000), 356; Stanley Aronson, "A Heart-Beat Is Amplified and Then Resonates in History," *Medicine & Health Rhode Island* 105, no. 6 (2012): 171.

3. "Rene Laënnec: Stethoscope," Lemelson-MIT, accessed November 12, 2023, https://lemelson.mit.edu/resources/rene-laennec.

4. John G. Leyden, "The Chance Invention That Changed Medicine," *Saturday Evening Post*, May/June 2001, 46–47.

5. This is the argument in Michel Foucault's *The Birth of the Clinic: An Archaeology of Medical Perception* (New York: Vintage, 1994).

6. Kristina Edvardsson, Rhonda Small, Margareta Persson, Ann Lalos, and Ingrid Mogren, "'Ultrasound Is an Invaluable Third Eye, but It Can't See Everything': A Qualitative Study with Obstetricians in Australia," *BMC Pregnancy and Childbirth* 14 (2014): 363.

7. Doyle, *Maternal Bodies*.

8. Ibid.

9. See, for instance, Ashe, "Law-Language of Maternity"; Armstrong, *Conceiving Risk, Bearing Responsibility*.

10. Michele Goodwin, *Policing the Womb: Invisible Women and the Criminalization of Motherhood* (Cambridge, MA: Cambridge University Press, 2020).

11. Sarah S. Richardson, *The Maternal Imprint: The Contested Science of Maternal-Fetal Effects* (Chicago: University of Chicago Press, 2021), 26–55; Karpin, "Legislating the Female Body."

12. Edith Wharton, "The Other Two," in *Roman Fever and Other Stories* (New York: Scribner, 1964), 75.

13. Wolf, *Cesarean Section*, 134.

14. Ibid., 128.

15. Quoted in Ibid., 134–35.

16. Albert D. Haverkamp et al., "The Evaluation of Continuous Fetal Heart Rate Monitoring in High-Risk Pregnancy," *American Journal of Obstetrics & Gynecology* 125, no. 3 (1976): 310–20.

17. Mary T. Paterno, Kathleen McElroy, and Mary Regan, "Electronic Fetal Monitoring and Cesarean Birth: A Scoping Review," *Birth* 43, no. 4 (2016), https://doi.org/10.1111/birt.12247.

18. Annelee Boyle, Uma M. Reddy, Helain J. Landy, et al., "Primary Cesarean Delivery in the United States," *Obstetrics & Gynecology* 122, no. 1 (2013), http://doi.org/10.1097/AOG.0b013e3182952242.

19. Jeff Denney et al., "Category III Fetal Heart Rate Tracings: A Rare Occurrence Strongly Associated with Adverse Neonatal Outcome," *American Journal of Obstetrics & Gynecology* 201, no. 6, supplement (2009), https://doi.org/10.1016/j.ajog.2009.10.426.

20. Marc Jackson et al., "Frequency of Fetal Heart Rate Categories and Short-Term Neonatal Outcome," *Obstetrics & Gynecology* 118 no. 4 (October 2011), http://doi.org/10.1097/AOG.0b013e31822f1b50.

21. Karin B. Nelson et al., "Uncertain Value of Electronic Fetal Monitoring in Predicting Cerebral Palsy," *New England Journal of Medicine* 334 (March 7, 1996), https://doi.org/10.1056/NEJM199603073341001.

22. Karin Nelson, Thomas Sartwelle, and Dwight Rouse, "Electronic Fetal Monitoring, Cerebral Palsy, and Caesarean Section: Assumptions versus Evidence," *BMJ* 355 (2016): i6405, https://doi.org/10.1136/bmj.i6405.

23. Thomas P. Sartwelle, James C. Johnston, et al., "Cerebral Palsy, Cesarean Sections, and Electronic Fetal Monitoring: All the Light We Cannot See," *Clinical Ethics* 14, no. 3 (September 2019), https://doi.org/10.1177/1477750919851055.

24. Nelson et al., "Fetal Monitoring, Cerebral Palsy, and Caesarean Section."

25. Quoted in Foucault, *The Birth of the Clinic*, 163.

26. Quoted in ibid., 163.

27. Andrea Mubi Brighenti, *Visibility in Social Theory and Social Research* (London: Palgrave Macmillan, 2010), 20

28. Jonathan M. Fanaroff, Michael G. Ross, and Steven M. Donn, "Medico-Legal Considerations in the Context of Neonatal Encephalopathy and Therapeutic Hypothermia," *Seminars in Fetal & Neonatal Medicine* 26, no. 5 (October 2021), https://doi.org/10.1016/j.siny.2021.101266.

29. Steven M. Donn, Malcolm L. Chiswick, and Jonathan M. Fanaroff, "Medico-Legal Implications of Hypoxic–Ischemic Birth Injury," *Seminars in Fetal & Neonatal Medicine* 19, no. 5 (October 2014): 317–21, https://doi: 10.1016/j.siny.2014.08.005.

30. Wolf, *Cesarean Section*, 165.

31. Marcus A. Banks, "Malpractice Suits Against Ob/Gyns Continue Downward Trend," *Medscape Medical News*, February 3, 2022, accessed September 6, 2023, https://www.medscape.com/viewarticle/967829#:~:text=Nearly%2080%25%20 of%20obstetrician%2Dgynecologists,Ob%2FGyn%20Malpractice%20 Report%202021.

CHAPTER 9: PAIN

1. Rich, *Of Woman Born.*
2. Joanna A. Kountanis, Robyn Kirk, Jonathan E. Handelzalts, et al., "The Associations of Subjective Appraisal of Birth Pain and Provider-Patient Communication with Postpartum-Onset PTSD," *Archives of Women's Mental Health* 25 (2022): 171–80.
3. Anne Drapkin Lyerly, *A Good Birth: Finding the Positive and Profound in Your Childbirth Experience* (New York: Avery, 2014).
4. Rachel Reed, Rachael Sharman, and Christian Inglis, "Women's Descriptions of Childbirth Trauma Relating to Care Provider Actions and Interactions," *BMC Pregnancy and Childbirth* 17, no. 21 (2017), https://doi.org/10.1186/s12884-016-1197-0.
5. Laura Y. Whitburn, Lester E. Jones, Mary-Ann Davey, et al., "The Nature of Labour Pain: An Updated Review of the Literature," *Women and Birth: Journal of the Australian College of Midwives* 32, no.1 (2019): 28–38.
6. Diane E. Hoffman and Anita J. Tarzian, "The Girl Who Cried Pain: A Bias Against Women in the Treatment of Pain," *Journal of Law, Medicine & Ethics* 29 (2001): 13–27.
7. Cecilia Tasca et al., "Women and Hysteria in the History of Mental Health," *Clinical Practice and Epidemiology in Mental Health* 8, 110–19, https://doi.org/10 .2174/1745017901208010110.
8. Quoted by Deborah Chambers, Linda Steiner, and Carole Fleming, *Women and Journalism* (Oxfordshire, UK: Taylor & Francis, 2004), 52.
9. Judith Butler, "Variations on Sex and Gender: Beauvoir, Wittig, Foucault (1987)," *The Judith Butler Reader* (Hoboken, NJ: John Wiley & Sons, 2004).
10. Ibid.
11. Stanley Joel Reiser, *Medicine and the Reign of Technology* (Cambridge, MA: Cambridge University Press, 1981), 171.
12. Ibid., 170–74.
13. American Pain Society Quality of Care Committee, "Quality Improvement Guidelines for the Treatment of Acute Pain and Cancer Pain," *JAMA* 274 (1995): 1874–80.
14. Oral History with Dr. Mitchell Max, March 1999, https://history.nih.gov/display /history/Max%2C+Mitchell+1999.
15. The Joint Commission, "Pain Assessment and Management Standards for Joint Commission Accredited Health Care Organizations," February 2020, accessed August 22, 2023, https://www.jointcommission.org/-/media/tjc/documents/corporate -communication/pain-management-standards-and-responses-to-myths-final -feb-2020.pdf.

16. Patrick Radden Keefe, *Empire of Pain: The Secret History of the Sackler Family* (New York: Doubleday, 2021), 189.

17. Ibid.

18. Claudia Avalos et al., "Opioid Prescription-Use After Cesarean Delivery: An Observational Cohort Study," *Journal of Anesthesia* 35, no. 5 (October 2021): 617–24, https://doi.org/10.1007/s00540-021-02959-z.

19. Ibid., 617–24.

20. Brian T. Bateman, Jessica M. Franklin, Katsiaryna Bykov, et al., "Persistent Opioid Use Following Cesarean Delivery: Patterns and Predictors Among Opioid-Naive Women," *American Journal of Obstetrics & Gynecology* 215, no. 3 (2016): 353.e1 -353.e18, https://doi.org/10.1016/j.ajog.2016.03.016.

21. Combined epidural and spinal anesthesia used during 2022 was 77 percent, according to Michelle Osterman, *National Vital Statistics Reports* 70, no. 17 (February 7, 2022), https://www.cdc.gov/nchs/data/nvsr/nvsr70/nvsr70-17-tables.pdf.

22. Whitburn et al., "The Nature of Labour Pain," 33.

23. Lauren Ann Gamble, Ashley Hesson, Tiffany Burns, "Sticking to the Plan: Patient Preferences for Epidural Use during Labor," *Medical Student Research Journal* 4, 59–65; A. B. Goldberg, A. Cohen, and E. Lieberman, "Nulliparas' Preferences for Epidural Analgesia: Their Effects on Actual Use in Labor," *Birth* 26, no. 3 (1999): 139–43.

24. Ellen D. Hodnett, Simon Gates, Justus Hofmeyr, et al., "Continuous Support for Women During Childbirth," *Cochrane Database of Systematic Reviews* 3 (2003), https://doi.org/10.1002/14651858.CD003766.

25. Jean Guglielminotti and Guohua Li, "Exposure to General Anesthesia for Cesarean Delivery and Odds of Severe Postpartum Depression Requiring Hospitalization," *Anesthesia & Analgesia* 131, no. 5 (2020): 1421–29, https://doi.org/10.1213/ANE.0000000000004663; Laurence Ring, Ruth Landau, and Carlos Delgado, "The Current Role of General Anesthesia for Cesarean Delivery," *Current Anesthesiology Reports* 11, no. 1 (2021): 18–27, https://doi.org/10.1007/s40140-021-00437-6.

26. Yu Chen, Xin Ye, Han Wu, et al., "Association of Postpartum Pain Sensitivity and Postpartum Depression: A Prospective Observational Study," *Pain Therapy* 10, no. 2 (2021), https://doi.org/10.1007%2Fs40122-021-00325-1.

CHAPTER 10: C-SECTIONS AND POSTPARTUM MOOD DISORDERS

1. Jon Cox, Jeni Holden, and R. Sagovsky, "Detection of Postnatal Depression: Development of the 10-Item Edinburgh Postnatal Depression Scale," *British Journal of Psychiatry* 150 (1987): 782–86, https://doi.org/10.1192/bjp.150.6.782.

2. Jon Cox, Jeni Holden, and Carol Henshaw, "Thirty Years with the Edinburgh Postnatal Depression Scale: Voices from the Past and Recommendations for the Future," *British Journal of Psychiatry* 214 (2019): 127–29, https://doi.org/10.1192/bjp.2018.245.

3. "Depression and Suicide Risk in Adults: Screening," The United States Preventative Services Task Force, June 20, 2023, accessed July 10, 2023, https://www.uspreventiveservicestaskforce.org/uspstf/recommendation/screening-depression-suicide-risk-adults.

4. "Optimizing Postpartum Care," ACOG Committee Opinion no. 736, The American College of Obstetricians and Gynecologists, May 2018, accessed July 10, 2023, https://www.acog.org/clinical/clinical-guidance/committee-opinion/articles/2018/05/optimizing-postpartum-care.

5. Karen Fratti, "This Mom Had the Cops Called on Her After Seeking Help for PPD & Her Story Is a Must-Read," *Romper*, January 21, 2018, https://www.romper.com/p/this-mom-had-the-cops-called-on-her-after-seeking-help-for-ppd-her-story-is-a-must-read-7969626; Aneri Pattani, "Silenced by Fear: New Moms Worry Postpartum Depression Could Mean Losing Their Children," *Philadelphia Inquirer*, April 5, 2019, https://whyy.org/segments/silenced-by-fear-new-moms-worry-postpartum-depression-could-mean-losing-their-children/.

6. "Using the EPDS to Screen for Anxiety Disorders: Conceptual and Methodological Considerations," MGH Center for Women's Mental Health, March 11, 2013, https://womensmentalhealth.org/posts/using-the-epds-to-screen-for-anxiety-disorders-conceptual-and-methodological-considerations/.

7. Claire Hilton, "Brice Pitt, MD, FRCPsych," *British Journal of Psychiatry Bulletin* 45, no. 6 (December 2021): 358–59, https://doi.org/10.1192/bjb.2021.56.

8. Brice Pitt, "Atypical Depression Following Childbirth," *British Journal of Psychiatry* 114 (1968): 1325–35.

9. Quoted by Natalie Feldman et al., "A Systematic Review of mHealth Application Interventions for Peripartum Mood Disorders: Trends and Evidence in Academia and Industry," *Archives of Women's Mental Health* 24 (April 2021): 881–92.

10. "Labile Definition & Meaning," Merriam-Webster.com Dictionary, accessed July 10, 2023, https://www.merriam-webster.com/dictionary/labile.

11. Pitt, "Atypical Depression Following Childbirth," 1327.

12. Rachel Cusk, *The Bradshaw Variations* (New York: Farrar, Straus and Giroux, 2009), 114.

13. Bruce Springsteen, "Dancing in the Dark" (1984), Sony/ATV Music Publishing LLC.

14. Pitt, "Atypical Depression Following Childbirth," 1332.

15. Chin et al., "Suicide and Maternal Mortality," 239–75.

16. Pitt, "Atypical Depression Following Childbirth," 1330.

17. Sarah Smithson et al., "Unplanned Cesarean Delivery Is Associated with Risk for Postpartum Depressive Symptoms in the Immediate Postpartum Period," *The Journal of Maternal-Fetal & Neonatal Medicine* 35, no. 20 (2022): 275–88; Valentina Tonei, "Mother's Mental Health After Childbirth: Does the Delivery Method Matter?," *Journal of Health Economics* 63 (2019): 182–96, http://doi.org/10.1016/j.jhealeco.2018.11.006.

18. Meralis Lantigua-Martinez et al., "Postpartum Depression, Mode of Delivery, and Indication for Unscheduled Cesarean Delivery: A Retrospective Cohort Study," *Journal of Perinatal Medicine* 50, no. 5 (2022): 630–33, https://doi.org/10.1515/jpm-2021-0575.

19. Hayden White, "The Historical Text as Literary Artifact," *Clio* 3, no. 3 (June 1, 1974).

20. S. Michelle Ogunwole et al., "Health Equity Considerations in State Bills Related to Doula Care (2015–2020)," *Women's Health Issues* 32, no. 5 (2022): 440–49, https://doi.org/10.1016/j.whi.2022.04.004.

21. "Annual Report 2001–2022," Health Child Manitoba, September 2002, accessed July 10, 2023, https://www.gov.mb.ca/healthychild/about/annual_report_2001_02.pdf.

22. Jennifer E. Enns et al., "An Unconditional Prenatal Income Supplement Is Associated with Improved Birth and Early Childhood Outcomes among First Nations Children in Manitoba, Canada: A Population-Based Cohort Study," *BMC Pregnancy and Childbirth* 21 (2021): 312.

23. Amina Zafar and Christine Birak, "$81 a Month Buys a Healthier Baby," CBC News, May 12, 2016, accessed July 10, 2023, https://www.cbc.ca/news/health/healthy-baby-prenatal-income-benefit-1.3578029.

24. "Health Department Announces Significant Contributions to the Philly Joy Bank from the William Penn Foundation and Spring Point Partners," Department of Public Health, City of Philadelphia, March 20, 2023, https://www.phila.gov/2023-03-20-health-department-announces-significant-contributions-to-the-philly-joy-bank-from-the-william-penn-foundation-and-spring-point-partners/.

25. Alexander J. Butwick, Cynthia A. Wong, Nan Guo, "Maternal Body Mass Index and Use of Labor Neuraxial Analgesia: A Population-Based Retrospective Cohort Study," *Anesthesiology* 129 (2018): 448–58, https://doi.org/10.1097/ALN.0000000000002322.

26. Yunefit Ulfa, Naoko Maruyama, Yumiko Igarashi, and Shigeko Horiuchi, "Early Initiation of Breastfeeding Up to Six Months Among Mothers After Cesarean Section or Vaginal Birth: A Scoping Review," *Heliyon* 9 (2023): https://doi.org/10.1016/j.heliyon.2023.e16235; Jane A. Scott, Colin W. Binns, and Wendy H. Oddy, "Predictors of Delayed Onset of Lactation," *Maternal & Child Nutrition* 3 no. 3 (July 2007), https://doi.org/10.1111/j.1740-8709.2007.00096.x.

27. Precious Fondren, "One State's Approach to Maternal Deaths: Free Nurse Visits After Birth," *New York Times*, July 29, 2021, https://www.nytimes.com/2021/07/29/nyregion/maternal-mortality-new-jersey.html.

28. Epworth Freemasons, "Relax at Park Hyatt Melbourne," https://www.epworth.org.au/-/media/project/epworth/epworthweb/documents/services/maternity/pi2374_mat_park-hyatt-brochure-web-v12.pdf.

CHAPTER 11: VBAC

1. S. Tahseen and M. Griffiths, "Vaginal Birth after Two Caesarean Sections (VBAC-2): A Systematic Review with Meta-analysis of Success Rate and Adverse Outcomes of VBAC-2 Versus VBAC-1 and Repeat (Third) Caesarean Sections," *BJOG: An International Journal of Obstetrics and Gynaecology* 117, no. 1 (2010), https://doi.org/10.1111/j.1471-0528.2009.02351.x.

2. Jeanne-Marie Guise, Karen Eden, Cathy Emeis, et al., "Vaginal Birth After Cesarean: New Insights," *Evidence Report/Technology Assessment* 191 (March 2010), https://www.ahrq.gov/downloads/pub/evidence/pdf/vbacup/vbacup.pdf.

3. Nathan Heller, "How Ayelet Waldman Found a Calmer Life on Tiny Doses of LSD," *New Yorker*, January 12, 2017, accessed August 23, 2023, https://www.newyorker.com/culture/persons-of-interest/how-ayelet-waldman-found-a-calmer-life-on-tiny-doses-of-lsd.

4. Rebecca Kukla, "Measuring Mothering," *Doing Feminist Bioethics* 1, no. 1 (2008): 67–90, https://www.jstor.org/stable/40339213.

5. Centers for Disease Control and Prevention, National Center for Health Statistics, National Vital Statistics System, Natality on CDC WONDER Online Database. Data are from the Natality Records 2016–2022, as compiled from data provided by the fifty-seven vital statistics jurisdictions through the Vital Statistics Cooperative Program. Accessed at http://wonder.cdc.gov/natality-expanded-current.html on November 12, 2023. Other sources put this number closer to six hundred thousand; see Bridget Basile Ibrahim et al., "Women's Perceptions of Barriers and Facilitators to Vaginal Birth After Cesarean in the United States: An Integrative Review," *Journal of Midwifery & Women's Health* 65 no. 3 (2020): 349–61, https://doi.org/10.1111/jmwh.13083.

6. "VBAC Ban Database Initiative," International Cesarean Awareness Network, accessed November 12, 2023 (2009), https://www.ican-online.org/vbac-ban-info/. See also: Erika Barth Cottrell et al., "Predictors of Hospital VBAC Policies," *American Journal of Obstetrics & Gynecology* 208, no. 1 suppl. (January 2013): S332–S333, https://www.ajog.org/article/S0002-9378(12)01214-8/fulltext; L. Indra Lucero, "Challenging Hospital VBAC Bans Through Tort Liability," *William & Mary Journal of Race, Gender, and Social Justice* 20 no. 2 (2013–2014), https://scholarship.law.wm.edu/cgi/viewcontent.cgi?article=1381&context=wmjowl.

7. Luna Zakiya, *Reproductive Rights as Human Rights: Women of Color and the Fight for Reproductive Justice* (New York: New York University Press, 2020), 48.

8. Bridget Basile Ibrahim, M. Tish Knobf, Allison Shorten, et al., "'I Had to Fight for My VBAC': A Mixed Methods Exploration of Women's Experiences of Pregnancy and Vaginal Birth After Cesarean in the United States," *Birth* 48, no. 2 (2021): 164–77.

9. Ibid.

10. Ibid.

11. The American College of Obstetricians and Gynecologists, "Practice Bulletin No. 184: Vaginal Birth After Cesarean Delivery," *Obstetrics & Gynecology* 130, no. 5 (2017), http://doi.org/10.1097/AOG.0000000000002398.

12. Christina Davidson, Patricia Bellows, Utsavi Shah, et al., "Outcomes Associated with Trial of Labor After Cesarean in Women with One versus Two Prior Cesarean Deliveries after a Change in Clinical Practice Guidelines in an Academic Hospital," *Obstetrics & Gynecology* (January 2018): S349, https://www.ajog.org/action/showPdf?pii=S0002-9378%2817%2931874-4.

13. Goodwin, *Policing the Womb*, 92–96.

14. Ibid., 94.

15. David Remnick, "Whose Life Is It, Anyway? Angie Carter Lived a Very Simple Life . . . and Died a Very Complicated Death," *Washington Post*, February 21, 1998, https://www.washingtonpost.com/archive/lifestyle/magazine/1988/02/21/whose-life-is-it-anyway-angie-carter-lived-a-very-simple-life-and-died-a-very-complicated-death/875f515e-64ab-4f93-af37-f6a4147e5189/.

16. Goodwin, *Policing the Womb*, 96.

17. Frank A. Chervenak, Laurence B. McCullough, and Judith Chervenak, "Perils of Miscommunication: The Beginnings of Informed Consent," *Donald School Journal of Ultrasound in Obstetrics and Gynecology* 10, no. 2 (April–June 2016): 125–30, https://www.dsjuog.com/doi/DSJUOG/pdf/10.5005/jp-journals-10009-1454.

18. Goodwin, *Policing the Womb*, 27–28.

19. Ibid., 6.

20. Ibid., 30.

21. Pregnancy Justice, "Who Do Fetal Homicide Laws Protect? An Analysis for a Post-Roe America," December 2022, accessed August 25, 2023, https://www.pregnancyjusticeus.org/wp-content/uploads/2022/12/fetal-homicide-brief-with-appendix-UPDATED.pdf.

22. United States Congress, "H.R.1997 - Unborn Victims of Violence Act of 2004," accessed August 25, 2023, https://www.congress.gov/bill/108th-congress/house-bill/1997.

23. Azi Paybarah, "Judge Dismisses Murder Charge Against California Mother After Stillbirth," *New York Times*, May 20, 2021.

24. Julie Rovner, "Woman Charged in Death of Fetus Is Out of Jail," NPR, May 22, 2012, https://www.npr.org/sections/health-shots/2012/05/22/153307529/woman-charged-in-death-of-fetus-is-out-of-jail.

25. Paybarah, "Judge Dismisses Murder Charge Against California Mother After Stillbirth."

26. Sam Levin, "She Was Jailed for Losing a Pregnancy. Her Nightmare Could Become More Common," *Guardian*, June 4, 2022, https://www.theguardian.com/us-news/2022/jun/03/california-stillborn-prosecution-roe-v-wade.

27. Edward B. Cragin, "Conservatism in Obstetrics," *New York Medical Journal* 104 (July 1916), https://babel.hathitrust.org/cgi/pt?id=nnc2.ark:/13960/t12n7td82&view=1up&seq=11&q1=cragin.

28. Ibid.

29. Wolf, *Cesarean Section*, 162.

30. Nancy Wainer Cohen and Lois J. Estner, *Silent Knife: Cesarean Prevention & Vaginal Birth after Cesarean* (New York: Bergin & Garvey Publishers, 1983).

31. Wolf, *Cesarean Section*, 4; "Cesarean Childbirth. NIH Consensus Statement Online 1980 Sep 22-24," *National Institute of Health* 3 (1980): 1–30.

32. The American College of Obstetricians and Gynecologists, "Vaginal Birth After Cesarean Delivery," ACOG Practice Bulletin 130, no. 5 (November 2017), https://portaldeboaspraticas.iff.fiocruz.br/wp-content/uploads/2021/02/Practice_Bulletin_No__184__Vaginal_Birth_After.48.pdf.

33. Mona Lydon-Rochelle, Victoria L. Holt, Thomas R. Easterling, et al., "Risk of Uterine Rupture During Labor Among Women with a Prior Cesarean Delivery," *New England Journal of Medicine* 345, no. 1 (July 5, 2001).

34. Cited in Wolf, *Cesarean Section*, 159–61.

35. Kim J. Cox, "Providers' Perspectives on the Vaginal Birth after Cesarean Guidelines in Florida, United States: A Qualitative Study," *BMC Pregnancy and Childbirth* 11, no. 72 (2011), https://doi.org/10.1186/1471-2393-11-72.

36. Sarah M. Nicholson, Kate C. O'Doherty, Niamh A. O'Halloran, and John J. Morrison, "VBAC over a 25-Year Period in Irish Obstetric Practice: Attempt, Success and Rates," *American Journal of Obstetrics & Gynecology* S348 (January 2018), https://www.ajog.org/action/showPdf?pii=S0002-9378%2817%2931874-4; Matias Vaajala, Rasmus Liukkonen, Ville Ponkilainen, et al., "The Rates of Vaginal Births after Cesarean Section Have Increased During the Last Decades: A Nationwide Register-Based Cohort Study in Finland," *General Gynecology* 308 (2023): 157–62, https://link.springer.com/article/10.1007/s00404-023-07010-y#Fig2.

37. Environmental Protection Agency, "Savannah River Site: Aiken, SC," https://cumulis.epa.gov/supercpad/SiteProfiles/index.cfm?fuseaction=second.Cleanup&id=0403485#bkground.

38. U.S. Department of Energy, "First Shipment of Downblended Surplus Plutonium from SRS's K Area Leaves South Carolina," *News from the Savannah River Site,* January 13, 2023.

39. "VAGINAL BIRTH AFTER CESAREAN (VBAC) GUIDELINES," Washington Alliance for Responsible Midwifery, 2018.

40. Brandy Zadrozny, "'I Brainwashed Myself with the Internet,'" NBC News, February 21, 2020, https://www.nbcnews.com/news/us-news/she-wanted-freebirth-no-doctors-online-groups-convinced-her-it-n1140096/.

CHAPTER 12: SOLUTIONS

1. Brittany M. Byerly and David M. Haas, "A Systematic Overview of the Literature Regarding Group Prenatal Care," *BMC Pregnancy and Childbirth* (2017): 17, 329–38.

2. Ebony B. Carter et al., "Group versus Traditional Prenatal Care in Low-Risk Women Delivering at Term: A Retrospective Cohort Study," *Journal of Perinatology* 37 no. 7 (July 2017), https://doi.org/10.1038/jp.2017.33.

3. Rhianon Liu, Maria T. Chao, Ariana Jostad-Laswell et al., "Does CenteringPregnancy Group Prenatal Care Affect the Birth Experience of Underserved Women? A Mixed Methods Analysis," *Journal of Immigrant and Minority Health* 19, no. 2 (2017): 415–22, https://doi:10.1007/s10903-016-0371-9; Tara E. Trudnak et al., "Outcomes of Latina Women in CenteringPregnancy Group Prenatal Care Compared with Individual Prenatal Care," *Journal of Midwifery & Women's Health* 58, no. 4 (July–August 2013), https://doi.org/10.1111/jmwh.12000.

4. Saraswathi Vedam et al., "Mapping Integration of Midwives across the United States: Impact on Access, Equity, and Outcomes," *PLoS ONE* 13, no. 2 (February 21, 2018): e019252, https://journals.plos.org/plosone/article/file?id=10.1371/journal.pone.0192523&type=printable.

5. Vivienne Souter, Elizabeth Nethery, Mary Lou Kopas, Hannah Wurz, Kristin Sitcov, and Aaron B. Caughey, "Comparison of Midwifery and Obstetric Care in Low-Risk Hospital Births," *Obstetrics & Gynecology* 134, no. 5 (2019): 1056–65, https://doi.org/10.1097/AOG.0000000000003521.

6. Saraswathi Vedam, Kathrin Stoll, Marian MacDorman, et al., "Mapping Integration of Midwives Across the United States."

7. Elliot K. Main et al., "Safety Assessment of a Large-Scale Improvement Collaborative to Reduce Nulliparous Cesarean Delivery Rates," *Obstetrics & Gynecology* 133 no. 4 (April 2019), https://doi.org/10.1097/aog.0000000000003109.

8. "Nowhere to Go: Maternity Care Deserts Across the U.S. (2022 Report)," March of Dimes, accessed November 13, 2023, https://www.marchofdimes.org/maternity-care-deserts-report#map.

9. Renee Y. Hsia, Yaa Akosa Antwi, and Ellerie Weber, "Analysis of Variation in Charges and Prices Paid for Vaginal and Caesarean Section Births: A Cross-Sectional Study," *BMJ Open* 2014 no. 4, https://doi.org/10.1136/bmjopen-2013-004017.

10. Margaret H. O'Hara, Linda M. Frazier, Travis W. Stembridge, et al., "Physician-Led, Hospital-Linked, Birth Care Centers Can Decrease Cesarean Section Rates without Increasing Rates of Adverse Events," *Birth* 40, no. 3 (September 2013): 155–63, http://doi.org/10.1111/birt.12051.

11. Alaska Federation of Natives, "Alaska Native Peoples," accessed November 13, 2023, https://www.nativefederation.org/alaska-native-peoples/.

12. Megan Hadley, Gretchen Day, Julie A. Beans, et al., "Postpartum Hemorrhage: Moving from Response to Prevention for Alaska Native Mothers," *International Journal of Gynecology and Obstetrics* 155, no. 2 (2021): 290–95, https://doi: 10.1002/ijgo.13883.

INDEX